THE
QUEEN CHARLOTTE'S HOSPITAL

Guide to Pregnancy & Birth

THE
QUEEN CHARLOTTE'S HOSPITAL
Guide to Pregnancy & Birth

All you have ever wanted to know – from preconception
to birth – from Britain's leading maternity hospital

Adriana Hunter

Vermilion
LONDON

9 10

Text © Adriana Hunter 1998
Cover illustration © Nicola Smee 1998
Text illustrations © Peter Cox 1998

The right of Adriana Hunter to be identified as the author of this book
has been asserted by her in accordance with the Copyright, Designs and
Patents Act 1988.

First published in the United Kingdom in 1998 by Vermilion
an imprint of Ebury Press
Random House
20 Vauxhall Bridge Road
London SW1V 2SA

Random House Australia (Pty) Limited
20 Alfred Street, Milsons Point, Sydney,
New South Wales 2061, Australia

Random House New Zealand Limited
18 Poland Road, Glenfield,
Auckland 10, New Zealand

Random House (Pty) Limited
Endulini, 5A Jubilee Road,
Parktown 2193, South Africa

Random House Group Limited Reg. No. 954009

www.randomhouse.co.uk

A CIP catalogue record for this book is available from the British Library

ISBN: 0 09 181595 9

Printed and bound in Great Britain by Mackays of Chatham plc,
Chatham, Kent

Contents

Introduction

This is not a book about having a baby at Queen Charlotte's Hospital; it is a book written by a mother for mothers-to-be about what to expect during – and how to cope with - pregnancy and childbirth. It comes with the backing and the expertise of the staff of Queen Charlotte's Hospital, one of the oldest and most respected maternity hospitals in the country.

It is widely recognised that women who read about pregnancy and childbirth and who learn about it from the experiences of other women are more likely to be more relaxed during pregnancy and to have a better experience of labour and delivery. This book is intended to help women understand the great physiological changes that take place during pregnancy, labour, delivery and the first few days postpartum, and to explain many of the physical and psychological effects of these changes. The book is written from a mother's point of view, and tries to address and answer the questions that may be raised during your pregnancy.

The case studies from 'real mothers' which appear throughout the book serve as very useful illustrations of what certain experiences really feel like. Where there is more than one case study on the same subject, the contradictions between them further prove that every woman's experience of pregnancy, labour and delivery is different: they help to build up a more complete picture.

Throughout the book, the word partner has been used to mean the woman's husband, the baby's father or the woman's partner who will be assuming the role of father. This general term is intended to embrace a number of different situations, and I hope that it will not cause offence to any readers. During the entire period of the pregnancy the unborn child is called the foetus for simplicity's sake (even though technically the foetus should be known as the embryo for the first two months). The foetus is referred to as 'it', because most women do not know the sex of their baby until the baby is born. In the chapters that deal with delivery and the postpartum period the baby is referred to as 'he' for the simple reason that it makes it easier for readers to distinguish between passages about the mother and the baby. I hope that this will not cause offence, especially as it is counterbalanced, purely by chance, by the fact that there are many more case studies from mothers of girls than of boys.

Doctors are usually referred to as he and midwives as she in this book. There are, of course, a significant percentage of female doctors, and there are a small number of male midwives; the terms he and she are used only to distinguish between references to doctors and midwives.

There are some sections in this book which may seem not to be relevant even to those who would like to read the book from cover to cover. Many women shy away from information on stillbirths and postnatal depression, for example, feeling that these are things that will not happen to them. Sadly, statistically, these things do happen; even if they do not happen to you, you may be better prepared to help a friend in need of support if you have read the relevant passages.

Any book on pregnancy is bound to be a little daunting to a first-time mother, describing as it does a great range of discomforts and problems which can arise during pregnancy, labour and birth. It may be reassuring for readers to know that for almost every woman I spoke to who had had a particular problem, there was another one who said 'I'm not the person to speak to, I've had a really easy time of it!'

Chapter 1

Preparing for Pregnancy

The very fact that you are reading this book probably means that you are already pregnant or that you have decided to start a family. If you are not yet pregnant, there are a number of things that you can do to improve your chances of conceiving quickly, and of having a safe pregnancy and a healthy baby with a good birth weight.

One of the first things you need to take into consideration is your partner's attitude to starting a family. Pregnancy and caring for a baby are great undertakings, and you will need the support of your partner and your family if you are to enjoy them. No one can tell you when is the right time to have a baby – whether it is your first or a second or subsequent one – but you might need to think about timing a pregnancy according to your job, your partner's job, your financial situation, moving house, a course of medication you may be on, illness in the family, and many other factors.

It goes without saying that your general state of health can have a great bearing on whether you conceive easily and have a trouble-free pregnancy. Your partner's state of health is also important: a number of factors can lower his sperm count, so that you may have difficulty conceiving; some aspects of your partner's health and lifestyle could even increase your chances of having a baby with certain abnormalities, however healthy you are yourself. The two most important elements in establishing a healthy lifestyle for both parents are nutrition and exercise.

Nutrition

If you have or can adopt a healthy balanced diet you will create the correct internal environment for conception and pregnancy. There are five main categories of ingredients that constitute a healthy diet:

Proteins: These are the building bricks for your body. The best sources of protein are meat, fish, eggs, cheese (and other dairy products), lentils, peas, beans and nuts. If you are a vegetarian – or more especially a vegan – you may need to read up in more specialised books to ensure that you have adequate sources of protein in your diet. Your requirement for protein rises markedly during pregnancy when you are literally 'building' a baby and a placenta as well as producing more blood. Dairy products are also important because they are a major source of calcium which is needed to build strong bones and teeth for your baby.

Starchy carbohydrates: Carbohydrates provide fuel for your body; the energy released from them maintains your metabolism and enables you to take exercise. Starchy carbohydrates are found in bread, pasta, rice, potatoes, breakfast cereals, semolina and other grain-based foods. Sugars contain another kind of carbohydrate from which the energy is more easily released by the body so that they give you a quicker 'buzz' of energy. The buzz is short-lived and brings with it many calories but little or no nutritional value.

Fibre: Fibre is the bulk in your diet which assists the passage of food through the digestive tract. This is particularly evident in the bowel, where fibre remains moist so that the stools are comfortably soft and are passed more easily. Most sources of dietary fibre also contain valuable amounts of vitamins and minerals. Good sources of fibre include wholegrain cereals and products made from them (such as wholemeal bread), green leafy vegetables, and fruit.

Fats and oils: Fats and oils are another source of energy, but they should not be the chief one. Most of the energy in your diet should be obtained from starchy carbohydrates, and you should limit the fatty foods in your diet and the fats that you use for cooking food. On the other hand, do not be tempted to have a diet very low in fat because fats and oils contain some much needed fat-soluble vitamins. Fats and oils are found in cooking oils, butter, lard and margarines as well as within other foods such as fatty meat, oily fish and nuts.

Fluids: Fluids are crucial to our health and survival; your body can survive longer without food than without fluid (not that you should be thinking of going without either at the moment!). If you are planning a pregnancy or are already pregnant you should try to drink about 1 litre (2 pints) of fluid a day. Spring water is the best and purest drink you can give your body; fruit juices and herbal teas are also good. Try to increase your intake of these and to reduce your consumption of coffee, tea and sugary drinks such as squash or cola.

Putting it all together: Try to eat a wide variety of foods and to have as many fresh and raw ingredients as possible; this will ensure that you are getting all the vitamins and minerals you need. Avoid processed foods (processing leaches out many of the vitamins and minerals in your food) whenever possible, and try to cut down on the salt that you use in cooking or add to food (too much salt in the diet can cause high blood pressure and fluid retention). It is also important to eat regularly, and to take time to sit down and eat meals slowly rather than grabbing them on the run.

Vitamins and minerals: If you follow the guidelines above you will probably have a full complement of vitamins and minerals in your diet, but it may be worth taking a multi-vitamin and -mineral supplement to ensure that you are not lacking in any of these vital micronutrients at a time when great demands are being made on your body. Supplements can be bought from chemists and health shops, and you may be able to find tablets specifically designed for pregnant women. Vitamin and mineral tablets should not be taken instead of a healthy diet; they should be used as a supplement to a healthy diet.

Folic acid: Folic acid is one of the B group vitamins, and research has shown that it plays an important role in ensuring that the fertilised egg implants in the uterine wall, in maintaining the pregnancy and even in the correct formation of the foetus's cells. If your diet is deficient in folic acid you could become anaemic, and your chances of conceiving and having a healthy baby may be compromised (folic acid deficiency in mothers has been specifically linked with an increased incidence of spina bifida in their babies). Dietary folic acid is found in green leafy vegetables such as cabbage and spinach: these should anyway feature regularly in your diet because they contain many other vitamins and minerals and are good sources of fibre. To ensure that you are consuming the recommended daily allowance of folic acid you may want to take a supplement of folic acid while you are trying to conceive and for the first three months of pregnancy. (Once you are pregnant and you have your first appointment with your doctor he may automatically prescribe you supplementary folic acid during your pregnancy.)

Exercise

If you already take regular exercise you will be aware of the benefits of exercise to your general health. Regular exercise improves your stamina and your fitness; your body repairs damage more easily, and is better prepared to take on extra demands such as those presented by pregnancy. You may notice that taking exercise makes you feel more energetic, helps you to sleep better, raises your morale and improves a number of minor complaints such as constipation and headaches.

When you are planning to start a family you need not make any changes to an existing fitness routine, except that – once you have stopped contraception – you should avoid very strenuous exercise at the time of each expected period (if you have conceived, the tiny fertilised egg is in greatest danger of being lost at this time and it can quite literally be dislodged if you take strenuous exercise).

If you do not take exercise regularly your planned pregnancy might be just the motivation you need to start. If you are not sure what sort of exercise you should take talk to your doctor or take advice from a local leisure centre. Walking briskly for 15 minutes three times a week would demand very little of your time and requires no special equipment but would make a noticeable difference to your level of fitness. Swimming is a very good form of exercise, using all the major muscle groups but not putting them under any strain, because your body is supported by the water.

It is important not to make too many demands on your body too quickly that might disturb your menstrual cycle, jeopardising your chances of conceiving easily. Start exercising gently and build up to a more demanding routine over a number of weeks. One of the problems with sticking to an exercise routine is maintaining the motivation and discipline; it may be easier for you if you exercise with your partner or a friend, or join a fitness class.

There are a number of other factors in your lifestyle that may affect your general health and these are outlined below and overleaf:

Smoking, Alcohol and Drugs

It has been established conclusively that smoking, alcohol and drugs are bad for the body and, taken excessively, can be fatal. The strains that they put on your body and your partner's could compromise your chances of conceiving. Even if you do not smoke, drink or use drugs but your partner does, there is an increased risk of many abnormalities in your baby. If you smoke, drink excessively or use drugs once you have conceived, you run a higher risk of miscarrying or of having a baby with abnormalities or a low birth weight.

Smoking: Smoking can reduce the fertility of both parents, so that smokers tend to have more difficulty conceiving. If a woman smokes when she is pregnant, she makes extra demands on her body, reducing her fitness during pregnancy, and sapping her energy for childbirth. During the pregnancy the nicotine and poor oxygen levels in her bloodstream are transmitted to her baby. Smokers have a higher incidence of bleeding during pregnancy and of miscarriage; and babies born to smokers tend to be smaller, less developed and more prone to breathing problems than the babies of non-smoking women. Smoking is also directly related to a higher incidence of cot death.

Alcohol: Alcohol in a pregnant woman's bloodstream is passed directly into the baby's bloodstream through the placenta. Excessive drinking, especially in early pregnancy, can lead to abnormalities in the baby and low birth weight; in really extreme cases the baby's life is threatened. Doctors have traditionally advised women to avoid alcohol altogether during pregnancy, but more recent research has shown that drinking in moderation – not more than a small glass of wine a day, for example – has no proven ill-effects on the baby. You should, however, never lose sight of the fact that alcohol is a drug and can be harmful to your baby.

Drugs: Using drugs can be damaging to the general health and the fertility of both parents, so that drug users (from the heroin addict to the social dope-smoker) may have difficulty conceiving. Drugs taken during pregnancy pass through the placenta into the baby's bloodstream and can have very damaging effects; drug use in pregnant women is associated with miscarriage, premature delivery, low birth-weight babies, and babies with a range of abnormalities. If the mother is addicted to a drug and uses it regularly, the baby may well suffer from withdrawal symptoms when his own 'supply' is cut off when the umbilical cord is severed after delivery.

Giving up: Many women and couples use a pregnancy or planned pregnancy as a really good reason to give up smoking, excessive drinking or using drugs. It is not easy to give up an addictive chemical such as nicotine, and you will need a lot of help and support from your partner, your friends and family. It may also be a long process, so it is best to try and stop or cut down even before you start trying for a baby. If you need help weaning yourself off smoking, drinking or using drugs, your own doctor may be able to give you some advice or to put you in touch with groups and organisations who specialise in this (the addresses of a number of such organisations appear at the end of the book).

CASE STUDY: *'It was easy giving up smoking at first because cigarettes just made me feel sick in the early weeks, but when I started feeling better it became quite hard. I really didn't want to smoke for the sake of the baby, but that doesn't stop you wanting them. It wasn't helped by the fact that [my husband] carried on smoking. At least he would go outside to do it, but I think there should be a law against fathers smoking when the mother's given up!'*

Current Medical Problems and Medication

If you have a medical problem – either a temporary one or a long term one such as diabetes or asthma – and you are planning to start a family, you may well need to talk to your doctor at length about the implications of the condition itself as well as the drugs used to treat it on your chances of conception, on your pregnancy and on the health of your baby.

In the first three months of pregnancy, the cells that make up the foetus begin to differentiate into the limbs and skeleton, the vital organs and the nervous system of your unborn child. While these crucial changes are taking place, the foetus is most sensitive to the chemical changes in the mother's bloodstream caused by medication. Some medicines can produce malformations in the foetus if they are taken at this stage in the pregnancy. If you need to take medication regularly it is important that you speak to your doctor before you become pregnant, so that he can ensure that you are treated in a way that will minimise the risk to your baby once you conceive.

If you do need regular medication and you suddenly discover that you are pregnant, do not give up the medication without consulting your doctor. It may be more dangerous to you and your baby for you to go without the medication than to carry on taking it.

If you have a physical disability or suffer from chronic back pain, you may need to consult with your doctor, an obstetric physiotherapist and other relevant specialists before trying to conceive. They will be able to advise you about how the strains of pregnancy are likely to affect you physically, and how to plan for your antenatal care and your labour and delivery.

CASE STUDY: *'I have always had problems with my back but nothing was going to stop me getting pregnant. I was told that I would be on bed rest from about four months onwards, and that's about when I did have to give up trying to pretend I could cope. It's been very boring and very painful, because I can't use anything stronger than paracetamol which has no effect on the pain at all, like putting a plaster on an amputated leg! I'm very nearly there now, and I'm getting plenty of help lined up because the next problem is going to be lifting the baby.'*

Work and Workplace

Your workplace may be a dangerous place for a pregnant woman: if your work is strenuous, especially if it involves lifting, it may compromise your chances of keeping your baby once you have conceived, and it will make unnecessary demands on your muscles and ligaments during pregnancy. A job that brings you in contact with X-rays, lead or other toxic chemicals could cause malformations in the unborn child. Working with cats or sheep can expose you to potentially dangerous micro-organisms: toxoplasmosis contracted from cats can cause foetal abnormalities; and chlamydia contracted from ewes and lambs can induce miscarriage.

If you think that the work you do is not compatible with pregnancy, you should speak to your doctor about the risks. He may advise you to leave your job before you even become pregnant. If you are not sure about the legal and financial implications of leaving your job because of a pregnancy or a planned pregnancy, contact your local Citizens' Advice Bureau (they should be listed in the telephone directory).

Travel and Vaccinations

If you are hoping to start a family you may need to think about whether the timing will fit in with existing or planned holidays. Vaccinations could be damaging to the foetus, so pregnant women are discouraged from travelling to countries for which vaccinations and malaria tablets are necessary. The stresses of travelling, especially long distance and to places that are very hot or at a high altitude, can make too many demands on your body when you are pregnant. If you have an exotic, long-haul holiday planned it would be better to go and enjoy it before embarking on a pregnancy.

In the early weeks of pregnancy you may feel too ill to travel, and in the last few weeks too tired – or wary of straying too far from your familiar hospital and midwife! (Most airlines will not, anyway, take passengers who are more than 36 weeks pregnant.) The second trimester (the middle months) is the best time for travel so long as you are not over-ambitious with your destination, and you check with your doctor before you leave. If you have had any complications with your pregnancy or suffer from high blood-pressure, your doctor may recommend that you stay close to home for your own and your baby's safety. Even if you are limited in this way, the middle trimester is a good time to have a break and spend some time alone with your partner before your baby arrives.

As there is no guarantee how soon you will conceive, or how you will be feeling when you do, it is better not to plan extravagant holidays when you are trying for a baby. On the other hand, if you do not conceive straight away you might regret having no plans to go away to take your mind off it. If you are planning to go away, strike a happy balance and book a reasonable holiday to a British or short-haul destination.

Older Parents

The age of both parents can affect how easily they conceive: older couples do not usually conceive as easily as younger ones. Women over 35 and men over 40 have an increased risk of having a baby with chromosomal abnormalities such as Down's Syndrome (this risk increases dramatically in a woman over 40 and a man over 55). Older women are also more likely to have multiple births, to develop problems – such as high blood pressure and diabetes – during pregnancy, and to need a Caesarean section.

If you are 35 or over and / or your partner is 40 or over, it may be worth talking to your doctor before you start trying for a baby so that he can give you advice about the special risks associated with conception, pregnancy and childbirth for older parents.

Rubella

If you are planning your first pregnancy, you should ask your doctor to check whether you are immune to rubella (German measles). If you are not immune to German measles and you contract it during the first few months of your pregnancy it can have a very damaging effect on your unborn child: it may cause blindness, deafness, brain damage and heart defects. It is very important to ensure that you are immune to rubella before becoming pregnant.

If you have had German measles or were immunised at school, you will still be immune; it is very rare to lose your immunity, but if you are in any doubt it is worth going ahead with the test. A simple blood test will assess whether or not you are immune, and if you are not, you can be immunised with a single injection. This immunisation should not be carried out if you are already pregnant as it could have some of the same effects as the illness itself.

If you discover that you are not immune to rubella but you are already pregnant, your doctor may recommend that you have tests regularly to check that you have not contracted German measles. The illness is, anyway, becoming increasingly rare in Britain as babies are now usually immunised at 13 months; but you should be aware that there may be an increased risk of catching rubella if you travel abroad.

Blood Groups

If you have the relatively rare Rhesus negative blood group you are likely to be aware of this already, but you may not know of its implications in connection with pregnancy and childbirth: a woman with Rhesus negative blood whose partner has Rhesus positive blood is likely to have a baby with Rhesus positive blood. This first baby is in no danger but, when it is delivered, the exchange of blood from the baby to the mother can cause the mother to build up antibodies to 'fight off' the Rhesus positive cells in her bloodstream. If she then has a second or subsequent Rhesus positive baby, that baby would be in danger of becoming anaemic because of the antibodies in the mother's bloodstream. This problem can be averted if the mother is given an injection after the birth of the first Rhesus positive baby.

If you are planning to start a family and you do not know what your blood group is, it is worth having a blood test. This can be done from the same sample as a test for rubella immunity.

Pelvic Floor Exercises

The pelvic floor is a part of your body that most women will not even know they have until they are well into their pregnancy, but many obstetricians and obstetric physiotherapists recommend doing pelvic floor exercises to strengthen this important group of muscles even before you conceive.

The pelvic floor muscles form a figure-of-eight configuration in your lower abdomen, supporting your uterus, bowel and bladder; you use them subconsciously to control the flow of urine from your bladder and to control your bowel movements. During pregnancy they help to support the growing uterus.

During pregnancy all your muscles loosen and relax under the effects of the hormone progesterone (this is to facilitate the process of childbirth), and this includes the pelvic floor muscles. Towards the end of your pregnancy you may find that you suffer from what is called stress incontinence. As the pelvic floor muscles relax, they can allow small amounts of urine to pass when they are put under sudden pressure, for example when you cough, sneeze, laugh or even just bend over. This can be embarrassing and, if you do not work on the pelvic floor muscles, it might continue long after you have had your baby.

Identifying and working on your pelvic floor muscles can help you to avoid what can turn into a long-term inconvenience and embarrassment. If you learn how to contract your pelvic floor muscles you will also know how to relax them and this could help you during the second stage of your labour, when you are actually pushing your baby into the world.

Identifying the Pelvic Floor Muscles

The simplest way to identify the pelvic floor muscles is to wait until you need to urinate and then to try and interrupt the flow of urine before you have finished. Although you only want to tighten the tiny but powerful sphincter muscle of your urethra (which releases urine from the bladder), you will actually feel the tightening throughout the pelvic floor, affecting your bowel, your vagina and your urethra. You can also identify the pelvic floor muscles by 'squeezing' your partner's penis with the muscles of your vagina when you are making love.

Exercising the Pelvic Floor Muscles

The ways of identifying the pelvic floor muscles are also good ways of exercising them. If you regularly interrupt your flow of urine, you will gradually increase the strength of your pelvic floor muscles. At first you may be able to hold only the last few drops for a second or so, but as the muscles become stronger your control will improve dramatically so that you can 'switch' the flow of urine on and off several times in one sitting.

Your partner can help and encourage you to strengthen your pelvic floor muscles – and he may enjoy it too – if you practise squeezing his penis during love-making. Again, at first, you will probably manage only short squeezes, but as the muscles develop and you become more conscious of them you may be able to hold and release a strong squeeze several times in succession.

Once you have become familiar with the feeling of contracting your pelvic floor-muscles, you need no longer wait until you are on the loo or making love to exercise them! You can work them when you are lying in bed reading a book: contract them for a count of three and then release. Or tighten them in stages (this is more difficult), as if you were tugging gently higher and higher before releasing.

Exercising your pelvic floor muscles need not take any time out of your day – you can do it when you are doing other things, even standing on the bus! – and it does not require any special equipment, but it could make your delivery easier and may well save you from the embarrassment of stress incontinence.

Posture and Back Care

It is very common for women to suffer from backache at some stage during pregnancy. Back pain might seem inevitable if you consider the extra demands that are made on your back: you put on weight, your entire shape and centre of gravity changes and the muscles and ligaments of the back are slackened by the effects of progesterone. A great deal of back pain could, in fact, be reduced or avoided altogether if more attention was paid to correct posture and to good back care (there is more information about posture and back care in the feature on **Backache** in **Week 28** of the **Your Pregnancy Week by Week** chapter).

Queen Charlotte's Hospital is one of several hospitals that have specialised obstetric physiotherapists, and they recommend that women think about their posture, and about how they lift things and bend over even before they become pregnant. It can take a long time to adapt and change postural habits, and the sooner you start the better. If you are prone to back pain, or are concerned about the effects that pregnancy might have on your back, speak to your doctor and he may be able to put you in touch with an obstetric physiotherapist. You may want to contact the Association of Chartered Physiotherapists in Women's Health (their address appears at the end of the book).

Discontinuing Contraception

Starting a family may not be as simple as you thought, you may already be astonished by how many things can affect conception, pregnancy and childbirth. Another factor that may affect when and how easily you conceive is the kind of contraception that you have been using.

If you use temporary barrier contraceptives – such as condoms, femidoms or a cap – your menstrual cycle will not have been disrupted, and you should be ovulating normally every month. You can simply stop using the contraceptive device and start trying to make babies. You may find that you conceive straight away, but you should not worry even if it takes several months.

If you use a more permanent barrier method – such as a coil – you will need to have the device removed by your doctor before you can conceive. Ask your doctor at which stage in your cycle it is best to have the device removed, and then make an appointment for the appropriate time. Once you have had the contraceptive device removed, your doctor may advise that you wait a couple of months before trying to conceive (you may be prone to infections of the cervix and even to miscarriage for a few weeks). In the intervening months you should use a barrier method of contraception, such as condoms, to ensure that you do not become pregnant.

If you use a chemical contraceptive – such as the pill, hormone injections or an implant – these actively disrupt your natural menstrual cycle, and you should talk to your doctor about discontinuing the contraceptive treatment. You will probably be advised to wait for about three months, or even up to six months, after discontinuing contraception before you start trying to conceive (some brands of implants claim that your cycle returns to normal as soon as they are removed). This will allow your own menstrual cycle to re-establish itself properly before you become pregnant. In order to ensure that you do not become pregnant, you should use one of the barrier methods, such as condoms, during these months.

You may resent the period of waiting after discontinuing contraception and before trying to conceive. If you do become pregnant very soon, there are few real risks to the baby but – because your cycle will have been disrupted – your pregnancy may be difficult to date. This not only means that you will not have a clear idea of your due date, it also means that medical professionals will not be able to judge whether the foetus is growing at the expected rate, because they will not know its exact age. Bearing in mind that many checks carried out on the foetus are directly related to its age and expected size, this could have even more serious implications.

The Menstrual Cycle and 'Fertile' Days

When you are trying to start a family, especially if you have been trying for a few months without success, it is just as well to have a good understanding of how your monthly cycle works, and when you are most likely to be fertile.

You will probably know more or less how long your cycle is and how regular it is. An average menstrual cycle is about 28 days long, but it may be as short as 25 days or as long as 35 days, and it can vary from one month to the next. Some women find that a very irregular cycle can be settled down permanently by taking the pill for a few months to establish a regular 28-day cycle. To assess when your fertile period is, you need to know when you are ovulating.

Ovulation and your Fertile Period

When you ovulate, a mature egg is released by your ovary and is wafted by tiny hairs called cilia into the end of your fallopian tube to begin its journey to the womb. Before this egg dies (up to two days later) it can be fertilised by your partner's sperm after love-making. The tiny spermatozoa travel all the way from your vagina, through your cervix and womb, and along your fallopian tube. This does not necessarily mean that fertilisation can take place only if you make love on the day of or the day after ovulation. Sperm can survive inside you for up to three days, so love-making can result in conception for a period of nearly a week, about three days on either side of the day on which you ovulate.

A small proportion of women are aware of a mild abdominal pain, known as the *mittelschmerz*, when they ovulate. Most have to do a simple calculation to work out when they ovulate and when their fertile period is.

Make a note of the day on which your next period is likely to start and then count back 14 days to establish approximately when you will ovulate. Most women ovulate 14 days before their period, regardless of the length of their cycle, although it can be between 12 and 16 days before.

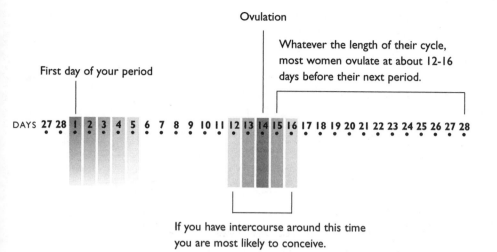

An average 28-day cycle. Yours may be longer or shorter

Vaginal Discharge

Once you are aware of when you are ovulating you may notice that your vaginal discharge changes during the course of the month (some women have very little vaginal discharge and will not notice a difference, others will have noticed the changes for themselves). For about the first five days of your cycle you lose menstrual blood, which is followed by a thick, whitish discharge for several days. About a week later the vaginal discharge changes: it becomes clearer, more fluid, and stringy or slimy. This is your natural lubricant which facilitates love-making during your fertile period. Another week later, when your fertile period is over, the discharge will thicken and become white again, drying up towards the end of your cycle. Your next period heralds the start of the next cycle.

If you notice that your discharge becomes clear and slippery earlier or later in the month than this, it could mean that you are ovulating unusually early or late in your cycle. It is possible to establish fairly precisely when you have ovulated by checking your body temperature.

Body Temperature and Ovulation

A woman's body temperature drops to about 36.2°C (97°F) just before she ovulates and then rises back above the normal 36.4°C (97.4°F) to about 36.7°C (98°F) after ovulation. The rise in temperature, which can

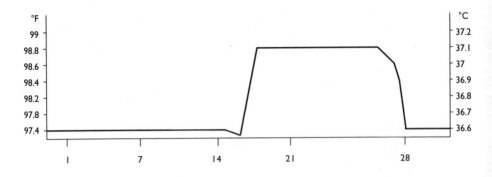

A noticeable rise in temperature indicates that you have ovulated.

last through to the end of the cycle, is caused by the hormone progesterone which is released with the egg and raises the body's metabolism.

If you want to pinpoint exactly when you are ovulating – either because you have a very irregular cycle or because you have been trying for a baby for several months without success – you can try to establish when you ovulate by taking your temperature daily. Take your temperature regularly at the same time of day for a whole cycle and you should see a pattern similar to the one shown in the graph above emerging. (You can buy ovulation kits from chemists: they include a thermometer and specially designed charts to fill in with your daily temperature readings.)

Your fertile period is on either side of the sharp rise in temperature, which immediately follows ovulation. The time to make love to give yourself the best chance of conceiving is when your temperature has dropped. That is, just before ovulation. This gives the sperm the time to begin their journey towards the fallopian tube so that they are there and still alive when the egg is released.

Obviously, if you have a fever, the readings for that time will be distorted and difficult to interpret. Your ovulation may also be affected by a number of other factors such as a sudden increase in the amount of exercise you are taking, a crash diet or stress.

If you do not see an obvious dip-and-rise in your temperature chart for two or three successive months this could mean that you are not ovulating at all, even though you may be menstruating normally. You should talk to your doctor who may advise that you have more detailed tests to establish whether or not you are ovulating. He may ask you many questions about your lifestyle, especially your eating habits, to discover whether your ovulation has been temporarily interrupted or whether there is an underlying problem of infertility.

When will you Conceive?

Some couples joke that they just have to sit on the same chair one after the other to conceive, whereas others can take up to a year, or longer, to conceive even if neither of them has any problems of infertility.

Making love at the right time of the month gives you the best chances of conceiving, but it certainly carries no form of guarantee. If you look at the mechanics of conception it can be a very 'hit and miss' affair: firstly the egg is released by the ovary, loose into your abdominal cavity. Admittedly, it is very near the end of the fallopian tube, but there is a chance that it will never enter the fallopian tube and will be lost in the abdominal cavity. Then it should be wafted into and along the tube by tiny finger-like projections called cilia. It only lives for about 24 hours, and if it is not fertilised in this time it will die. The dead egg will be wafted on into the uterus and washed away with your next period.

If you do make love at this time, your partner's ejaculation will release around 200 million microscopic spermatozoa into your vagina. They are chemically programmed to head for the cervix, through the uterus to the egg in the fallopian tube. They are produced in their millions in order to increase the chances that just one will eventually fertilise the egg. Millions of them can be lost if the ejaculate drains out of your vagina. The same number may never reach further than the neck of the womb, and millions more may travel into the 'wrong' fallopian tube (your ovaries usually release an egg alternately each month; in the example illustrated below the egg has been released by the left ovary).

A few thousand spermatozoa will start the journey along the correct fallopian tube but only about 200 (1 in 1,000,000 of the original number released) will reach the egg and swarm around it until one manages to penetrate the outer layer of the egg and fertilise it. The outer layer of the egg immediately changes its chemical make-up, acting as a barrier to the other spermatozoa, protecting the genetic information which will become your baby. This whole process can happen in the space of an hour, but sometimes even the law of averages fails.

A doctor probably would not question your fertility unless you had been trying unsuccessfully to conceive for at least a year. This is because there

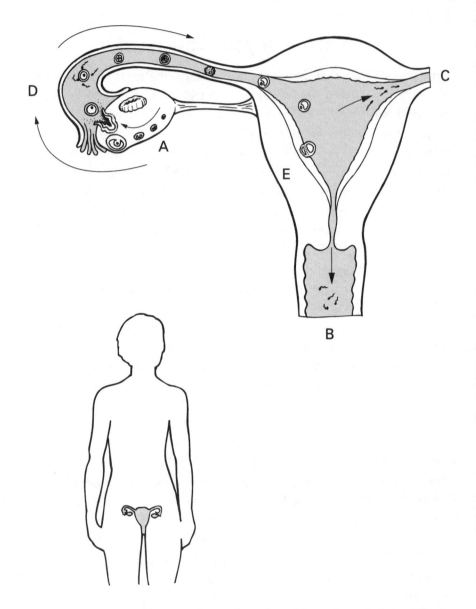

The egg matures in the ovary (A) and is released into the end of the fallopian tube. Sperm is ejaculated into the vagina (B); thousands of spermatozoa may drain out of the vagina and thousands more may be lost in the 'wrong' fallopian tube (C). A few hundred may reach the ripe egg, and one single spermatozoa may fertilise the egg in the fallopian tube (D).

are so many things, apart from the purely mechanical ones, that affect your chances of conceiving. The fertility of both partners can be temporarily compromised by changes to their lifestyle, and especially by stress.

If you have been trying to conceive for more than three months, have a good look at your lifestyle, at what you eat, whether you smoke or drink, and how much pressure your job or your financial circumstances put on you, to see whether any of these factors could be reducing your chances of conceiving. Try to improve your chances by following the guidelines laid out at the beginning of this chapter, and by working out when you are ovulating as explained above. Make an appointment to see your doctor to discuss factors that could be affecting your fertility. He will probably reassure you that it is quite normal for conception not to take place straight away, and it can take up to a year for a healthy couple to conceive. He may arrange for you to have another appointment in about six months if you still have not conceived.

CASE STUDY: *'We conceived our first baby very quickly but we tried for over a year before the second one came along. The disappointment of not conceiving is indescribable. Every month you have this terrible strain, and every day you worry: "shall I have a gin and tonic or will it hurt the baby?" and then every month you're disappointed, you've taken all these precautions for nothing.'*

Frequency of Love-making

If you are trying to help your chances of conceiving in every way, you can make a point of having intercourse when you know that you are ovulating. Some doctors advocate making love as often as possible at this time, but this might actually work against the law of averages. The sperm-producing cells in the man's testicles cannot replenish the average 200 million spermatozoa per ejaculate if he is ejaculating several times a day. If each ejaculate contains a lower than average number of spermatozoa, the chances of conceiving after any one ejaculation are lowered.

On the other hand, if you abstain from love-making in the hopes of building up a large number of spermatozoa, the sperm-producing cells will not be stimulated to keep producing new cells so rapidly. You may well have a larger than average number of sperm in that one ejaculation, but they may not be replenished so quickly for the next time. It is a simple question of supply and demand, and although it varies from one man to another, your chances of conceiving are probably highest if you make love about once a day during your fertile period.

We are genetically programmed to enjoy sex in order to ensure that we propagate the species, but it is alarming how many couples who are having difficulties conceiving find that intercourse can become a chore, something that has to be done to order when the temperature chart says so. Try not to be obsessive about temperature charts and having intercourse at exactly the moment that your temperature drops. If you are familiar with your cycle, you should know in advance when your fertile period is likely to be. Far from spoiling your love-making by robbing its spontaneity, planning ahead for the days when you 'should' have intercourse can add its own element of fun. Do not lose sight of the fact that sex itself is pleasurable and not just a necessary step to having a baby.

HELPING CONCEPTION

By looking at the diagram of the vagina and the uterus in the section **When will you Conceive?** you can see that if you are in an upright position (for example, sitting astride your partner) during or immediately after making love, much of the ejaculate can be lost as it drains out of the vagina. If you make love in the missionary position or face-down with your bottom in the air (or if you move into a similar position immediately after your partner has ejaculated), the force of gravity will help the ejaculate to pass through your cervix and to the top of the womb where it can enter the fallopian tubes.

Chapter 2

Your Pregnancy Week by Week

Some women say that they are aware of the moment of conception, whereas others can go through an entire pregnancy without realising it, and are astonished to produce a baby at all. These are obviously extremes, but your experience could be anywhere along the spectrum in between.

I f you have been planning a pregnancy, especially if you have kept a note of your periods and have made love at your most fertile time of the month, you will be on the look-out for tiny clues in the days preceding your next period.

There are a number of different early warning signals that women may notice in the first few days after conception. A small minority say that they can feel a little twinge or just 'something different' in the area of the uterus; others notice changes to their sense of smell and taste, or experience tiredness or nausea as the hormones released by the fertilised egg kick in. Many women say that the first sign of pregnancy is a tingling feeling in their breasts, or that their breasts feel heavy.

EARLY SIGNS OF PREGNANCY

Tingling, heavy breasts   **Acute sense of smell**
Unexpected tiredness   **Frequent urinating**
Changes to sense of taste   **Feelings of nausea**

CASE STUDY: *'One morning I realised there was a tugging feeling in my breasts, as if a thread was attached behind the nipple and it was being pulled ever so gently backwards. They felt a bit heavy too, like just before a period, except that it was about a week until my next period was due.'*

Most women first realise they are pregnant when they miss a period, but this is not conclusive proof of pregnancy: you can, for example, miss a period if you are under a lot of stress or if you suddenly start taking more exercise than usual. On the other hand, you may not actually miss your first period after conceiving; you may have what appears to be a period or some light bleeding at the time of your expected period.

You can confirm a pregnancy with a home testing kit as early as the first day of a missed period (some kits can give a positive result even before the first day of a missed period).

Home Testing Kits

Pregnancy testing kits can be bought from most chemist shops, and they are very simple to use. They are urine tests designed to detect the presence of a hormone called human chorionic gonadotrophin (HCG). HCG is present in the mother from conception and is excreted in the urine.

The way kits work and display their results varies, so does their accuracy and the time when they should be used. You should check the manufacturer's instructions and follow them carefully. Most kits are over 90% accurate if they are used in the early morning (when the urine is concentrated) on or later than the first day of a missed period. If the results of the test are positive, you should make an appointment to see your doctor. If you have a negative result after the first test, wait about a week and, if you still have not had a period, take a second test.

Testing kits can be costly, and free pregnancy testing is available from the NHS. Your local surgery or hospital will provide a sample bottle for your urine, and test it for HCG (if the urine test is not conclusive they may run a blood test for HCG). Results are available in one or two days.

Letting Your Doctor Know

You should arrange to see your doctor as soon as you think that you are pregnant. This is especially important if you are on any sort of medication, which might be dangerous for your baby. Your doctor will be able to give you advice about medication and other drugs, smoking, alcohol, exercise and nutrition in connection with your pregnancy.

You will probably not be examined if you are in the very early stages of pregnancy, but your GP will discuss any questions or anxieties that you might have. He will be able to tell you about antenatal care in your area, and he will help you to think about whether you want your antenatal care to be handled by the surgery, the local hospital or a midwife.

Choosing Your Antenatal Care

Most women attend all or most of their antenatal clinics at their local doctors' surgery. If your GP's workload allows, you may be offered the choice of seeing a midwife or your own GP for your antenatal check-ups.

In some areas a Domino Scheme (**Dom**iciliary – **in** – **o**ut) is operated; in the Domino Scheme your antenatal check-ups are handled by one of a team of community midwives, often in your own home. One of thesm will accompany you to hospital for the birth of your baby, and will oversee your early transfer from hospital. The same midwives continue with your check-ups at home for at least the first ten days of your baby's life. Queen Charlotte's Hospital has piloted a one-to-one midwife scheme in which a woman sees the same midwife throughout her pregnancy, and is then delivered by her. Research has shown that this sort of continuity of care they feel more relaxed and confident during their pregnancy, and they may even need less intervention for labour and delivery.

Your doctor will ask you to make a 'booking appointment' – your first official antenatal check-up – for about the twelfth week of your pregnancy. In order to establish when that will be, he will ask you the date of the first day of your last period to date the pregnancy.

Dating Your Pregnancy

Even though pregnancy knows no national frontiers, and is recognised the world over as being just over nine months long, health professionals in different countries once used a number of different ways of calculating your estimated date of delivery (EDD), the date that your baby is due to be born. It is now internationally recognised that pregnancy lasts about 40 weeks from the first day of your last menstrual period (LMP).

January	October	February	November	March	December	April	January	May	February	June	March
1	8	1	8	1	6	1	6	1	5	1	8
2	9	2	9	2	7	2	7	2	6	2	9
3	10	3	10	3	8	3	8	3	7	3	10
4	11	4	11	4	9	4	9	4	8	4	11
5	12	5	12	5	10	5	10	5	9	5	12
6	13	6	13	6	11	6	11	6	10	6	13
7	14	7	14	7	12	7	12	7	11	7	14
8	15	8	15	8	13	8	13	8	12	8	15
9	16	9	16	9	14	9	14	9	13	9	16
10	17	10	17	10	15	10	15	10	14	10	17
11	18	11	18	11	16	11	16	11	15	11	18
12	19	12	19	12	17	12	17	12	16	12	19
13	20	13	20	13	18	13	18	13	17	13	20
14	21	14	21	14	19	14	19	14	18	14	21
15	22	15	22	15	20	15	20	15	19	15	22
16	23	16	23	16	21	16	21	16	20	16	23
17	24	17	24	17	22	17	22	17	21	17	24
18	25	18	25	18	23	18	23	18	22	18	25
19	26	19	26	19	24	19	24	19	23	19	26
20	27	20	27	20	25	20	25	20	24	20	27
21	28	21	28	21	26	21	26	21	25	21	28
22	29	22	29	22	27	22	27	22	26	22	29
23	30	23	30	23	28	23	28	23	27	23	30
24	31	24	1	24	29	24	29	24	28	24	31
25	1	25	2	25	30	25	30	25	1	25	1
26	2	26	3	26	31	26	31	26	2	26	2
27	3	27	4	27	1	27	1	27	3	27	3
28	4	28	5	28	2	28	2	28	4	28	4
29	5			29	3	29	3	29	5	29	5
30	6			30	4	30	4	30	6	30	6
31	7			31	5			31	7		

January	November	February	December	March	January	April	February	May	March	June	April

The duration of a pregnancy is, however, not unlike the length of a piece of string, because there are so many contributory factors that can affect it. It is considered normal for a pregnancy to be as short as 37 weeks or as long as 42 weeks. To add further confusion, a woman may have some bleeding at the time of her expected period for one or even several months after conception. Other smaller considerations can alter the due date by a few days: the 40-week dating system is based on a 28-day menstrual cycle, whereas many women have shorter, longer or irregular menstrual cycles.

July / April		August / May		September / June		October / July		November / August		December / September	
1	7	1	8	1	8	1	8	1	8	1	7
2	8	2	9	2	9	2	9	2	9	2	8
3	9	3	10	3	10	3	10	3	10	3	9
4	10	4	11	4	11	4	11	4	11	4	10
5	11	5	12	5	12	5	12	5	12	5	11
6	12	6	13	6	13	6	13	6	13	6	12
7	13	7	14	7	14	7	14	7	14	7	13
8	14	8	15	8	15	8	15	8	15	8	14
9	15	9	16	9	16	9	16	9	16	9	15
10	16	10	17	10	17	10	17	10	17	10	16
11	17	11	18	11	18	11	18	11	18	11	17
12	18	12	19	12	19	12	19	12	19	12	18
13	19	13	20	13	20	13	20	13	20	13	19
14	20	14	21	14	21	14	21	14	21	14	20
15	21	15	22	15	22	15	22	15	22	15	21
16	22	16	23	16	23	16	23	16	23	16	22
17	23	17	24	17	24	17	24	17	24	17	23
18	24	18	25	18	25	18	25	18	25	18	24
19	25	19	26	19	26	19	26	19	26	19	25
20	26	20	27	20	27	20	27	20	27	20	26
21	27	21	28	21	28	21	28	21	28	21	27
22	28	22	29	22	29	22	29	22	29	22	28
23	29	23	30	23	30	23	30	23	30	23	29
24	30	24	31	24	1	24	31	24	31	24	30
25	1	25	1	25	2	25	1	25	1	25	1
26	2	26	2	26	3	26	2	26	2	26	2
27	3	27	3	27	4	27	3	27	3	27	3
28	4	28	4	28	5	28	4	28	4	28	4
29	5	29	5	29	6	29	5	29	5	29	5
30	6	30	6	30	7	30	6	30	6	30	6
31	7	31	7			31	7			31	7

July / May		August / June		September / July		October / August		November / September		December / November	

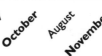

Finally, any system of dating assumes that conception takes place approximately half way through the cycle, which is not always the case. In any event, it is important to understand that the estimated date of delivery is just that – an estimate.

> CASE STUDY: *'I breastfed my first baby for a year and didn't have a period for that whole year. When I stopped feeding her we went away for a holiday and were … a bit careless, and, well, I just kept not having a period. I soon realised I was pregnant again, and we worked out that the baby was conceived on the holiday. I did a sort of guestimate of my due-date. When the scan gave me a date it was only two days out.'*

If it is difficult to date a pregnancy using the criteria above, an ultrasound scan can be used to estimate the baby's due date. The scan can check the exact size and stage of development of the baby, and this information can be used to establish how old your baby is and when your EDD will be.

Telling Friends and Family

Only a generation ago many women did not have their pregnancy officially confirmed until the third month, and they waited for this confirmation before announcing the pregnancy to friends and family. Many feel that, however soon you yourself know that you are pregnant, it is better not to announce a pregnancy until the end of the first twelve weeks; this is the period when the pregnancy is at greatest risk of miscarriage. Others would question this approach, saying that if a woman miscarries she will need the help and support of those around her, and it will be easier for her to talk to them and ask for their help if they knew about the pregnancy in the first place.

One minor consideration is the fact that nine months is actually a very long time. Although you may be terribly excited about your pregnancy and the arrival of your baby, it might be difficult for other people to share this excitement and sustain it for nine months. If you tell people on the first day of a missed period, they may have to wait three months before you even have a tiny bump to show for it, and then it will still be another five months before your baby is born.

The most important thing is for you to announce the pregnancy at a time that is right for you. You should think about it and discuss it with your partner. You may feel that you want to keep it to yourself until after the three month threshold or you may want to share your happiness straight away. If you are not happy about the pregnancy, or worried about its implications you might need to discuss it with friends and family as well as you midwife and your GP as soon as possible.

Even if you do decide to wait a few weeks before telling people you could suffer from such obvious symptoms that they guess anyway. Close girlfriends, mothers and women who have recently had babies themselves are particularly good at picking up tell-tale signs.

Telling your Employer

If you work, you need to think about when you are going to let your employer know that you are expecting a baby, so that he or she can make arrangements to cover for your absence. Every woman is entitled to 14 weeks maternity leave and to return to the same job on the same hours after that time, no matter what hours she has worked or how long she has been in her present job. Your employer should also allow you time off for antenatal care: your check-ups and antenatal classes.

Many employees wait until the third month to tell their employers that they are pregnant, but you may decide to tell your employer earlier, and it could work to your advantage: if you feel very tired or nauseous in the early weeks, an understanding employer may be more lenient with you if he or she knows that you are pregnant.

The earliest that your maternity leave can start is the twenty-ninth week of your pregnancy. If you intend to start your maternity leave then, you should have written to your employer to tell him or her by the end of the twenty-sixth week. Whatever your plans concerning maternity leave, your employer will probably ask you for a certificate of pregnancy (Mat B1), which you can obtain from your GP, midwife or hospital when you have a check-up.

Week 3

Although pregnancies are dated back to the first day of the last period, conception does not actually take place until about two weeks later, at the beginning of the third week of the cycle. The pregnancy, therefore, actually starts in week three.

When the head of one spermatozoa penetrates the outer surface of the egg, that egg has been fertilised. The egg and the sperm each contain a half set of genetic information; those two halves make up the whole that will be your child. Once the egg has been fertilised it begins the process of cell division: one cell divides to form two, then four, then eight and so on. At the same time, the fertilised egg travels along the fallopian tube towards the uterus, wafted by tiny hairs called cilia.

The Foetus

By the end of week three (about seven days after fertilisation has taken place) the fertilised egg has developed into a ball of about 100 cells known as a blastocyst. It measures a tiny 0.15mm, and is just visible to the naked eye.

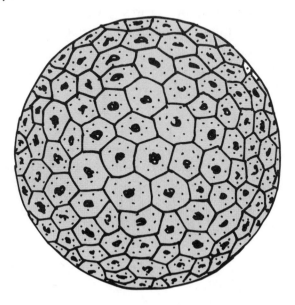

One week after conception, the fertilised egg has divided repeatedly to form a ball of about 100 cells known as a blastocyst.

What is Happening to the Foetus

At about this time the fertilised egg arrives in the uterus and implants itself in the endometrium, the lining of the uterus. This site will eventually become the placenta, the sophisticated organ that filters oxygen and nutrients into the foetus from the mother's bloodstream, and removes waste products from the foetus's bloodstream. When the blastocyst has successfully implanted itself in the uterine wall the exchange between the mother and baby has truly begun: the human chorionic gonadotrophin (HCG), which is released by the rudimentary placenta, passes directly into the mother's bloodstream and begins to trigger the hormonal activity in the mother which is necessary to maintain the pregnancy. It is at this stage that some women begin to feel early symptoms of pregnancy, and that HCG can be detected in the urine.

How you Feel

You could remain oblivious to the momentous events inside your womb for some weeks yet, or you may be experiencing early signs of pregnancy such as tingling, heavy breasts, tiredness and nausea. If you are aware that you are pregnant, your emotional reaction to the pregnancy could take you by surprise. You may be overjoyed and excited with a tremendous feeling of importance and achievement, even at this early stage.

Conversely, some women – even those who have been very keen to conceive and have been trying for several months – suddenly feel unsure of themselves when they realise they are pregnant. Pregnancy is usually the biggest physical and emotional undertaking of a woman's life, and it can be daunting. There is nothing wrong with you if you are not glowing with pride and enthusiasm from the word go; having a baby will change your life dramatically, and you may be apprehensive about the implications to yourself, your job and your relationships. The system allows for this: it gives you nine months to adjust!

CASE STUDY: *'It felt incredibly unreal. It was two days before I could tell anyone, even my partner. We'd been trying for six months but I suddenly went from not having anything to having this thing in my hand [the pregnancy testing kit] and I felt everything else might change. I needed some time to come to terms with it.'*

Things you Should Avoid in Early Pregnancy

Heavy Lifting – Stretching Up – Strenuous Exercise

There are a number of things that can jeopardise your baby, especially in the early weeks of pregnancy. In the first few weeks, when the fertilised egg has just implanted itself in the uterine wall, it is at risk of becoming detached from the wall which provides its supply of nutrients and oxygen. To give the foetus the best chance of implanting itself securely you should avoid activities which use your abdominal muscles, such as heavy lifting, repeated stretching, and very strenuous exercise.

Your fitness and general health are important to the growing foetus, but you should try to establish a fitness routine before conceiving, rather than rushing out to get fit once you know that you are pregnant. Sudden changes to the requirements you make on your body can compromise your chances of keeping the baby.

Medicines and Other Drugs

In the first three months of pregnancy the cells that make up the foetus begin to differentiate into the limbs and skeleton, the vital organs and the nervous system of your unborn child. While these crucial changes are taking place, the foetus is most sensitive to the chemical changes in the mother's bloodstream caused by medication and other drugs. Some medicines can produce malformations in the foetus if they are taken at this stage in the pregnancy. Tell your doctor or pharmacist that you are pregnant before they suggest any medication for you. Always read labels carefully before taking any kind of medicine, even alternative remedies can contain powerful ingredients which may be harmful to the foetus.

Smoking

If a woman smokes when she is pregnant, the nicotine and poor oxygen levels in her bloodstream are transmitted to her baby. Smokers have a higher incidence of bleeding during pregnancy and of miscarriage; and babies born to smokers tend to be smaller, less developed and more prone to breathing problems than the babies of non-smoking women. Smoking is also directly related to a higher incidence of cot death.

Smoking is bad for your baby before and after birth. Smoking also makes extra demands on the mother's body, reducing her fitness during pregnancy and delivery. If you do smoke you should try to use your pregnancy and your baby's health as motivation to give up. It is not easy to give up smoking, and you will need a lot of help and support from the baby's father, your friends and family, as well as your GP who may be able to suggest ways of 'weaning' you off cigarettes.

Alcohol

If a pregnant woman has an alcoholic drink, the alcohol will be passed on to the baby's bloodstream through the placenta. This sounds alarming and it can indeed have alarming consequences. Excessive drinking, especially in early pregnancy, can lead to abnormalities in the baby and low birth weight; in really extreme cases, the baby's life is threatened.

Doctors have traditionally advised women to avoid alcohol altogether during pregnancy, and this is no hardship for many women because a sizeable proportion of women loose any desire to drink alcohol, at least in the early weeks. More recent research has shown that drinking in moderation – not more than a glass of wine a day, for example – has no proven ill-effects on the baby.

Many GPs will consider that it is safe for pregnant women to consume about 1 unit of alcohol a day (this is the equivalent of a single measure of spirits, a small glass of wine or half a pint of ordinary strength beer, lager or cider). Some may even say that, ironically, the baby might benefit indirectly: if the mother is used to having a drink in the evening and finds that it helps her to relax, the baby will benefit from the physiological differences produced by her relaxed state. You should, however, never lose sight of the fact that alcohol is a drug and can be harmful to your baby: moderation is essential.

Pâté – Soft Cheese – Uncooked Meat

Certain foods are potential sources of bacteria which can harm your baby. Even if they are things that you normally eat and you feel that your 'system' is used to coping with them, the pregnancy may be compromised. Pâté and soft cheeses (including goat's and ewe's milk cheeses) should be avoided altogether when you are pregnant. They can contain the listeria bacterium which is known significantly to increase the risk of miscarriage or stillbirth.

Always make sure that pre-prepared meals are cooked right through and piping hot, and make sure that eggs and meat are cooked thoroughly. Raw egg and undercooked meat can also contain harmful bacteria. Make sure that the milk that you drink is pasteurised; and clean fruits and vegetables well before eating them.

Many doctors advise pregnant women to avoid eating liver and liver products altogether, but this is another instance where moderation is advisable. Liver is a good source of a number of nutrients including iron and vitamin A, which means that it is good for you and the baby. Too much vitamin A, however, could be harmful to your baby. Vitamin A is what is called a fat-soluble vitamin, and excesses of fat-soluble vitamins are not easy for the body to excrete. If you eat a lot of liver and liver products, you could accumulate harmful amounts of Vitamin A in your bloodstream. If, on the other hand, you eat no liver at all, you are denying yourself a useful source of iron (and iron is so important to a healthy pregnancy that many women have to take iron supplements).

X-rays – Sun-beds

X-rays, and other tests which use forms of radiation, could be extremely harmful to the unborn child. If you have had this sort of test in the early weeks of a pregnancy before you knew that you were pregnant, discuss it with your doctor or specialist and he will be able to implement tests such as an ultrasound scan to establish whether your baby has been affected in any way. If you need to have a radiation test performed when you are pregnant, always tell the doctor or specialist that you are pregnant. X-rays are not only performed by doctors, they may also be carried out by dentists … and vets. If your pet needs an X-ray when you are pregnant, tell the vet, and he will find someone else to hold the animal.

Sun-beds, and the ultra-violet rays they emit, could also harm your baby. Little is known about the possible harmful effects of concentrated ultra-violet rays on the foetus, but the heat of a sun-bed alone could be damaging, so do not use sun-beds when you are pregnant.

Week 4

The end of the fourth week of your pregnancy, when the foetus is two weeks old, is an important time. The blastocyst has implanted itself in the uterine wall and has started 'signalling' its presence to the mother's physiology with human chorionic gonadotrophin. The mother's glands, including the ovary from which the egg was released in the first place, respond to this by producing and excreting hormones that create the correct environment to sustain the pregnancy. One of the first things these hormones have to do is to suppress the menstruation which would otherwise happen after four weeks.

If the hormones have not reached high enough levels, normal menstruation will take place and the tiny foetus will be 'washed out' of the uterus. Even without losing the foetus, it is possible to have a light period or to have a show of blood two weeks after conception, when your next period was due. In most cases there will be no bleeding, and this will be the first concrete evidence that conception has taken place.

The Foetus

In one week the foetus has more than doubled in size, although it is still only about half a millimetre in length. The foetus is no longer just a ball of cells, it is slightly elongated, and is becoming separate from the cells that will form the amniotic sac (which surrounds and protects the baby inside the womb) and the placenta.

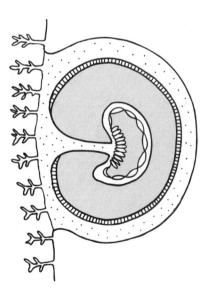

What is Happening to the Foetus

The foetus has 'designated' some cells to specialise and become the amniotic sacs and the placenta. It was once believed that the uterus provided these, but research has now proved that

The two-week old blastocyst attaches itself to the uterine wall, and the cells begin to specialise into the embryo itself, the placenta and the amniotic sac.

they come from the growing foetus. It is, in fact, possible – although extremely rare – for the foetus to imbed itself in the wall of another abdominal organ, such as the large intestine, and to grow to term safely. It has even been suggested that an implanted foetus could gestate successfully in a man's abdominal cavity.

The structure of the foetus itself is also changing. The cells are beginning to form three distinct groups known as germ layers. These groups are the foundations for every part of your baby's body including the skeleton, the nerves and the vital organs.

How you Look
On the outside you will not look any different, unless you are a little pale and nauseous. There will certainly be no physical evidence of the tiny but tumultuous changes taking place inside you. The uterus is still tucked inside the pelvis, and you will not have a 'tummy' for a number of weeks yet.

How you Feel
It is very early days yet and you may feel nothing at all or you may be experiencing some of the early symptoms of pregnancy, such as sensitive breasts, an altered sense of taste and smell, tiredness and passing urine frequently.

Talking to Your Partner

Pregnancy is a tremendous undertaking. Women have been doing it for millions of years, and it should be a very happy and exciting time, but that does not make it any less of a drain on your physical and emotional resources. Not only does it make huge demands on your body, it also has a number of far-reaching psycho-social implications: it will certainly change your life but it might also alter the equilibrium of many relationships; it could mean giving up work or moving house; or it could cause financial difficulties.

The physical changes are going on inside your body alone, but all the other changes will affect your partner too. Even right at the very beginning it is important to discuss how you feel with him, and to let him know what sort of support you need from him. It is often difficult for the father to feel involved in the very early stages, and you may resent him if you feel that he is just carrying on as before, oblivious to the momentous

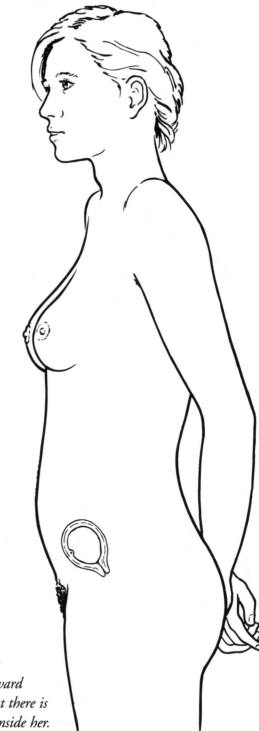

*At four weeks there are
unlikely to be any outward
signs in the mother that there is
a new life developing inside her.*

event your body is building up to. Speak to him about your feelings, but listen to what he has to say about his feelings too. If you can both get used to talking about the baby and the way that your lives are going to change it will make the whole process easier.

CASE STUDY: *'I was annoyed with my husband because he seemed so tied up in his work and hobbies, and I was feeling really ill and very excited that I was pregnant. He just didn't seem to notice. I was so upset. I thought it was because he wasn't excited about the baby, and I just started crying when a friend asked me what was wrong. She said I should just talk to him about it. It was difficult starting the conversation, but once we got talking he said that he felt a bit strange and cut off, as if I was listening to someone talking inside me and he wasn't involved. He was excited about the baby but I think it made him feel insecure. We were both going around worrying about completely stupid things and we probably would have carried on like that if my friend hadn't said to talk to him.'*

Week 5

By the time a period is a week late, many women have taken a pregnancy test, so the fifth week of pregnancy is the one in which many pregnancies are confirmed. This also means that the foetus has overcome three of its greatest hurdles: it has travelled down the fallopian tube into the uterus, attached itself successfully to the uterine wall, and triggered sufficient hormonal activity to suppress a period.

The Foetus

The foetus has again more than doubled in size in the space of a week. It is now approximately 1.5mm long, about half the length of a grain of rice. It is developing at an astonishing rate: the elongated body already has a tiny series of ridges along its 'back', these will eventually form the spine. The head is beginning to differentiate from the rest of the body, which curls round to a tail at the other end. At this stage your baby looks rather like a tiny sea-horse.

What is Happening to the Foetus

Two of the three germ layers which developed in week four have now started to specialise into different cells. The outer layer, known as the ectoderm, is developing most quickly at this stage: it forms a rudimentary brain and the beginnings of a spinal cord, running the length of the foetus. The middle layer, the mesoderm, is forming the early foundations of your baby's spinal column, which appear as the ridges along the foetus's 'back'.

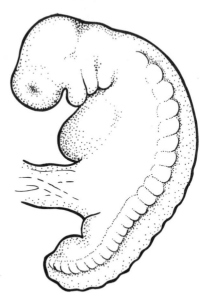

The head is now distinguishable from the body and the beginnings of the spine form a line of ridges along the back.

How you Feel

This is probably the first week in which you really know that you are pregnant. It is no longer a hunch or a suspicion, it has probably been confirmed by a test. Your emotions could well be running pretty high, and you may be feeling both elated and unsure of yourself. Some women say they have a tremendous feeling of importance when they first know that they are pregnant, a feeling that nothing else matters as much as the tiny foetus they are carrying.

LETTING YOUR DOCTOR KNOW / FREE PRESCRIPTIONS

As discussed in the introductory chapter of the **Your Pregnancy Week by Week** chapter, you should arrange to see your doctor or midwife as soon as you think that you are pregnant. He or she will advise you about medication and other drugs, smoking, alcohol, exercise and nutrition in connection with your pregnancy. You will also be able to discuss the antenatal care available in your area.

Your doctor can give you a signed form to say that you are pregnant (Mat B1). Your employer may need to see this form before granting you time off for antenatal check-ups and parentcraft classes. You should also ask your doctor for a free prescriptions form to fill in. You are entitled to free prescriptions throughout your pregnancy and for the first year of your baby's life.

Your Teeth and Gums

There is an old wives' tale which claims that a woman loses one tooth for every child she bears, because the baby takes the calcium from the mother's teeth to form its own bones and teeth. You will be relieved to know that the calcium cannot be leached out of your teeth. Women may well, however, have lost teeth during pregnancy, but this was probably due to gum infections or disease.

One of the many side-effects of the hormones circulating in the mother's bloodstream during pregnancy is to make the gums, especially the edges of the gums directly in contact with the teeth, softer than usual.

They bleed more readily when you brush your teeth and they are also more prone to infection (their softness means that it is easier for tiny particles of food to become trapped under the gum).

Gum infections can be painful and can, ultimately, lead to the loss of teeth. Treatment of gum infections may involve medication, such as antibiotics, which might be harmful to your baby. It is, therefore, very important to try and prevent them by paying special attention to oral hygiene when you are pregnant. Make sure that you brush your teeth at least twice day, and use dental floss at least once a week.

If you are registered with a NHS dentist, you are entitled to free dental treatment during your pregnancy and for one year after the birth of your baby. Make an appointment to see your dentist as soon as you know that you are pregnant; he may ask to see a signed certificate from your doctor to say that you are pregnant. He will probably tell you to arrange one or two more check-ups during the pregnancy, and he can advise you on an oral hygiene routine which will benefit your teeth.

Pregnancy does not alter the fact that the best way of looking after your teeth is to clean your teeth after meals and to avoid sugary foods. Pure sugar is the 'favourite food' of the bacteria that cause gum infections and tooth decay. If your mouth is a sugary environment they will thrive and multiply more rapidly. If you do eat a lot of sugary foods, brush your teeth afterwards or chew a sugar-free gum (this stimulates the production of saliva which has natural antibacterial qualities).

Week 6

At around the sixth week of pregnancy the foundations for your baby's entire body have been or are being laid down, not only the physical structure but also the vital organs and glands. Their most crucial period of development takes place over the next few weeks. It is during these weeks that the normal development of the growing foetus can be threatened or compromised by 'foreign' chemicals, such as those present in medicines, that may be introduced from the mother's bloodstream through the placenta.

The Foetus

The foetus is now about 4mm long and it has metamorphosed from the tiny 'sea-horse' of week five into a strange creature, still with a curved tail but with a bulbous head and another bulge which will form the thorax to house the heart and lungs. Slight depressions on the head indicate where the eyes and ears will form, and the lower jaw is already beginning to distinguish itself from the rest of the head. Four tiny protrusions have appeared on the body; they are called limb buds and they will grow into the arms and legs of your baby. A slender network of blood vessels now connects the foetus to the growing placenta, and this will become the umbilical cord.

What is Happening to the Foetus

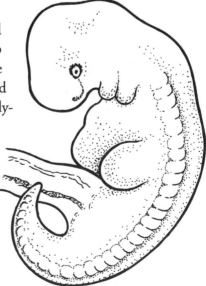

The ectoderm and mesoderm mentioned in week five are continuing to develop and specialise. The blueprint for the baby's nervous system is now established and the brain, which occupies the newly-formed head, divides into chambers. The cardio-vascular system is also beginning to develop. Inside the 'bulge' that will become your baby's chest is a simple tube which already

The eye can be seen beneath the skin now, and buds of the arms and legs appear.

contracts regularly to pump the first blood cells through the first blood vessels. This tube will develop into your baby's heart. Cartilage is laid down in the ridges along the foetus's spine and in the limb buds. The third germ layer, the inner layer known as the endoderm, begins to specialise into the internal organs: the lungs, stomach, intestines, liver, bladder and some of the glands.

How you Feel

By the sixth week of pregnancy the placenta has begun one of its many functions, the production of the hormones necessary to maintain the pregnancy and to prepare the mother's body for birth and lactation. The levels of these hormones in the mother's bloodstream now rise, and she begins to experience some or all of the symptomatic side-effects associated with pregnancy.

Many women feel tired at this stage of their pregnancy – this might be a direct effect of the relaxant hormone progesterone or it might be an indirect effect: the body's way of asking for sleep at a time when it is undergoing great upheaval. You may be suffering from morning sickness (which can happen at any time of day), and you are likely to notice that you need to pass urine more frequently. Your sense of taste and smell may have changed, and your appetite may be diminished or unpredictable.

If you suffer from some of these uncomfortable physical responses to pregnancy, this may alter your psychological response as well. Some women feel a little afraid of the pregnancy because it is now that they realise that it is out of their control; they may be feeling awful, but they cannot make it stop. This is one of the first steps to realising that your baby – although like a part of you during pregnancy – is a totally separate individual. This discovery can be alarming, but it should also make you feel proud: you are in the process of making an entire human being.

Sense of Smell and Taste / Diminished Appetite

One of the most common symptoms of early pregnancy is an alteration to the sensitivities to taste and smell. The sense of smell can change so that the pregnant woman is suddenly nauseated by smells, such as cooking smells or cigarette smoke, to which she might otherwise have been indifferent. The sense of smell may also be heightened, which can be a distinct disadvantage for the pregnant woman: she is more likely to pick up the smells she can no longer tolerate.

CASE STUDY: *'We used to go to a Sunday market every week to buy fruit and veg. and bits and bobs, and I had to stop going for a few weeks because the smell of the hot dog stand made me feel like I wanted to be sick. And it was no good trying to stay away from that area, I really could smell it from miles away, and I'd never really noticed it before.'*

A woman's sense of taste changes too. In some cases it is deadened so that food seems to taste of nothing, and this contributes to the fact that women often have less appetite in early pregnancy. Others say that food takes on a metallic taste, or that they permanently have a metallic taste in their mouth which makes their food taste unpleasant. This might mean that a woman is less interested in food in general, or that she 'goes off' particular foods or drinks. A great many women say that they no longer feel like drinking tea, coffee or alcoholic drinks at least in the first two or three months of pregnancy.

CASE STUDY: *'I've always been a great tea drinker, but I suddenly found I didn't want tea. It wasn't just that I didn't feel like it, the thought of it made me sick. Then I came up against this big problem: what did I feel like drinking? I was actually quite thirsty for a couple of days while I tried to work out what I wanted to drink. It was orange juice in the end. I wouldn't call it a craving, just the one thing that I didn't not want!'*

Many women find that they lose their appetite or their appetite becomes unpredictable for a few days or weeks in early pregnancy. This may be while they adapt to their altered sense of taste and smell or may be as a result of suffering from morning sickness. Some complain that they are very hungry but – like the case study of the woman who was thirsty above – they cannot identify anything that they feel like eating.

As a result of this altered appetite, you may actually lose some weight at this stage. Unless you were very underweight when your pregnancy began, your baby will not suffer at all if you lose a couple of pounds while you adjust to your new sense of taste and smell, and while you learn which foods your altered palate finds acceptable! Whatever your appetite, try to ensure that you eat a good balanced diet and that you eat regularly (see the section on nutrition in the chapter **Preparing for Pregnancy**).

Morning Sickness and Dealing with it

Morning sickness is the most widely recognised symptom of pregnancy and perhaps the one with the most misleading name. Although a lot of women suffering from nausea and sickness in pregnancy find that it is at its most acute when they get up in the morning, it can be experienced regularly at any other time of day or throughout the day.

Morning sickness, like the altered sense of taste and smell, is a reaction of the digestive system to the hormones in the mother's bloodstream. The sickness may be at its worst when your stomach is empty (hence the tradition that it occurs first thing in the morning), and this can become something of a vicious circle: as soon as you feel hungry you start feeling nauseous so you cannot eat and, therefore, continue to feel hungry. The trick here is to try to overcome the first hurdle of nausea; some women will actually vomit before they feel any better, others may not, and they may be able to settle their stomach with a dry biscuit (ginger biscuits are meant to be especially effective). It is often recommended that you keep a tin of biscuits by the bed and eat one or two before you get up to try to overcome early-morning sickness.

In other instances, the sickness seems to be directly related to tiredness. Many women experience 'morning' sickness in the early evening when they have been busy all day. This sort of sickness is best overcome if you can rest in the middle of the day: you may not need to sleep, but just put your feet up for half an hour, and avoid the temptation to rush off shopping in your lunch hour. It may also help to have a little snack mid-afternoon, a banana or a couple of biscuits to raise your blood sugar level.

Some women feel quite well in themselves most of the time, but are spontaneously sick during or after a meal. This is usually as a reaction to a particular food and, although it is not always easy to isolate the culprit, you should try to work out what it is that has triggered the sickness. Oily and spicy foods are common triggers but this varies from one woman to another.

Even if you suffer none of the morning sickness described above, you may find that in the early weeks of pregnancy you suddenly become prone to car-sickness or – if you travel anywhere by sea – sea-sickness (morning sickness is often described as being like sea-sickness). Do not be tempted to take travel sickness pills because they might contain ingredients which could harm your baby.

Happily, most women find that morning sickness wears off by about the end of the third month. Unfortunately, in some cases, it can last the entire pregnancy. Morning sickness can actually cause women to lose weight in the early weeks of their pregnancy. This will do the foetus no harm at all (the foetus will take from your body the nutrients that it needs) but if it is a long time before you gain weight it could be harmful to you. If you are worried about continued morning sickness, you could try keeping a record of what you eat and when you eat it, and of when you feel nauseous and when you are actually sick. It may be possible to establish a link between certain foods and your sickness, then you can eliminate the trigger foods.

Another knock-on effect of morning sickness is possible damage to your teeth. If you vomit frequently the acid in your vomit causes the enamel of your teeth to disintegrate; over a prolonged period this can cause you to lose your teeth. The best way to avoid this is to put a teaspoon of bicarbonate of soda (an alkali which counterbalances the acid) into a glass of water, and to gargle and sloosh the mouth out with it. Do not swallow the mixture because it will upset the delicate acid-alkali balance in your stomach.

CASE STUDY: *'It wasn't morning sickness with me, it was evening sickness. It came on in the early evening, and I just felt exhausted and very, very sick. I wanted to be sick but I was only actually sick about three times. It just made me feel terrible, and it meant I couldn't do anything about preparing an evening meal. I found just sitting doing nothing for about quarter of an hour, with my eyes closed and taking slow deep breaths helped. It seemed to wear off more quickly if I could find the time to do that.'*

CASE STUDY: *'When I was carrying the twins I was sick every single day of the pregnancy. At the beginning I really felt awful, and I went around groaning waiting to be sick. After the fourth month it was like a routine … I would get up and sick up a little bit of bile before I could start the day.'*

Zinc

Research has shown that women whose diets are rich in zinc are less prone to morning sickness, and that a diet deficient in zinc can cause nausea and alterations to the sense of taste and smell even in people who are not pregnant. Zinc supplements have been used successfully to combat morning sickness in some cases. Natural sources of zinc in the diet include dairy products, meat, liver, eggs, fish, shellfish, maize, nuts and pulses. Ginger is also a good source of zinc (making the traditional tin of ginger biscuits kept by the bedside doubly effective).

Week 7

Your growing baby is now over a month old and has undergone an extraordinary period of development with many of its internal organs almost complete.

The Foetus

The foetus now measures up to 1.5cm (just over ½in), and at this stage almost half its length is taken up by the disproportionately large head. The head is not only growing very quickly it is also developing at an incredible rate: the beginnings of the eyes are now visible under the surface, there are tiny holes where the nostrils will be, and the lower jaw is becoming more defined.

The thorax and abdomen form two distinctly separate bulges now, housing the heart and lungs, and the digestive tract, respectively. The limbs, especially the arms, are lengthening. The ends of the arms are rounded into rudimentary hands, with indentations where the fingers will be. The tail is beginning to thin and recede.

What is Happening to the Foetus

Rapid developments are going on in every part of your baby's body. In the head, the brain has now divided into the two cerebral hemispheres and is growing very quickly; the eyes and the inner ears are well formed too, although the external structure of the ear has not yet appeared.

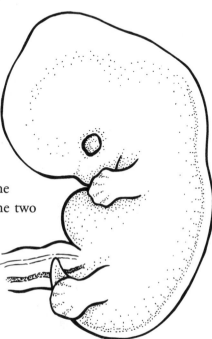

Inside the thorax, the heart has divided into two chambers and the lungs have formed, complete with the two major airways, the bronchi. The lungs are compact and solid at this stage, and will not fully

The outline of the body becomes more rounded and the tail begins to recede.

develop until much later in the pregnancy. The abdomen now contains a virtually intact digestive tract.

Along the spine and in the limbs the first bone cells are laid down in the cartilage structure which marked the beginnings of your baby's skeleton.

How you Feel

You almost certainly know that you are pregnant by the seventh week of your pregnancy, and you will very probably have a number of early symptoms. You may have feelings of elation, but they could be tempered with an element of surprise at just how terrible you can feel if you suffer from morning sickness. If you are feeling tired and ill, try to get plenty of rest and use the advice given about morning sickness in **Week 6**.

Tiredness and Sleep in Early Pregnancy

Everyone knows that women in the last few weeks of pregnancy feel tired; and they have such a visible reason to feel tired that it is easy for others to sympathise. What is less widely known, and therefore elicits less sympathy, is the fact that you can feel inexplicably tired in the early weeks of pregnancy too. It is a completely different kind of tiredness, and it can be quite overwhelming; it may be constant or it may wash over you in waves at particular times of day.

This tiredness is caused by hormonal upheaval. The body may simply be 'asking' for sleep at a time when it is being expected to adapt to a great many physiological changes, or the tiredness may be a direct effect of the hormone progesterone which is produced by the placenta.

One of the many properties of progesterone is its sedative effect. This accounts not only for the tiredness but also for the facility for sleep. Women experiencing this tiredness find it easy to drop off to sleep even if they cannot normally sleep at that time of day. This sedative effect of progesterone is also associated with the serene, other-worldly look of some pregnant women, a feeling of being slightly detached from the frenzy of everyday life.

It may not be practical to indulge your every desire to sleep, especially if you are working. It is, however, important that you get enough sleep, particularly as a number of other symptoms of pregnancy, such as nausea and morning sickness, can be directly related to tiredness. You will learn your new limits, and you must respect them: if you are working, you may find that you are too tired to go out in the evenings, or that you need a rest in the early evening.

If there are particular times of day when you feel tired, try to make time for a little rest. Even if you do not actually sleep, make a point of sitting down quietly. You can feel rested after just ten minutes of 'time out', sitting with your feet up and your eyes closed. It may help if you try some calming breathing exercises: try breathing in slowly for a count of ten, and then exhaling on a count of ten; or inhaling, holding for a count of ten, and exhaling.

CASE STUDY: *'I was amazed by this feeling of tiredness. It was an absolutely constant, nagging urge to sleep. We went away for what was supposed to be a fun weekend with some friends, and I spent the whole time wondering when I could next legitimately sneak off to bed.'*

Difficulty Sleeping

If you have difficulty sleeping in the early weeks of pregnancy, it may help to work out what is stopping you sleeping. It could be physical factors such as discomfort from indigestion, or psychological ones such as worrying about money or relationships. It might be helpful to establish the same routine of winding down for sleep every day, making sure that you eat a light meal in the evening well before going to bed, having a hot bath and a soothing drink such as cocoa or camomile tea, and using the breathing exercises described above.

Do not use any kind of sleep aid without consulting your doctor or pharmacist first. Remember that even 'natural' remedies can contain powerful ingredients which could harm your baby.

FREQUENT URINATING

A frequent need to pass urine is another of the slightly unexpected and inconvenient symptoms of early pregnancy. This has two causes: firstly the hormone progesterone acts as a muscle relaxant, so that the muscles of the bladder signal the need to urinate long before the bladder is full. Secondly, in the early weeks the growing uterus is competing for space in the pelvic girdle with the bladder. Once the uterus begins to 'pop' out of the pelvis – at about 12 weeks – pressure on the bladder should ease. (In the final weeks of pregnancy when the baby's head is engaged it puts pressure on the bladder).

This need to pass urine should be no more than inconvenient. If you have any pain in your lower abdomen, especially when you pass water, speak to your doctor because you could have an infection of the urinary tract. Always make sure that you empty your bladder before going to bed to minimise the chances of being woken in the night by a full bladder. Do not be tempted to cut down on your fluid intake to counteract this; it is important that you drink plenty of fluids in pregnancy.

CASE STUDY: *'You definitely notice that you go to the loo more often. I even started having to get up in the night. I'd expected that at the end but not right at the beginning.'*

Week 8

The growing baby inside you is now officially called a foetus. Although for the purposes of this book the word foetus has been used from the point when the fertilised egg implanted itself in the uterine wall, the baby is usually called an embryo up until the end of the eighth week or the second month of pregnancy. In this last week, the foetus has again changed dramatically and it is beginning to look like a mammal; soon it will be like a miniature baby, perfectly formed and growing by the day.

The Foetus

The foetus is now about the size and shape of a cashew nut. It measures about 2.2cm (just under 1in) from the top of its head to the curve of its bottom. This is known as the 'crown-rump' measurement, and it is used even after the legs have grown beyond the 'rump' because the legs are often bent, making a crown-to-toe measurement more difficult to establish.

The head is now taking on a more mammalian rounded shape. The ears, eyelids and nose are beginning to form. The body is lengthening into a smooth trunk incorporating the thorax and abdomen. The limbs have changed most dramatically in this last week: the arms and legs have grown longer with obvious elbow and knee joints. The fingers are becoming more clearly defined, although they are still joined together, and the ridges that will form the toes are just appearing. Finally, the tiny genitals have grown, and at this stage male and female genitalia look remarkably similar.

Webbed fingers and toes are now clearly visible, and the arm has an elbow joint.

What is Happening to the Foetus

Inside the tiny foetus the major structures of all the internal organs have been laid down. The heart now has valves preventing a back-flow of the blood that it pumps round the developing circulatory system. The spine and limb bones contain more bone cells now and are attached to the first strands of muscle tissue. The foetus can make tiny movements, although it will be several weeks before they are strong enough for you to feel them.

How you Look

In the eighth week of pregnancy you are still unlikely to look any different to the casual observer. You may well have noticed some changes, though. Your tummy will probably not have grown at all, but you may have a slight thickening of the waist and you might have put on a couple of pounds. The most obvious changes are likely to be in your breasts. Some women find that their breasts grow quite quickly, even in early pregnancy, and this can mean that bras become tight and uncomfortable. You may need to buy new bras more than once during your pregnancy. Even if your breasts have not grown, they are likely to be changing subtly: blood vessels under the surface become more obvious and the nipples grow larger and darker.

Libido and Sex in Early Pregnancy

It is difficult to generalise about a woman's libido in early pregnancy because, as with so many other things, it varies enormously from one woman to another. Some women notice little difference in their libido, others feel too tired or nauseated to be interested in sex, yet another group have a burst of sexual energy and enjoy better sex in early pregnancy than at virtually any other time (this is attributed to the surge of hormones in the woman's bloodstream and the hypersensitivity of the breasts and vagina).

Whatever your physical appetite for sex, you may be worried that intercourse could be harmful to the baby. There is no reason why a normal pregnancy should be jeopardised by intercourse, but if you have a history of bleeding in pregnancy or of miscarriage your doctor may advise you to avoid intercourse at least in the first 12 weeks. Some couples find that, even if they have been told that intercourse will not harm the baby, they still do not feel that it is safe or quite right.

The important thing to remember is that you both have sexual appetites as well as feelings on the subject. This can be a testing time if both partners have very different feelings. It is not always easy to talk about sex, but try to talk to your partner and to let him know how you feel; you may both discover new ways of being intimate and finding gratification without having vaginal sex, if one or other of you is troubled by the idea.

CASE STUDY: *'It did make me feel guilty, but I was just too tired to make love. Even the thought of it made me feel a bit sick. I'm afraid I got into the habit of going to bed really early so that I was sound asleep when he came to bed. It got better after the first three months ... but not much.'*

CASE STUDY: *'Initially my libido increased, probably because my breasts became larger and so I felt sexier ... it was definitely hormonal as well, but part of it was because I've always been very flat-chested and I suddenly had these breasts, and it just made me feel sexy.'*

CONSTIPATION IN PREGNANCY

Constipation is another of the unpleasant symptoms of pregnancy and, like many other symptoms, it is caused by the muscle relaxant effect of progesterone. The muscles of the intestines, including the bowel, slow down so that stools spend longer in the bowel. Fluids are drawn out of the stools in the bowel, making them drier and harder and, therefore, more difficult to pass.

In order to minimise this effect, make sure that you drink plenty of fluids and that you have a fibre-rich diet. Wholegrain cereals, green leafy vegetables, and fresh and dried fruits are good sources of dietary fibre. It is also important to eat regularly and to empty your bowels whenever you feel the need. Consult your doctor or pharmacist before taking any kind of laxative because they may contain ingredients which could be harmful to your baby.

Week 9

Another important threshold has been passed: this would have been the time of your second period. You are now three quarters of the way through the vital first 12-week period of your pregnancy.

The Foetus

By the ninth week of the pregnancy the foetus is about 3cm (just over 1in) long from crown to rump. In the last week the limbs have grown significantly, with ankle and wrist joints beginning to appear and much clearer definition in the hands and feet. The head is taking on a more human form with an obvious neck. The ears, nose and mouth are developing gradually, and the eyelids have nearly closed over the eyes. The tail has all but disappeared.

What is Happening to the Foetus

Underneath the beginnings of the external ear the baby's hearing mechanism is now almost fully formed. The organs are continuing to develop and grow, and more bone and muscle tissue are being laid down.

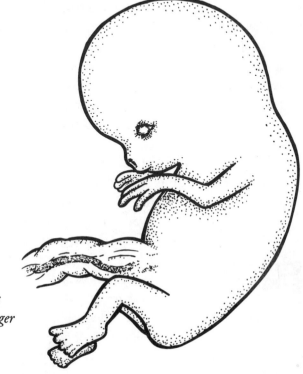

The webbing between the fingers and toes is receding, and the arms and legs are becoming longer and finer.

How you Feel

You could well be at the height of your morning sickness in the ninth week. Many women find that the sickness begins in the sixth week, rises to a peak in the ninth and then begins to dwindle, tailing off in the twelfth week. If you are feeling very tired and nauseous, make sure that you get plenty of sleep and try to eat regular meals. Remember that it does not go on for ever, but if you are worried about how ill you are feeling, talk to your doctor or midwife.

Thinking Ahead About Leaving Work

If you are in permanent work, you need to start thinking about when you will want to take your maternity leave. You may well have told your employers that you are expecting a baby, but you will need to let them know when you will be leaving work so that they can make arrangements to cover for your absence. Every woman is entitled to 14 weeks maternity leave and to return to the same job after that period, no matter what hours she has worked or how long she has been in her present job. (If you have worked for the same employer for two or more years, and if it is a company of more than five people, you could be entitled to extended maternity leave of up to 29 weeks from the week your baby is born.)

The earliest that your maternity leave can start is the twenty-ninth week of your pregnancy, but many women choose to start their leave much later than this so that they can spend as much time as possible recovering from the birth and being with the baby. If you do not take your leave until the last minute, however, it could be a false economy: if your job is demanding and tiring, you may exhaust yourself by carrying on working in the latter stages of pregnancy. Some rest and relaxation may be useful preparation for labour, delivery and motherhood.

You need to think carefully about how you are coping with the pregnancy, what demands your job makes on you, and when it would be best for you to leave work. You also need to take into consideration whether or not you want to breastfeed your baby and for how long, because breastfeeding is not really compatible with full-time work. You may want to discuss all these factors with your partner, your doctor, your employer and other colleagues.

You may be planning to stop work altogether when your baby is born, in which case your employer needs plenty of warning. Or you may be hoping that you can return to work part-time after you have had your baby, for example as part of a job-share scheme. Discuss these ideas with your employer, and do not be afraid of suggesting this sort of scheme even if it has not been done before in that company – it could work to everyone's benefit, but particularly yours and your baby's.

CHANGES TO EYESIGHT

The amount of fluid retained by the body changes during pregnancy. If the amount of fluid retained in the eye increases enough to alter the shape of the eyeball this can cause temporary long or short-sightedness, and it can make the wearing of contact lenses uncomfortable. If you are aware of changes in your eyesight, or if you get a headache when you read, arrange to have your eyes tested.

Week 10

Your baby is now looking very much like a little person: although the proportions are all wrong, it could no longer really be confused with the foetus of any other animal.

The Foetus

By the tenth week of pregnancy, when the foetus is nearly two months old, it measures around 4cm (1½in) from crown to rump, about the length of the top two joints of your little finger. Although the head is still very large, it is taking on the refined shape of a human head; and the definition of the features contributes to its increasingly human appearance. The limbs are also becoming longer and finer with clear fingers and toes.

What is Happening to the Foetus

The internal organs of the baby are now virtually intact. They will develop further and grow considerably during the rest of the pregnancy, but most of the 'groundwork' has been done.

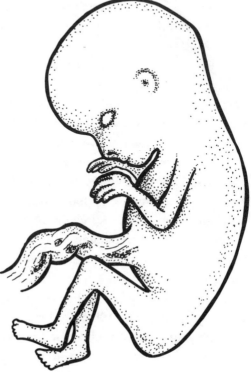

The structure of the external ear is now visible on the side of the foetus's head.

How you Feel

You are now one quarter of the way through your 40-week pregnancy, and this should give you a sense of achievement. You are also coming to the end of the period in which your baby is at most risk of miscarriage and malformation, and – with luck – your uncomfortable symptoms should be beginning to diminish.

Weight Gain in Pregnancy

By the tenth week of pregnancy you may have noticed your waist line thickening a little and you are likely to have put on a couple of pounds. It is normal for a woman to gain between 7.5 and 13.5kg (17 and 30lb) during her pregnancy, although it may be acceptable for her to gain more or less than these guideline figures. The amount of weight a woman should gain in order for her and her baby to be healthy depends to some extent on her frame and her weight before the pregnancy. A woman who is underweight will need to gain more weight to nourish herself and her baby than one who has a normal weight or is overweight before the pregnancy starts.

There are more problems associated with poor weight gain in pregnancy than with excessive weight gain, and pregnancy is definitely not a time to think about dieting and losing weight. On the other hand, really excessive weight gain – to the point of obesity – can cause complications in later pregnancy and is associated with an increased incidence of Caesarean section. The old adage of 'eating for two' is a dangerous one, implying that a woman has free rein to eat as much as she wants. She may have a huge and capricious appetite, but she is certainly not feeding two fully grown adults.

To ensure that you gain an acceptable amount of weight in pregnancy, you should try to eat three or four regular meals a day, and you should avoid snacking on sugary foods which are very calorific but have little nutritional value. It is especially important to have a well-balanced diet during pregnancy, providing your own metabolism and your growing baby with the full complement of nutrients, vitamins and minerals (see the section on **Nutrition** in the chapter **Preparing for Pregnancy**).

You will probably be weighed regularly once you start having antenatal check-ups so that your GP or midwife can monitor your weight gain. You can ask your GP or midwife for advice on nutrition and exercise in pregnancy if you feel that you are gaining too much or too little weight.

Where the Weight Goes

You may be a little alarmed at the prospect of putting on around 12.7kg (2 stone) in weight, but the weight gained in pregnancy is not exclusively laid down as fat. The baby itself is likely to account for about 3.4kg (7lb 8oz), with the placenta and amniotic fluid accounting for about half as much again. This means that over 4.5kg (10lb) of your weight gain will drop off when you have your baby.

Some of the weight gain is attributable to the growing uterus and to the increase in the amount of blood circulating in your body during pregnancy. The uterus and the blood supply will diminish fairly quickly in the first few weeks after pregnancy.

The third element of weight gain is fat stores that are laid down during pregnancy to prepare the mother's body for lactation. These fat stores should break down gradually in the months following delivery, especially if you breastfeed your baby and if you take regular exercise.

Women carry the weight gained in pregnancy in different ways and these differences begin to emerge when the bump becomes more obvious in the sixth month. In some women the weight is spread fairly evenly over the body so that the bump itself is less apparent, but there may be comparatively more fat stores to burn off after pregnancy. Others will have a more obtrusive bump but very little weight gain to the rest of their bodies, so that the weight that they gain is 'all baby'.

When the Weight Goes On

Some women gain very little weight early in pregnancy and do not appear to be pregnant at all until as late as the sixth or seventh month, others may gain weight quickly at the beginning of the pregnancy and feel as if they need to be in maternity clothes by the fourth month. Neither of these extremes should be cause for concern. Pregnancy is not a beauty competition; it is not a competition of any kind. So long as the mother's weight is acceptable for her height, and so long as her doctor or midwife is happy with the rate at which she is gaining weight, it does not matter when the weight goes on.

Usually, a woman will put on only about 10% of her eventual total weight gain in the first three months – say 0.9 or 1.3kg (2 or 3lb). The weight gain will step up in the second trimester: she is likely to gain a further 2.3 or 2.7kg (5 or 6lb) by the end of the fifth month. The most significant increase in weight usually occurs between weeks 24 and 32 of the pregnancy when the baby and the uterus are growing most rapidly. By the end of the seventh month a woman may have gained another 5.5 or 5.9kg (12 or 13lb) (a total weight gain of 8.7-10kg [19-22lb] so far). In the last two months weight gain usually slows down again, and may constitute another 2.3 or 2.7kg (5 or 6lb) (these examples give a total weight gain of 10.9-12.8kg [24-28lb]).

BREAST SIZE AND BRAS IN EARLY PREGNANCY

The tingling, heavy feeling in a woman's breasts is often the first sign that she is pregnant, and many women find that their breasts grow quite quickly in the early weeks of pregnancy. They may well change, too: the nipples become larger and darker, and the blood vessels under the surface may become more visible. If your breasts grow sufficiently to make your bra feel tight, you should be properly fitted for a new bra. Depending on how early in your pregnancy you need to be refitted for a bra it might be worth considering buying a nursing bra straight away to economise. However much you resent buying new underwear that may only be worn for a few weeks, it is better to do so than to be uncomfortable.

If your breasts do not grow significantly in the early stages of pregnancy, this is nothing to worry about, and it certainly does not mean that you will not be able to breastfeed your baby. Breast size is directly related to fat stores in the breast and not to the size of the milk producing structures. Small breasts are just as good at producing milk as large ones.

Nuchal Fold Test

In the tenth week of pregnancy you may be offered a test known as the nuchal fold or nuchal translucency test to screen for chromosomal abnormalities such as Down's Syndrome in the foetus. Although the test cannot prove conclusively whether a baby has Down's Syndrome, the advantage of this test is that it can indicate an increased probability of Down's Syndrome much earlier than a blood test (see **Testing for Abnormality in the Foetus** in **Week 16**).

The test is performed during an ultrasound scan (see **Your Ultrasound Scan** in **Week 18**) by measuring the size of a fold at the back of the foetus's neck, the nuchal fold. In babies with Down's Syndrome, fluid retention in the area makes the fold larger; if the fold measures more than a certain amount your baby is more likely to have Down's Syndrome.

CASE STUDY: *'I was offered a nuchal test by my GP because I am just 35. The result showed that I had a much lower probability of having a Down's Syndrome baby than expected for my age: 1 / 1900 instead of about 1 / 330. It's very reassuring, but I know that it is only part of the picture. I will still have the blood tests at 16 weeks.'*

Week 11

The most critical period of development is now over and your baby is much less likely to be damaged by harmful drugs or infections after this point. It will now begin a period of remarkable growth.

The Foetus

In the eleventh week of pregnancy the average foetus is about 5cm (2in) from crown to rump, it would fit snugly in the palm of your hand. The head, which houses the rapidly developing brain, is still disproportionately large, but the neck is now longer and stronger, and the foetus can actually move its head. The external genitalia are also growing fast, although it is difficult to distinguish between male and female.

What is Happening to the Foetus

All the baby's organs are formed, and the sexual organs are developing internally: testicles in a baby boy and ovaries in a baby girl. The heart is now divided into right and left atria, and right and left ventricles, complete with valves; and it pumps the baby's own blood around the baby's body (it may be possible to hear the baby's heartbeat with ultrasound equipment by now). The bones are growing too, not only in the spine and limbs but also in the skull, and tiny ribs are visible under your baby's skin.

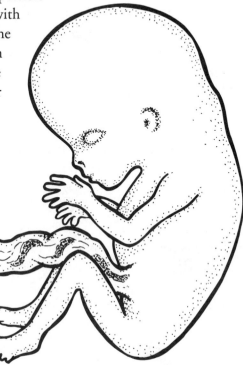

The foetus's face and outline is now unmistakably human, although the head is still disproportionately large.

How you Feel

You may have your booking appointment in the next couple of weeks, and you may well be feeling excited and apprehensive about that. Some women do not really believe that they are pregnant until they are past the threshold of the first three months and have had their first antenatal check-up.

Thinking about How you will Feed your Baby

It is important to start thinking early on about how you want to feed your baby. If you put some thought into it before you have your booking appointment you can then ask your GP or midwife for advice, and they may be able to recommend leaflets or books about feeding that will help to inform your choice.

In an ideal world, no one would ever have to think about how they want to feed their baby: there is only one food that is specifically designed for the human baby, perfected over hundreds of thousands of years of evolution, and that is human breast milk.

Breast milk contains the exact balance of fluids, proteins, fats and other nutrients as well as antibodies that your baby needs to survive and grow. It is available at the correct temperature at any time of day, and your body is so finely tuned to your baby's needs that the milk not only changes over the weeks as your baby grows, it changes during the course of a single feed: the foremilk is more watery and thirst-quenching, whereas the hindmilk is richer and more nutritious. The milk-producing cells are even sensitive to atmospheric differences; on a very hot day they will produce more foremilk to compensate for the fact that your baby may be sweating.

It is not a perfect world, however, and many women may want or have to return to work or other commitments soon after the birth of their baby. If this is the case, they may prefer not to breastfeed at all than to start and then stop. Before making this sort of decision you should consider the benefits to your baby of breastfeeding even for two or three weeks ... or just a few days. In the first few days after a baby is born, the mother produces colostrum, a particularly rich milk spiked with vital antibodies which will help 'jump start' your baby's growth and the development of his immune system. Even if you feed your baby just for these few days he will have benefited enormously.

Although breastfeeding is obviously the most natural way of feeding a baby, we, as animals, are so far removed from our natural state that it can feel very unnatural indeed: our chins were surely not designed to clamp layers of clothing to our chests when we have pulled them up in haste to feed a screaming baby! Breastfeeding can be a huge pleasure for the mother as well as the baby, but no one is pretending that it is always easy right from the first feed. It can be frustrating, exhausting and painful, and it can take several weeks to establish a good supply of milk. You should not let these factors put you off, but you need to bear them in mind when you are thinking about how you want to feed your baby.

If you are expecting twins, you should not let this discourage you from wanting to breastfeed your babies. Feeding any baby can be demanding and tiring, and feeding twins is especially so: you will certainly need a lot of help and support looking after your babies if you are to feed them successfully. You may also need help finding a comfortable position in which to feed the babies or advice on how to juggle the needs of both babies. (The addresses of organisations that can give you specialised advice on looking after twins and on breastfeeding appear at the end of the book.)

When your baby is born the midwives and nurses will try to give you all the advice and support you need to start feeding your baby. If you have difficulty establishing feeding or if you feel that you are not coping with the physical and psychological demands of breastfeeding, there may be more specialised support available. Queen Charlotte's Hospital is one of a number of hospitals that have breastfeeding counsellors and run breastfeeding workshops. If you want more information about breastfeeding and want to know about the support available in your area, ask your GP or midwife whether they can put you in touch with a local breastfeeding counsellor. (The addresses of some nationwide organisations specialising in advice and support for breastfeeding mothers appear at the end of the book.)

For the sake of her baby, every mother should try to breastfeed. But if you decide against it, the decision not to breastfeed is yours to make. You will not achieve anything by feeling guilty or inadequate if others criticise your decision, or by letting them persuade you to carry on breastfeeding against your will.

Entire books have been written about the choice between breast- and bottle-feeding babies. From a woman's point of view, there may be advantages and disadvantages to both, which make it difficult to choose between the two. From the baby's point of view there is no contest: breast milk is the best food for the human infant.

CASE STUDY: *'I feel there's a lot of pressure on women to breastfeed … from hospitals, the media and from other women. I didn't have any strong urge to do it, but I felt I should give it a go. I had a really awful delivery with forceps and a third-degree tear. I was just so uncomfortable and feeding the baby hurt so much because of my stitches and because my nipples were sore. On the third day I just said to [my husband] "I'm sorry, I can't do this, I just don't want any more pain."'*

CASE STUDY: *'I knew I wanted to breastfeed all along. I felt it physically and emotionally, as well as knowing that it was the best thing for the baby. She is very good at it, she latched on straight away. My milk came in two days ago, and I am very uncomfortable at the moment, but feeding her gives me the most incredible feeling of fulfilment, it's the ultimate way of nurturing her.'*

Changes to Your Skin in Pregnancy

You may notice a number of changes to your skin during pregnancy. You may find red, threadlike raised patterns of veins on your upper body; these are known as vascular spiders. They are harmless and will disappear once you have had your baby. Some women notice that the palms of their hands appear red or that areas of skin become darker, especially the nipples and a line from the pubic hair up to the navel, known as the linea negra. Darker patches of skin, called chloasma, can appear on or near your face during pregnancy. You may find some of these changes unsightly, but they will not do you or your baby any harm, and they will fade when you have had your baby.

Women who suffer from acne sometimes find that their skin improves dramatically when they are pregnant. Others may find that it is aggravated by pregnancy, and even women who do not normally have acne may develop acne, or be subject to spots. You may be able to control acne and spots by taking regular light exercise and cutting down on fats in your diet, and they should, anyway, wear off by the middle of the pregnancy. If you develop bad acne, ask your doctor for advice about treating it, and always speak to your doctor or pharmacist before using medication to treat acne: it might contain ingredients which could be harmful to your baby.

Week 12

The twelfth week of pregnancy is seen as a major watershed. The foetus is now less likely to be harmed by infections and medication, and you should be experiencing fewer discomforts associated with early pregnancy. You have come to the end of the first trimester (the first third of your pregnancy), and you may well have your booking appointment this week.

The Foetus

It is now ten weeks since your egg was fertilised, and the foetus measures approximately 6.5cm (2½in) from crown to rump, and it weighs up to 14g (½oz). The face is still changing rapidly: the chin is becoming more clearly defined and the eyes, nose, mouth and ears are continuing to develop. The fingers and toes are no longer webbed and tiny nails are beginning to grow at the flattened ends of the digits. The genitals have developed sufficiently to distinguish male from female.

What is Happening to the Foetus

Most of the bones in your baby's body have bone cells laid down in the cartilage structures, and there are growing muscles attached to the bones. The nervous system has also developed so that the muscles receive messages from the brain by the twelfth week. The baby is now capable of a number of movements, including curling its toes and swallowing amniotic fluid.

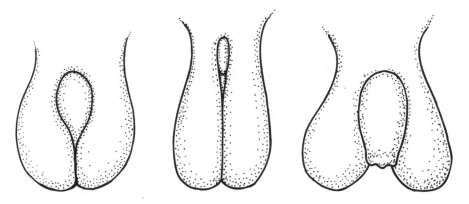

Until the twelfth week, male and female foetuses look very much alike (left). From then on they are more easily distinguishable as baby girls develop the long, thin protective labia and the small clitoris (centre) whereas baby boys develop the more rounded scrotal sacs and the larger penis (right).

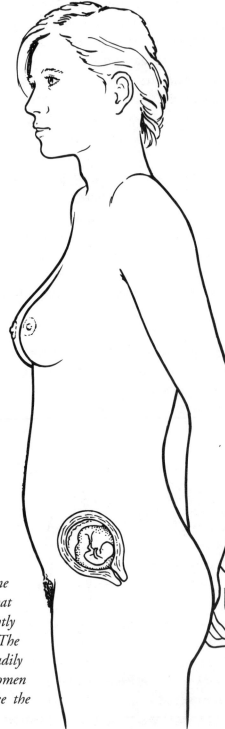

By the twelfth week some women will notice that their breasts are slightly enlarged and tender. The uterus is growing steadily upwards into the abdomen and may start to make the mother's tummy swell.

The digestive tract is like a miniature version of your own, and it can already absorb some nutrients, such as glucose. The baby's glands are beginning to develop and the pituitary gland has already begun to produce the baby's own hormones.

How you Look

Your uterus has grown considerably since conception: it not only has to accommodate the growing foetus but also the placenta and the amniotic sac containing amniotic fluid. In about the twelfth week the uterus has grown beyond the pelvic girdle and can be felt by a trained doctor or midwife just by putting gentle pressure on your abdomen (abdominal palpation). In a first pregnancy, many women change little in the first 12 weeks, although their breasts may have grown; but in second and subsequent pregnancies the uterus may be forming a bit of a 'tummy' already at this stage.

Your Booking Appointment

Your booking appointment is the first of your antenatal check-ups and it will probably be your longest. You may have many things to discuss with your doctor and midwife, and it might be worth making a list of the questions that you want to ask.

Your Questions

The questions you want to ask might include:

Who will be looking after you antenataly?
Where can you have the baby?
What tests are available and what are they for?
What should you be eating?
What exercise should you be taking?
What active hobbies can you carry on doing, such as horse-riding and cycling?
Can you go abroad and which inoculations can you have?
What antenatal classes are available locally? (Classes run by independent organisations such as the NCT may be oversubscribed and you may need to think about booking a place at this stage.)
How you want to feed your baby.
Who you might want with you for the birth of the baby.

The doctor may well be able to answer some of your questions immediately, or he may refer you to leaflets or other sources to find the answers. Many of the issues raised by these questions are tackled in this book.

Background Questions

The doctor in turn will ask you a number of questions about your health, lifestyle and family history to try and build up a picture of any factors that might be relevant to your baby. The questions he asks will be about:

Your age
Your general health
Illnesses you have had
Illnesses for which you are currently receiving treatment
Previous pregnancies you have had
Abnormalities in previous pregnancies
Your partner's health
History of twins or inherited diseases in both families
Ethnic origins of both families (some inherited diseases are more common in certain ethnic groups)
Whether you are related to your partner
Where you live
Where you work

Physical Examination

Height: Your height will be measured on your first visit and you may be asked your shoe size. This is to give the doctor an idea of the size of your pelvis: if you have a particularly small pelvis, the size of the growing baby will be monitored more closely during your pregnancy and you may have to have a Caesarean section.

Weight: You may be weighed regularly throughout your antenatal visits. The amount of weight that you gain and the rate at which you gain it are useful indicators as to how your pregnancy is progressing. A sudden increase in weight gain, for example, could indicate excessive fluid retention which is a symptom of a dangerous condition called pre-eclampsia (see the chapter **When Things Go Wrong**).

Heart, lungs and blood pressure: The doctor will listen to your heart and lungs, and check your heart rate and blood pressure. Your blood pressure will be taken at every visit because it is a useful indication of how your body is coping with the demands of pregnancy. You may find that your blood pressure rises or falls during pregnancy.

Urine sample: You should bring a urine sample with you to every antenatal appointment. Your urine will be tested for the presence of sugars and proteins. If a woman regularly has sugar in her urine during pregnancy, she may have developed a form of diabetes known as gestational diabetes, which disappears again after delivery. This condition need not pose any threat to the mother or the baby if it is detected by such tests and controlled by altering the mother's diet and, in some cases, by prescribing insulin. Proteins in the urine could imply that the mother has an infection of the urinary tract or that she has pre-eclampsia.

Blood sample: On your first visit you will be asked for a blood sample. This is firstly to establish your blood group. (If you have the rare Rhesus negative blood group this will be picked up now. If a mother with Rhesus negative blood has two consecutive Rhesus positive babies, the second baby is in danger of being anaemic because of antibodies in the mother's blood, unless she is treated with an injection after the birth of her first baby.)

Your blood test will also assess whether or not you are anaemic (have a low red blood cell count). During pregnancy the total amount of blood circulating in your body increases and this makes considerable demands on your metabolism which can result in anaemia. If you suffer from anaemia you will feel tired and drained, you will have lower resistance to infection and your body will recover more slowly from the loss of blood when you have your baby. Your haemoglobin level – a guide to your red blood cell count – will be checked periodically, and if you are anaemic you may be prescribed iron and folic acid supplements.

Your doctor will also check your blood sample for your immunity to rubella, and for syphilis and hepatitis B infection. All these conditions have very serious implications for the unborn child. If you are not immune to rubella, or if you are infected with syphilis or hepatitis B your doctor will be able to advise you about what action you should take. He will probably recommend that you have an ultrasound scan immediately to assess how the foetus has been affected. You may also be offered HIV testing.

Abdominal palpation / physical examination: Your doctor or midwife may check your breasts and ask you to lie down to check your abdomen, to feel the position of the uterus and the 'height of the fundus' (how high up your abdomen the top of the uterus is – this is often a useful guide to dating a pregnancy). If there is some discrepancy about the dating of the pregnancy he or she may do an internal examination to assess the size of the uterus. By putting two fingers inside your vagina and the other hand firmly on the abdomen, the doctor or midwife can gauge the size of the uterus and likely age of the foetus. Most doctors prefer to use an ultrasound scan to clear up such discrepancies.

Your doctor may also ask to look at your hands, wrists and ankles, and he may ask whether any rings that you wear regularly have felt any tighter recently. This is to check whether you have excessive fluid retention, or oedema, which can be cause for concern in pregnancy.

Baby's heartbeat: The doctor will probably listen for your baby's heartbeat using an ultrasound instrument called a Doppler device. The heartbeat can usually be picked up by the twelfth week, and you will be able to hear it too: a strange, unexpectedly fast percussion sound. You may feel quite emotional when you hear your baby's heartbeat for the first time; this is concrete evidence of a whole new life growing inside you. If you are carrying twins, the doctor may be able to pick up the two distinct heartbeats with the Doppler device; he may recommend that you have an ultrasound scan to check whether or not you are carrying twins and that they are growing well (see the feature on twins in **Week 13**).

CASE STUDY: *'Just hearing that heartbeat was wonderful. When I had my first pregnancy test it was negative, so I was never really confident until I heard that heart beat. This little tiny heart rattling away inside me.'*

On your first visit you will probably see a doctor and a midwife. At a later stage you may have one or several appointments with the consultant overseeing your pregnancy, but most of your antenatal check-ups from now on will be carried out by a midwife.

You will come away from your booking appointment armed with your dossier in which all your antenatal check-ups will be recorded. You may well have a number of other leaflets and booklets about pregnancy, childbirth and breastfeeding ... as well as advertising material from companies who manufacture childcare equipment. You will definitely feel pregnant now: excited but a little daunted too, perhaps.

Understanding Your Antenatal Notes

The way that information is stored on antenatal notes varies from one clinic to another, but you are likely to come across the same headings whatever the format. Some of them are self-evident, others may seem like a foreign language to you, and this section is to help you understand the headings and remarks in your antenatal notes.

Date: The date on which you have a check-up.

Weeks: The number of weeks since the first day of your last period, or the estimated age in weeks of your pregnancy.

Weight: Your weight.

Urine: The results of your urine test. With any luck this will always read 'nil' or 'NAD' (no abnormalities detected). If sugars have been detected 'glucose' or 'gluc' may be entered here; and if proteins have been detected the abbreviation 'Alb' may be entered (Albumin is one of the proteins detected in urine during pregnancy).

BP: Your blood pressure.

Height of fundus/ H o F / Fundus height: The height in centimetres of the top of the uterus measured from your pelvis. The uterus grows upwards by about 1cm (½in) for every week of the pregnancy (reaching the navel by about the middle of the pregnancy). The height of fundus figure should, therefore, be similar to the number of weeks, and it can act as a guide as to whether the baby is developing at the expected rate.

Presentation / position / lie: The presentation or lie of the baby means the position in which it is lying within the womb at the time of your check-up. In the early weeks this may not be felt or recorded and in the middle months the baby moves around a great deal and may change presentation frequently.

In the latter stages of the pregnancy, the baby usually settles into the head-down position ready for delivery: this is indicated in your notes as 'vertex', 'Vx', 'Cephalic', 'ceph' or 'C'. If the baby is lying across you this is known as a transverse lie and will be indicated as 'transverse' or 'Tr'. A breech baby, lying with its head up will be noted as 'breech' or 'Br'.

Towards the end of the pregnancy your doctor or midwife might use even more detailed abbreviations about the lie of your baby, depending on which way the baby is facing in the womb, towards your front, your side or your back. These may include abbreviations such as 'ROA' (right occiput anterior, meaning the right side of your baby's head is to the front), and your doctor or midwife will explain them to you.

Relation of PP to brim: This refers to how close the presenting part (PP, the part of your baby which will be born first, usually the head) is to the brim of the pelvis. The letters 'NE' may be entered here to mean that the presenting part is not 'engaged' in the pelvis. If your baby moves down in the last weeks of the pregnancy, your notes will indicate the degree of engagement in the pelvis, that is, how far into the pelvis the baby has passed. Engagement is often indicated in fifths: if, for example, your notes said 2/5 this would mean that two fifths of the baby's head (or other presenting part) was engaged and three fifths was not. If the presenting part becomes fully engaged, your notes will probably say 'eng.' or 'E'.

FH: This stands for foetal heart. If the foetal heart has been heard during your check up the entry may read 'FHH' (foetal heart heard) or just 'H' for heard. The letter R may be used to indicate a regular heartbeat.

FM: This stands for foetal movement. If the foetus has been felt to move during the check-up, the letters 'FMF' (foetal movement felt) should appear in this column.

Oedema / Oed: Oedema means fluid retention. Some women find that they retain more fluid during pregnancy, causing puffiness in the fingers, wrists and ankles. If oedema is noticed, it may be indicated as 'oed.' in your notes. Excessive oedema can cause complications in pregnancy and may be a sign of other more serious conditions.

Hb: Hb stands for haemoglobin, and your haemoglobin level is an indication of your red blood cell count. An acceptable haemoglobin level would be indicated as 12gm or over. If your level drops below 11.5gm you may be prescribed iron supplements.

Next visit: The date of your next visit. Unless there are any complications in your pregnancy, you will probably have a check-up every four weeks until week 28. You will then have check-ups fortnightly until week 36, and then once a week until delivery. (The spacing of antenatal check-ups may vary from one hospital to another, and you may need more frequent check-ups if there are any complications in your pregnancy.)

Signature / sig: The signature or initials of the doctor or midwife who carried out your check-up.

Notes / comments: There is usually a column in your notes for your doctor or midwife to make any special comments about your check-up. These notes could be an indication of some possible complication in your pregnancy. If you do not understand or are not sure about anything that they have written here or in any other part of your notes, ask your midwife or doctor to explain it to you.

Week 13

In the first 12 weeks of your pregnancy the skeleton, organs and nervous system of your baby were laid down. Now the foetus begins to grow more rapidly in size, and its organs continue to mature and develop.

The Foetus

As you come into the second trimester of pregnancy in week 13, the foetus measures about 7cm (nearly 3in) from crown to rump, and it still weighs around 17g (less than 1oz). The limbs and digits are continuing to lengthen, and the body is becoming longer too. At this stage, your baby's body is quite thin looking because no fat stores have been laid down.

What is Happening to the Foetus

Much of your baby's internal development is now complete, but important changes are still taking place. The intestine is maturing and beginning to function more like an adult intestine. The section of intestine, mentioned in **Week 7**, which protruded into the umbilical cord, begins to recede back into your baby's abdomen.

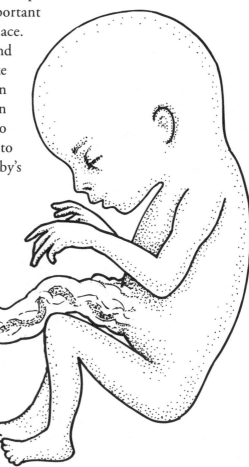

The foetal intestines have begun developing in a swelling in the umbilical cord. Around the thirteenth week this swelling subsides as the intestines shift into the foetus's abdomen.

How you Feel

You should be shaking off any morning sickness and other early symptoms of pregnancy by now, and you may just be beginning to have a bit of a tummy. You may not need to wear different clothes yet because your growing uterus is still well below your waistline, but you should avoid wearing tight fighting clothes across your tummy.

Telling People You Are Pregnant / Changing Relationships

Many women choose to wait until the end of the first three months, around the thirteenth week, before announcing to their friends, employers and possibly even relations that they are pregnant.

Once you have decided to tell people your momentous news, it can be surprisingly difficult to find an opportunity to slip it into conversation. It is an important piece of news so you do not want it to be swallowed up in a more immediately pressing conversation, but it is not easy throwing it out as an opening gambit either. You may also have to bear in mind that there could be some people in your circle of friends who need to be told particularly sensitively: someone who has been trying for a baby for a long time, for example, or someone who has recently had a miscarriage or lost a baby.

Whenever and however you announce your news, you may well be surprised by people's reactions. People will suddenly see you in a new light and it can dramatically change the dynamics of many relationships. Your partner may suddenly become more proud, attentive and protective (although pregnancy certainly does not come with any guarantee to this effect); and you could get the same sort of treatment from male friends and colleagues too. On the other hand, people at work might feel a little embarrassed and unsure how to deal with you, especially if they are younger than you and have not reached the same stage in their lives: it can feel like an intrusion of your private life into your work environment. Your employer might even view your pregnancy as an inconvenience if he or she relies on you heavily and will have to replace you at least temporarily when you take your maternity leave.

Relationships with parents and siblings can alter too. Many women feel closer to all the members of their family, but especially their mothers, when they start having children themselves. In some cases, though, it may drive them apart: if a mother and daughter have very different attitudes to the pregnancy and how the daughter should behave during her pregnancy, the pregnancy itself can aggravate existing disagreements. If your parents are young to be grandparents – or even if they are not! – they may find that their initial elation is tempered with concerns about their own changing identity. Just as you are grappling with the idea of being a mother and getting used to nappies and feeds, they have to come to terms with being a grandparent and being perceived as old.

When you announce the news to other women who have had children themselves – whether they are friends, colleagues or just women waiting in a bus queue with you, you may feel as if you have passed the initiation ceremony into a special club. You immediately have something in common with other women all over the world, whatever their social and financial circumstances, their race or their religious belief. You are doing something that they have done, that they understand and on which they can advise.

CASE STUDY: *'I was quite young when I had my first baby, and lots of my friends weren't even in steady relationships. Once they knew I was pregnant, and even more so when I had the baby, there was this sort of distance between me and them. I felt as if they were saying "well, we can't ask [her] now, she's got a baby". I met lots of new friends through the baby, but I lost touch with some of my old friends.'*

CASE STUDY: *'Being pregnant and having children brings you so much closer to other women. It's funny, for the first time in my life I really wish I had a sister. It would just be so brilliant to show her my children and to see hers. It's not quite the same with my brother.'*

Where to Have Your Baby

As recently as two generations ago, almost all babies were delivered at home, and hospital beds were really only available for very high risk deliveries and those who could afford private hospitals. The advent of the National Health Service, and a massive programme of hospital building in the 1960s, meant that one generation ago a huge percentage of deliveries took place in hospital. It was assumed that hospital was the best and safest place to have a baby.

In the last ten years the emphasis has shifted, partly as a result of research and partly because of women's own experiences. It was found that women felt less in control in a hospital environment, and that hospital care could deny them the sort of continuity of care that could contribute to a trouble-free pregnancy, and could make a significant difference to the amount of intervention needed in labour and delivery.

You have a choice about where you have your baby. The very fact that you are reading a book about pregnancy and childbirth shows that you want to understand for yourself what is happening to your body and what choices are open to you for every aspect of pregnancy and delivery. The more informed you are, the more likely you are to be able to make the most of the choices available to you.

Delivery in Hospital

There is no denying that if there are any complications or causes for concern in a pregnancy, a hospital is very much the best place for the delivery to take place. A hospital offers the specialist and emergency care that may be needed on-site. A recent swing towards midwife-only care has sometimes vilified the medical profession, saying that hospitals tend to use intervention for intervention's sake, but it is important to strike the right balance between midwifery care for the normal pregnancy and medical attention should there be any need for it. If you have your baby in hospital, you can be assured that specialist teams and expertise will be on hand should you need them.

There are, however, drawbacks to hospital care. Hospitals are large and busy places: they can feel impersonal and the sheer numbers of people and quantity of equipment can be a little overwhelming. There is a large staff dealing with an even larger number of women at any one time, and the probability that you will be delivered by a midwife that you have never met before is fairly high. This does not always matter, but if this is not what you expected it could make a difference to your experience of childbirth and your feeling of control.

The argument about intervention for intervention's sake does have some value too: because of the facilities available in hospitals, intervention can become something of a self-perpetuating myth. If, for example, a woman's labour is perceived to be advancing too slowly, she may be given a syntocinon drip to accelerate the labour. The contractions induced by syntocinon are so sudden and so powerful that she may need far more pain relief than she would had her labour been allowed to progress naturally. She may resort to an epidural, and the use of epidural is linked directly to an increased need for Caesarean section. If that same woman had been able to discuss how her labour was progressing with a midwife she knew well and – perhaps more importantly – who knew her well, she might never have agreed to have the syntocinon drip. Even if she went on to need an emergency Caesarean for another reason, at least she would feel that decisions had not been taken out of her hands right at the start.

In the United Kingdom, about 90% of births do take place in hospitals, and having your baby in hospital should not mean that any of the decisions and choices are taken out of your hands. For one thing, you are not obliged to go to your nearest local hospital; you can ask your GP for advice on this matter, and he should be able to help you apply to another nearby hospital if you prefer it for whatever reason.

There is also no need for you to 'take pot luck' on the midwife who delivers you. If you attend antenatal clinics at your local surgery, especially if you are on a Domino Scheme, you may be able to elect for one of the doctors or midwives from that local surgery to attend you and deliver you in hospital. You then have the best of both worlds, benefiting not only from the continuity of care but also the medical expertise on hand should you need it.

Neither should a hospital delivery mean that you are bulldozed into having intervention or pain relief that you do not want. There are accounts of women having their labours speeded up by induction for the convenience of the hospital, but the doctors and midwives in hospital will probably only suggest pain relief or intervention to help you or if they think that there is any threat to your baby's wellbeing. If you read books such as this one which explain the physiological process of labour and delivery, and give you details of the various forms of pain relief and intervention, you will be better equipped to make informed choices during your own labour and delivery.

Home Delivery

In recent years, home deliveries, which were once the norm, have become more common again. Women who feel confident about the completely natural process of childbirth sometimes decide that the benefits of being in their own home – a private, relaxing and familiar environment – outweigh the disadvantage of having no emergency care immediately on hand should it be needed.

Statistics show that there is a massively reduced incidence of intervention of any kind (and of infant and maternal mortality) in home deliveries. This is partly because women who have had any sort of complication in their pregnancy are actively discouraged from having a home delivery. It is also due to the fact that women who choose to have home deliveries are necessarily more confident and feel in control of the birth process.

Every woman has the right to have a home delivery if she elects to do so. If you think you would like to have your baby at home, you should discuss the idea as soon as possible with your partner as well as your doctor and midwife. In some areas there is still resistance to the idea of home delivery, but a doctor has no legal power to stop you making this choice, and a midwife is legally bound to attend you if you choose to have your baby at home.

If your doctor recommends that you do not have a home delivery on medical grounds – either when you first enquire or at a later stage in your pregnancy – it is advisable to respect his recommendations. It is important to remember that, whatever the benefits of home delivery, they are not worth risking your life or your baby's.

CASE STUDY: *'I planned to have my first baby at home, and I was going to have no pain relief. But nothing had prepared me for how painful the labour would be. After 18 hours I gave up, went to hospital and had an epidural. The relief of the pain going away and not worrying about "what if something goes wrong" was incredible.'*

CASE STUDY: *'I decided to have my second baby at home, and it was just wonderful. I did most of the labour by myself and the midwife arrived just 40 minutes before he was born. I was dilating very quickly and the contractions were very painful and powerful, but I felt so normal in between them, I was just sitting at home on my sofa! He was born at 4.30 and at 6.00 our daughter woke up to find she had a little brother. I'll never forget her face coming downstairs and seeing him there.'*

Twins or More

One of the biggest surprises that can come out of a booking appointment can be the news that you are carrying twins. If you conceived with the help of fertility treatment, when the likelihood of multiple births is higher, you would probably have had scans by now and you would know whether or not you had more than one baby. Natural twins occur in just over 1% of pregnancies (this percentage rises as a woman gets older), and many women are not aware that they are expecting twins – or the much rarer triplets – until their booking appointment or even their first scan.

How and Why Twins Happen

Identical and non-identical twins are conceived in completely different ways.

Identical twins: The sometimes remarkable similarities between identical twins exist because both babies arise from the same single fertilised egg which spontaneously divides into two, and the two foetuses develop according to one set of genetic information. Identical twins are, therefore, always of the same sex and look very alike. Statistics do not suggest that there is any connection between the incidence of identical twins and the mother's age, race or family history of twins; the division of the fertilised egg seems to be an 'accident of nature' which happens once in about 275 pregnancies.

Fraternal twins: Fraternal or non-identical twins occur when two eggs are fertilised at the same time and both implant successfully in the uterus. This happens if the woman's ovaries have released two or more ripe eggs in one cycle.

Fraternal twins occur in just under 1% of births, but the incidence is considerably higher in certain groups of women: if there is a history of fraternal twins in a woman's family she is more likely to have fraternal twins herself – the predisposition to releasing more than one egg at a time is probably hereditary. As women get older their chances of having twins increase slightly, and this may be the body's insurance policy against the onset of the menopause, increasing the odds in favour of fertilisation. Women from African countries have a higher incidence of twin pregnancies, and women from Middle Eastern countries have a lower incidence.

How Triplets Occur

Natural triplets are much more rare – occurring in about one in 9000 pregnancies – and they can occur in three ways: either three separate eggs are fertilised at once, or two eggs are fertilised and one of them spontaneously divides to create identical twins, or one egg may spontaneously divide into three.

What to Expect in a Multiple Pregnancy

A twin pregnancy obviously makes greater demands on a woman's body than a single pregnancy. If you were fit and healthy before the pregnancy started, and if you eat well and get a lot of rest during your pregnancy you will be best equipped to cope with these extra demands.

Some of the expected problems of early pregnancy are aggravated in a twin pregnancy; you are even more likely to need to pass urine frequently, for example, because the uterus will be growing more quickly to accommodate both babies. Morning sickness is often worse in twin pregnancies; this may be to do with the extra surge of hormones produced by the two placentae, but there is also often a direct correlation between morning sickness and tiredness. You must not underestimate the value of sleep and rest if you are carrying more than one baby – the pregnancy is making enormous demands on your body and its resources. A well-balanced diet is, therefore, essential too. You may need to supplement your diet with multi-vitamins and minerals: women carrying twins are at greater risk of becoming anaemic and / or having a deficiency of folic acid during pregnancy.

There is also an increased incidence of vaginal bleeding and of miscarriage in twin pregnancies. It is perfectly possible to lose one foetus, but for the other to go to term and be delivered quite safely. This probably happens in more pregnancies than we realise: ultrasound scans taken very early in pregnancy show a much higher incidence of twins than the average incidence at birth. It has been suggested that a higher proportion of pregnancies start out as twin pregnancies but that one of the foetuses is lost – either in bleeding or re-absorbed by the uterus – in the early weeks.

As the pregnancy progresses you may be more likely to suffer from high blood pressure and fluid retention, and to suffer from them comparatively early in the pregnancy. If you do have problems with blood pressure and / or fluid retention you may be asked to attend clinics more frequently so that you can be monitored more closely. These are both symptoms of the dangerous condition pre-eclampsia which is more common in twin pregnancies.

Even though twins are usually smaller than single babies, their combined weight is often well in excess of the average single baby's birthweight. Your uterus not only has to accommodate the two foetuses but also two placentae and two amniotic sacs. As the uterus grows very large in the last trimester of the pregnancy you may be more prone to the problems associated with the last weeks of pregnancy: back pain, sciatic pain, round ligament pain, stress incontinence, shortness of breath, heartburn and indigestion.

Whatever the extra demands and potential complications of a twin pregnancy, you should never lose sight of the fact that it is still a natural process – you may just need to take a little extra care of yourself and to be monitored that bit more frequently to ensure that everything goes smoothly.

Twin pregnancies usually last an average of between 37 and 38 weeks (as compared to 40 weeks for single pregnancies); twins are, therefore, usually not only smaller than the average single baby but also less mature (see the section on **Premature Labour** in the chapter **When Things Go Wrong**). If you threaten to go into labour before the thirty-sixth week your consultant may try to subdue the contractions with drugs to prolong the pregnancy so that the foetuses have a chance to mature more fully.

CASE STUDY: *'I did get very tired when I was carrying the twins, but then I'd got the other two children to look after already.'*

CASE STUDY: *'I'm very prone to morning sickness. I was bad enough with my daughter, but with the twins I was sick every single day of the pregnancy. Not badly sick, but I would be sick every morning without fail.'*

There is more information about labour and delivery in twin pregnancies in the chapter **Labour and Delivery**, and the addresses of organisations who can give you more specialised advice about multiple pregnancy appear at the end of the book.

Week 14

You are now a third of the way through your pregnancy, and this fact alone should give you a sense of achievement. You are entering the second trimester of pregnancy, the middle months in which many women 'blossom' and feel full of energy.

The Foetus

By the end of the fourteenth week of pregnancy your baby measures about 8.5cm (3½in) from crown to rump, and weighs around 30g, just over 1oz. It has grown appreciably and has put on half its own bodyweight in the last week. The fingers and toes are becoming finer and the tiny fingernails and toenails are well in evidence. The head now has a more human face, as the eyes come further towards the front of the head and the ears move up and to the side.

What is Happening to the Foetus

As your baby begins to grow and put on weight more rapidly the bones and muscles develop further. The baby now makes quite strong movements with its limbs (although you will not feel it yet). The internal and external genitalia are continuing to mature: a baby boy now has the structures which will produce sperm throughout his adult life; a baby girl will have not only both her ovaries but all her eggs by the time she is born.

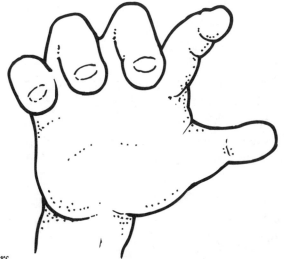

Soft nails begin to emerge on the fingers.

How you Feel

You could well be feeling happier and more relaxed about your pregnancy now than at any other stage so far. You are likely to be feeling much better physically by the fourteenth week, you may well have had your booking appointment and you may have told everyone you know that you are pregnant. This is a time to try and enjoy being pregnant, to make sure that you eat well, drink lots of fluids, take regular exercise and get plenty of sleep. The fitter and healthier you are in the middle months of your pregnancy, the better equipped you will be for the demands of the final trimester, delivery and motherhood.

Correct Posture and Back Care

As your muscles and ligaments loosen under the effects of progesterone and as your centre of gravity is altered by your changing shape, you may find that you suffer from a number of aches and pains. Most of these pains are mild, but some women suffer from more serious and persistent pain which cannot be ignored. Many of the aches and pains experienced in pregnancy can be eradicated or alleviated by altering your posture, following simple exercises and learning relaxation techniques. Queen Charlotte's Hospital is one of a number of hospitals that have obstetric physiotherapists on hand to deal with these problems.

Many obstetric physiotherapists give an advisory session at around the fourteenth week to prevent possible problems. They would cover back care, posture, pelvic floor exercises and relaxation techniques; and they would address any specific problems raised at this stage in the pregnancy.

Posture

Your balance changes subtly during pregnancy as you put weight on your tummy and your breasts, and it is not uncommon for women to compensate for this by sticking their bottoms out. This exaggerates the curve of the spine and puts unnecessary strain on the vertebrae, causing back pain; the effect is exaggerated still further if you wear high-heeled shoes. Even at this early stage, before your bump has become large or heavy, it is important to try and stand up straight, making a conscious effort to tuck your bottom in so that your spine makes as straight a line as possible.

Back Care

It is very important that you look after your back during pregnancy because the pregnancy makes considerable demands on it. Part of back care is adopting the correct posture when you are standing, but you should also think about how you sit, how you walk, how you get in and out of cars, what you carry and how you carry it, and how you lift things. Even if you do not suffer from back pain at this stage in your pregnancy, it is common for women to have backache later on. If you start thinking about your back now, you are far more likely to avoid trouble later (for more detailed information about how to look after your back see the feature on **Backache** in **Week 28**).

Pains and Treatment

The loosening up of muscles and ligaments in early pregnancy can give rise to a number of specific pains that may be remedied with physiotherapy. One example is a condition called symphysis pubis dysfunction when the tiny cartilaginous link at the front of the pelvis becomes slightly loose. This can be very painful, and could be aggravated by the growing uterus if it is not dealt with early on. This problem can usually be improved with the help of an obstetric physiotherapist who can teach you correct posture and some simple pelvic tilt exercises, and may be able to recommend a support girdle if necessary.

If you are interested in finding out more about posture, back care and physiotherapy during pregnancy, ask your GP or midwife whether there is an obstetric physiotherapist attached to your local hospital or contact the Association of Chartered Physiotherapists in Women's Health (their address appears at the end of the book).

I'm not Fat, I'm Pregnant

However excited you are about your pregnancy, you may have a tweak of troubled vanity when your 'tummy' first appears. Once the uterus has popped above the line of the pelvic girdle around the twelfth week, it continues to grow up towards the navel and outwards. At this stage in the pregnancy some women have already lost their waistline and put weight on their breasts, others will look just the same except for the slightly protruding tummy.

Few women actually look pregnant to the casual observer at this stage, and you may feel that you just look fat to them. The pressure on women in our society to be slim is so great that even this tummy can have a demoralising effect; but you can easily disguise the not-yet-a-proper-bump tummy with looser clothes: a loose shirt, jumper or jacket over your skirt, dress, trousers or leggings. You also need to get things in perspective: you must remember that what your tummy is doing is far more important than some unrealistic expectation of what women's bodies should look like.

CASE STUDY: *'I usually weigh myself and look at myself in the mirror every morning. I know it's a bit obsessive, but being slim mattered and I always used to pride myself on having a flat tummy in the morning. Then this little podgy belly started appearing. I thought I was going to mind and try to cover it up, but it was ridiculous, I went all sort of gooey over it. "That's my baby," I used to think.'*

Caring for Your Hair and Nails During Pregnancy

You may notice that your hair has changed since you became pregnant, and this may be a change for the better or for the worst. Progesterone increases the activity of the glands in your scalp that produce oils, so hair is likely to be more greasy, especially towards the end of your pregnancy.

Your hair is likely to become thicker too. More hair grows and less is lost in pregnancy, and many women find that their hair is thicker and sometimes more luxuriant when they are pregnant. The excess hair does come out quite naturally after you have had your baby; it may feel as if you are then losing an alarming amount of hair, and it may feel comparatively thin afterwards, but it will return to its normal thickness by the time your baby is about a year old.

Some women notice that the very structure of their hair changes during pregnancy: it may become more or less curly, silkier or coarser, and these are changes that might persist even after the end of the pregnancy. Body hair can become darker and more abundant too, especially in women who develop patches of darker skin colour during pregnancy.

Caring for your Hair

You may find that you have to change your shampoo, your hair-washing routine or even the way that you style your hair to accommodate the way that it has changed. Many books advise that pregnancy is not a good time to have hair dyed, highlighted or permed because your hair is not in its normal condition, but if you are frustrated or demoralised because your hair is not behaving the way it usually does, there is no reason why you should not give it a little artificial help.

Changes to your Nails

Fingernails and toenails are made of the same protein as hair. It is called keratin, and the keratin in your nails can alter during pregnancy just as much as the keratin in your hair. Some women find that their nails become tougher during pregnancy, others complain that their nails are prone to brittleness and flaking.

Caring for your Nails

If you notice that your nails are tending to break more easily, you can minimise this by keeping them warm and dry. Wear gloves outside in cold weather, wear rubber-gloves if you need to get your hands wet, and apply hand lotion – rubbing it well into your nails and cuticles – after washing your hands.

Week 15

It is now three months since the egg was first fertilised, and in those weeks your foetus has really become a miniature human baby.

The Foetus

The foetus is now into its period of growth; it measures approximately 10cm (4in) from crown to rump. It has put on more than half its bodyweight again in the course of a week: it now weighs 50g (just over 1½oz). The face is still changing by the day, the eyelids, nose, lips and external ears are becoming better defined. Hair is also beginning to grow, not only ordinary head hair, eyelashes and eyebrows but also tiny hairs called lanugo appear all over your baby's body. It is not known why babies are covered in lanugo during the middle and latter months of pregnancy. Some are born with this fine, fluffy coating of hair which rubs off the new-born infant rather like the fluff of a peach.

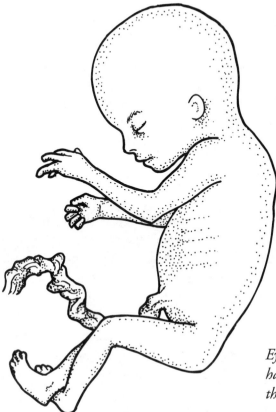

Eyebrows and eyelashes have begun to grow on the foetus's face.

How you Feel

You should not be troubled by so many unpleasant symptoms of pregnancy during the middle months. If you are worried about any aches and pains that you have or by continued morning sickness, talk to your doctor or midwife who may be able to help you deal with them or at least reassure you that they are normal.

The 'Bloom' of the Middle Months

Once your body has adjusted to the great hormonal upheavals at the onset of pregnancy, you may come into a period of unusual wellbeing. Some women say that they never feel better than in the middle months of pregnancy (there are others who suffer morning sickness through their entire pregnancy and find they would rather forget even the middle months). However well or otherwise you feel, you may appear to have a bloom during pregnancy: your skin retains fluids making it firmer and smoother, and the increased blood circulation can give you a healthy glow.

As your baby begins to put on weight more rapidly you may find that you have an increased appetite. Your metabolic rate will be higher than normal, making you feel warm and full of energy. Progesterone is causing your muscles to relax and your ligaments to slacken (this is to facilitate the passage of the baby through your pelvis for the delivery), and this means that most women are more supple during their pregnancy than at any other time. This too can give you a feeling of wellbeing, but you should not abuse it: slackened ligaments can easily be damaged by overuse and strain. Listen to your body and do not do things that cause aching or pain.

The sedative effect of progesterone coupled with the natural pain-killers endorphins which circulate in your bloodstream during pregnancy may make you feel unusually relaxed, comfortable and at ease with the world. If you do not feel energised and well at this stage in your pregnancy, you should not worry; it does not mean that there is anything wrong with your or your baby. It may simply be that your body has not adapted so well to the hormonal changes of pregnancy, or it could be that the demands of your job and other commitments are not giving your body a chance to 'bloom'. If this is the case, make sure that you eat regularly and get plenty of rest.

CASE STUDY: *'Oh, don't talk to me about the middle months! If you ask me, pregnancy is highly over-rated: I was sick at the beginning, incontinent at the end and fat in the middle. Next question?!'*

CASE STUDY: *'I must admit I did feel very well after the first three months were over. I bounced out of bed in the mornings – not normal! – and had a sort of "what does it matter" attitude to anything that went wrong. I slept very well ... I was full of beans and had the most colossal appetite! ... And people kept saying it, they kept saying: "pregnancy really suits you".'*

Exercise in the Second Trimester

If you are feeling very well in the second trimester of your pregnancy you may feel that you want to take up or go back to an exercise routine. Although it is important that you remain fit during your pregnancy, you should be careful not to make too many demands on your body or to do anything that could harm your baby.

Your body is changing gradually, and if you already take exercise regularly, you will notice that some activities might cause you pain or result in aches later. You should respect these signals and avoid activities which cause pain. If you have not been taking regular exercise and you feel that you would like to, talk to your doctor about what sort of exercise you should take. There may be a trained fitness instructor at your local leisure centre who will be able to advise you. Walking and swimming are both good forms of exercise which use the major muscle groups and improve cardio-vascular fitness, without putting too much strain on the muscles and ligaments.

If you go to fitness classes there is no reason why you should not continue these classes during your pregnancy so long as you do not do anything that causes you pain. Make sure that your instructor has been properly trained, and let him or her know that you are pregnant. Your instructor will be able to advise you which exercises you should not do during pregnancy: abdominal exercises are not recommended at any time in pregnancy, and exercises which mean lying on your tummy are discouraged after the 12-week watershed when the uterus has come up out of the pelvis.

For the sake of your muscles and ligaments you may be advised to adapt to a low-impact routine instead of a high-impact one. If you are used to running or using a running machine, remember that brisk walking up a slight gradient has just the same benefits for cardio-vascular fitness as running on the level, but it causes fewer injuries to muscles and ligaments.

If you usually take part in a hazardous sport such as riding, ski-ing or canoeing, you have to weigh up the enjoyment that you get from it with the possibility that you could lose your baby. Many enthusiasts of hazardous sports will argue that they are competent and experienced, and that the risk to their baby is very small. It is important to remember that, however competent you may be at the sport, circumstances beyond your control can cause an accident which may have tragic repercussions. If, for example, you are an experienced skier and you ski especially carefully because you are pregnant, you still cannot guarantee that someone else on the slopes would not cause you to fall. If you are travelling abroad your medical insurance company may not agree to cover you for hazardous sports when you are pregnant.

Week 16

The sixteenth week of pregnancy is often an important one because a number of tests can be performed on the foetus at this stage.

The Foetus

By the end of the sixteenth week of pregnancy the foetus measures about 11.5cm (4½in) from crown to rump and weighs nearly 80g (just under 3oz). The lanugo hair is growing abundantly, and a fine network of blood vessels can be seen through the thin skin all over your baby's body. The fingers are longer with fully formed nails and their own individual fingerprint. The baby's lips are also much clearer now, and the face is becoming even more defined as the eyebrows grow.

What is Happening to the Foetus

Your baby's muscles are growing in strength every day and the foetus makes quite vigorous movements. It can curl up its toes, make a tiny fist with it hand, and even suck its thumb.

The foetus's skin is so fine that the blood vessels are visible under the surface.

How you Look

By the sixteenth week of pregnancy some women have already changed sufficiently to warrant wearing proper maternity clothes. Most women will at least have noticed that their breasts are bigger, their waistline has thickened and their tummy has grown. Your hair and skin may have changed too; you may look well with glowing skin thanks to the increased blood circulation.

Testing for Abnormality in the Foetus

There are a number of tests which can establish whether your foetus has any abnormalities and which are available at around the sixteenth week of pregnancy. Some hospitals carry out one or more of these tests routinely on all pregnant women in their care; in other areas only women who are perceived to be at high risk of having babies with abnormalities are offered these tests as a matter of course. In all but a very few areas, the tests are all available to women who ask to have them performed. If you are keen to have a particular test ask your doctor or midwife well in advance whether it can be arranged. If any test that you want is not available locally on the National Health, you may be able to have the test performed privately.

Before you decide to have any tests for your unborn child, you need to think about why you are having them performed. Few of these tests are 100% reliable and some carry a small risk of causing a miscarriage. Are you having these tests to reassure yourself that the baby you are carrying is normal and, if so, are the risks worth taking? If you discover that your baby has some kind of abnormality, what action would you take? You may be faced with the decision to consider terminating your pregnancy, or you may use this early warning to prepare for a baby with special needs and find out as much as possible about your baby's condition.

Alpha-fetoprotein (AFP) test: This test is carried out routinely in many hospitals in the sixteenth week of pregnancy. A blood sample is taken from the mother (causing no risk to the foetus) to test for the presence of a protein known as AFP. AFP is produced by the foetus and should be present in the mother's bloodstream; if the amount of AFP detected is higher or lower than normal this may indicate that the baby has Down's

Syndrome or spina bifida. AFP testing can only indicate the likelihood that the foetus has this sort of condition and further testing is necessary to prove conclusively whether or not it has.

Triple test: The triple test is another blood test (again posing no risk to the foetus) performed at about 16 weeks to check the levels of three chemicals, including AFP, in the mother's bloodstream to compute the probability that the foetus has Down's Syndrome. The results of the test are usually given as a ratio, for example you may be told that you have a 1 in 900 or a 1 in 125 chance of having a Down's Syndrome baby. If the probability is high, 1 in 100 or less (but this will depend on your age), you may decide to have an amniocentesis to establish whether or not your baby has Down's Syndrome.

Amniocentesis: Amniocentesis is a more sophisticated and invasive test which is usually performed at about 16 weeks and can be used to establish conclusively whether the foetus has Down's Syndrome, spina bifida or a number of genetic disorders such as cystic fibrosis or muscular dystrophy. There is no guarantee that the baby will be normal even if the amniocentesis establishes that the baby is not suffering from one of these conditions. The test itself carries a small risk element: just under 1% of amniocentesis tests result in miscarriage.

Amniocentesis may be offered systematically to women over 35 who have an increased risk of having a Down's Syndrome baby; to women who have a family history of genetic disorders; or it may be offered to you if the results of your AFP or Triple blood test suggested an increased risk of any of these conditions.

A woman having amniocentesis will be given an ultrasound scan (see **Your Ultrasound Scan** in **Week 18**) to check the lie of her baby. Then she will be given a local anaesthetic to her abdomen, and a hollow needle will be passed through her abdominal wall and into the amniotic sack to draw out a sample of the amniotic fluid. You should know within a few days whether your baby has spina bifida, but it can take up to two weeks to get a result for Down's Syndrome and genetic disorders. The amniocentesis will also establish the sex of your baby, which could be important if you are a carrier for a sex-linked genetic disorder. Otherwise, you can choose whether or not you want to know the sex of your baby before it arrives.

Chorionic villus sampling (CVS): Chorionic villus sampling can be performed as early as the tenth week of pregnancy to establish the presence of Down's Syndrome and a number of genetic disorders of the blood such as sickle cell anaemia. CVS is an invasive test and it carries a comparatively high risk of miscarriage (about 2.5%).

A hollow needle is passed through the abdomen under general anaesthetic or a fine tube is passed into the uterus through the cervix and a tiny sample of the placenta is removed (the doctor uses an ultrasound scan as a map of where the placenta is). The procedure takes about 15 minutes and the results are usually available in about a week. The advantage of CVS is that it can give a woman early warning of abnormality in her baby, allowing her more time to make very difficult decisions.

Understanding Test Results

If you do not understand the results of a test or the implications of these results, make sure that you speak to your doctor or midwife. They can explain to you exactly what the results mean and what courses of action are open to you. If tests confirm that your baby has some sort of abnormality, there are many organisations that can give you advice and support whether you choose to terminate your pregnancy or to keep your baby. Their addresses are listed at the back of this book.

Week 17

You are now nearly half way through your pregnancy and you probably have an obvious bump to show for it.

The Foetus

The foetus now measures about 12.5cm (5in) from crown to rump and weighs about 100g (3½oz). It may be not only kicking but actually moving about within the uterus, touching its toes and moving its hands about its face and head. You may not feel any foetal movement yet if this is a first pregnancy, but you may well have recognised its movements already if this is a second or subsequent pregnancy.

What is Happening to the Foetus

In about the seventeenth week of pregnancy the first tiny fat stores are laid down in your baby's body and the muscles are continuing to fill out, although your baby still appears quite long and thin.

Less than half way through the pregnancy the foetus already looks very much like a tiny baby and it can even suck its thumb.

How you Feel

You may feel a little apprehensive if you are waiting for the results of any tests for abnormalities. If you have any concerns about these tests and their implications, discuss them with your partner as well as your doctor or midwife.

Libido and Sex in the Second Trimester

Some couples find that their libido dwindles dramatically in pregnancy and during the early weeks of parenthood; others find that they are very sexually active during pregnancy; yet another group find it difficult to synchronise their sexual appetites.

Any discrepancy in when and how often you want to make love can cause frustration and resentment, feelings that you can ill afford at a time when you and your partner need support and reassurance. Whatever your feelings about sex, it is important that you discuss them with your partner. Tell him what you need and want to do or do not want to do, but also listen to him and his needs.

You may be feeling full of energy at this stage in your pregnancy, and the increased circulation in your vagina and nipples means that they are more sensitive and may be more easily stimulated. Even if you feel like making love, you might think that it could harm the baby. There is no danger of this and if your partner worries that he could hurt the baby with his penis, you should reassure him that he cannot.

If you have quite a big 'bump' you may find that the missionary position is uncomfortable and you might be concerned that the baby is being crushed under your partner's weight. On the other hand, if your partner is slight and you have put on a lot of weight you may feel as if you are crushing him if you sit astride him. This could be a time to experiment with different positions for love-making. If you feel shy about discussing ideas, there is no need to talk: just move yourself and guide him!

CASE STUDY: *'Our sex life has just gone dead. I think we are both scared, it just doesn't seem quite right. But we're not bothered; I mean he doesn't seem bothered and I'm not bothered. We haven't actually talked about it, but it has never been a problem.'*

CASE STUDY: *'It was odd, because suddenly I was the one that was asking to make love. I really felt very good, but he was funny about it. He said he was worried about the baby, but I actually think there was more to it than that. I think it turned him off, I think he just found the whole idea of me being pregnant a bit of a turn-off.'*

LOSING YOUR HEAD

Many women complain that they 'lose brain cells' when they are pregnant, and most would say that they never recoup them. You may find that you become forgetful, you have difficulty concentrating and that you are simply not as efficient as usual during your pregnancy.

This relaxing of concentration is another side-effect of the hormones circulating in your bloodstream rather than an irretrievable depletion of your brain cells! It can be inconvenient, and you may find that you need to keep lists of things that really need doing. It may also be a good incentive to cut down on commitments at a time when there are so many demands on you physically and psychologically.

You may continue to feel less efficient in the first weeks after your baby is born when you will be too physically tired for mental acuity, but the hormonal effect on your concentration will wane rapidly after delivery.

CASE STUDY: *'I really do feel as if my brain has turned to porridge.'* *[said in the fifth month of pregnancy]*

Week 18

This is likely to be the week in which you have your ultrasound scan (although this varies from one hospital to another), when you will be able to see your baby moving inside you.

The Foetus

By the end of the eighteenth week of pregnancy the foetus has come to the end of its first major growth spurt (it will begin another growth spurt in about week 24). The crown-rump measurement is now about 13.5cm (5½ inches) and the foetus weighs about 150g (just over 5oz). The eyes are now right at the front of the baby's head, forming a proper face. The face looks a little condensed in the lower third of the head. The upper two thirds of the head are taken up with the huge forehead behind which the brain continues to develop.

What is Happening to the Foetus

The human brain is one of the most sophisticated and complex structures in the natural world, and your baby's brain is growing and developing throughout your pregnancy. By this stage the brain is already sending messages to many parts of your baby's body, triggering the heartbeat, movements, digestive process and the production of hormones. The brain also receives and acts upon external stimuli: a very loud noise, for example, can make the foetus jump.

The eyes have travelled round the head since they first appeared under the skin, and the features now form a true face.

How you Feel

You are likely to be excited about your forthcoming scan when you will be able to see an image of your baby moving on a screen. You may be wondering whether you want to know what sex your baby is and whether the staff will let you know the sex of the baby.

Your Ultrasound Scan

Most hospitals offer all pregnant women at least one ultrasound scan in about the eighteenth week of their pregnancy. If there is any doubt about the dating of your pregnancy, the rate at which your baby is growing or any abnormalities that you or the baby may have, you may be offered more than one scan or regular scans throughout your pregnancy.

What the Scan is For

The scan will be used to take critical measurements of your baby to confirm the dating of the pregnancy and check that the baby is growing at the expected rate. The scan can be used to ensure that the baby's skeleton, nervous system and vital organs as well as the placenta are developing normally (some abnormalities such as spina bifida and heart defects can be picked up on ultrasound scan). The scan will also show if you are carrying two or more babies – which can come as a great surprise – and it can usually show fairly conclusively what sex your baby is.

How the Scan Works

The scan will not hurt you or your baby. About half an hour before having the scan you may be asked to drink up to 0.5 litre (1 pint) of water so that your bladder pushes the uterus well up into the abdomen. This makes it easier for the scan to build up a picture of the baby and the placenta. You will lie down and pull your clothes away from your tummy; the radiologist will cover your tummy in a cool slippery gel to facilitate the movement of the ultrasound equipment and to keep it in contact with your abdomen.

A piece of equipment about the size of a fist is swept over your abdomen. It is called a transducer and it sends a series of very high frequency, inaudible sound waves into your abdominal cavity. The sound waves bounce off certain tissues, back up to the transducer, building up a picture of the pattern of tissues inside you. This information is relayed through a flex to a screen where the live image of your baby inside the womb can be seen.

What you can See

The image projected on the screen is in black and white; it may be static or there may be a great deal of movement depending on how active your baby is at the time. To the untrained eye, it is not always obvious what is going on on the screen: make sure that you ask the staff what you are seeing if you do not understand the picture. They should be able to alter the position of the transducer so that you can see the baby from many angles, seeing its head and features, its spine, tummy, bottom and limbs. You may even be able to watch your baby sucking its thumb or making kicking or waving movements. In most hospitals you can ask for a picture to be taken from the scan for you to keep (you may be charged for this service).

The Baby's Father

If your partner has the time, he might really enjoy accompanying you for your scan. He may be conscious of your growing tummy, but he cannot feel pregnant and excited about the baby in the way that you do: the scan will make the baby seem very real to him, and it might make it easier for him to talk about the pregnancy and the baby. If your partner is not free to come with you, you may like to have a friend or relation to accompany you.

Asking the Baby's Sex

It is usually possible for trained staff to tell the sex of a baby if an ultrasound scan is performed after about the fifteenth week of pregnancy. You may decide that you would like to know the sex of your baby, or you may feel that this is a surprise you want to save until the birth. If you have a family history of sex-linked genetic diseases you will certainly be told the sex of the baby because it could have serious implications. If not, the hospital staff will very probably tell you the sex of your baby if you ask them, although they will warn you that telling a baby's sex from an ultrasound scan is not 100% reliable. Some hospitals are not willing to tell you your baby's sex. If you feel very strongly that you would like to know your baby's sex, speak to your doctor or consultant and he should be able to arrange for the information to be disclosed to you.

Causes for Concern

If the ultrasound scan raises any causes for concern, such as showing that your baby has some abnormalities, or that your placenta has implanted unusually low in your uterus, you will be referred to your consultant immediately. He will explain to you the findings of the scan and their implications. In some cases, for example if the baby has been found to be very severely handicapped, he may recommend that you consider terminating the pregnancy. You will need to think about this carefully and discuss it thoroughly with him, with your partner and possibly your own parents and your own doctor or midwife.

Week 19

The top of your uterus, the fundus, should be just under the level of your navel by the nineteenth week of pregnancy. Press the tips of your fingers gently around your navel, and you should be able to feel the rounded shape of the fundus.

The Foetus

By now the foetus measures 14.5cm (just under 6in) from crown to rump and weighs 200g (7oz). It still looks thin for its length, but will fill out and grow in the second half of the pregnancy. The head and face of the foetus are continuing to develop and the muscles of the neck are growing stronger. It can now move its head backwards and forwards.

What is Happening to the Foetus

Inside your baby's jaw the beginnings of tiny teeth are being laid down. Most babies do not cut their first tooth until they are four to six months old, but they are born with a full set of milk teeth formed in their jaws.

The foetus now has enough muscle development to kick and move about quite vigorously. It is still very small and well cushioned by amniotic fluid, but most women will feel their baby's first kick at about this time.

How you Feel

Now that your tummy is getting bigger and you have seen the baby on your scan you probably feel as if you are entering a whole new phase of your pregnancy. The baby seems real to you now, and – if you have not already – you might start thinking about names for the baby and about shopping in preparation for your baby. Although some people are superstitious about shopping too much in advance of a baby's arrival, it is advisable to start planning what you want and need, and seeing what is available in the shops before the very end of the pregnancy when you may feel too tired to shop.

Nutrition in the Second Trimester

During the second trimester, when your baby is growing rapidly and making considerable demands on your metabolism, you may find that you are very hungry. You are likely to have got over any morning sickness and lack of appetite, and your uterus has not yet grown high enough to push up on your stomach, making you feel full more quickly. There should be little to stop you eating to meet your hunger.

You do need to eat more than usual by this stage in your pregnancy, partly to feed the growing baby but mostly to fuel your own metabolism which is working at a higher rate. At this point in your pregnancy you may be needing 200-400 more calories a day. (A slice of bread or a banana each provides about 100 calories.)

There are two important things to remember: you need only eat to satisfy your hunger, and you and your baby are what you eat. Try to stick to the principles of good nutrition laid out in the chapter on **Preparing for Pregnancy**. You need plenty of protein rich foods (meat, fish, eggs and cheese) to build up your baby's muscles and your own strength; starchy carbohydrates (bread, pasta, rice and potatoes) to give you energy; and fresh fruit and vegetables to provide fibre and the full complement of vitamins and minerals. Fats and oils are also valuable parts of your diet, bringing with them some fat-soluble vitamins and providing a good source of energy, but remember that most of your energy requirement should be supplied by the carbohydrates in your diet, not the fats.

You may find that you feel hungry between meals, but try to avoid snacking on fatty and sugary foods. Sugary foods give you a surge of energy – and a surge of calories too – but it is a short-lived supply of energy and it usually brings few essential nutrients with it. If you like sweet snacks, try nibbling dried fruits which contain natural sugars as well as lots of fibre and some vitamins.

Iron Tablets and Other Supplements

If you suffer from anaemia during pregnancy, you will be prescribed an iron supplement to bring your haemoglobin levels back up to normal. Iron tablets can cause constipation, but there are various different preparations of iron, and your doctor or midwife may be able to recommend one that is less likely to cause constipation. As pregnancy itself often causes constipation, you should make sure that you eat plenty of fibre (wholegrain cereals, fruit and green leafy vegetables) and drink plenty of fluids to try and make your bowel movements easier. Do not use any sort of laxative without consulting your doctor or pharmacist (they could contain ingredients which might be harmful to your baby).

Some doctors systematically prescribe iron supplements for all the pregnant women in their care. If you are already having trouble with constipation and you are worried about the effects of the tablets, ask to have your haemoglobin levels checked before agreeing to take them. If your haemoglobin levels are normal, the supplements would be wasted on you.

The best way to ensure that you keep your haemoglobin levels up is to eat lots of iron-rich foods. The best sources of iron are black puddings, mussels, kidneys, game, lentils, haricot beans, wholemeal bread and meat. Liver is also a very good source of iron, but liver products should be eaten not more that once a week to avoid a harmful build up of vitamin A. Avoid drinking tea with or just after a meal, because tea can significantly reduce the absorption of iron from your food.

If you are in any doubt about what vitamins and minerals are or are not present in sufficient quantities in your diet, there are a number of multi-vitamin and -mineral tablets available from chemists and health shops. Some of these tablets are specifically designed for pregnant women, and they can be useful supplements to a well-balanced diet.

Week 20

You are now half way through your 40-week pregnancy. You have probably put on up to about 4.5kg (10lb) in the first 20 weeks, and should have an obvious tummy. You will probably have felt your baby moving, and will think of yourself as carrying a baby rather than being pregnant.

The Foetus

When you are half way through your pregnancy the foetus's crown-rump measurement is about 16cm (nearly 6½in). It weighs about 250g (about 9oz), and is only a fraction of your baby's likely birthweight. The foetus is now covered in the fine lanugo hair, which began to appear in week 15, and it may already have some growth of hair on its head. The proportions of the head and body are beginning to change slowly as the body grows more quickly and catches up with the head.

What is Happening to the Foetus

Your baby's digestive system is still developing and changing. The foetus is known to swallow amniotic fluid from as early as the twelfth week, but by the twentieth week the digestive tract is sufficiently developed to absorb not only the water but certain nutrients and enzymes from this fluid. The repeated action of swallowing stimulates the developing muscles all along the baby's digestive tract, so that they expand and contract regularly. Your baby may sometimes give itself hiccups by swallowing amniotic fluid, although you are unlikely to feel them this early. They will do the baby no harm, and will provide amusement for you and anyone else who cares to feel your tummy at the time!

How you Look

The top of your uterus, the fundus, is probably on a level with your navel by the middle of the pregnancy, and you may now have to wear loose-fitting clothes to accommodate your bump. Your breasts may have become larger too, and you may notice that the nipples have become darker. Your waist has probably all but disappeared and you may be aware that you have gained some weight on your thighs and buttocks. However, a fair proportion of women still do not look obviously pregnant until the sixth month of their first pregnancy; in subsequent pregnancies the weight seems to go on more quickly and to make the pregnancy obvious earlier.

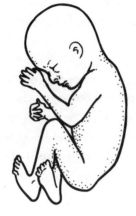

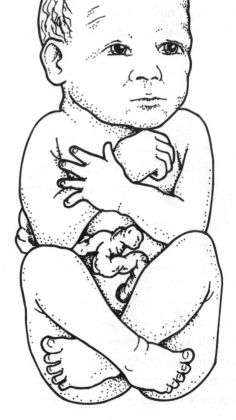

Compared to the full-term baby,
the 20-week foetus still has a lot
of growing and filling out to do.

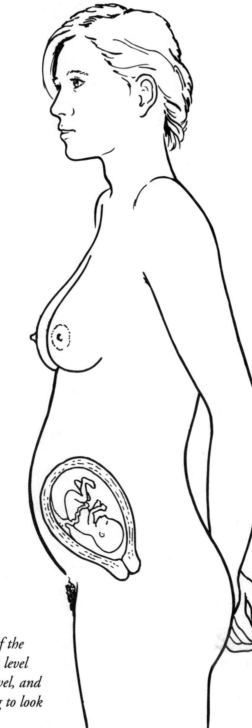

By week 20 the top of the uterus is usually on a level with the mother's navel, and she may be beginning to look obviously pregnant.

Feeling Your Baby Move

You are likely to feel your baby move at around the twentieth week of your pregnancy if this is your first pregnancy (in later pregnancies women tend to recognise a baby's movements a little earlier). The first movements you feel are very slight and can easily be mistaken for wind! Here are some descriptions of those first sensations: 'like a bubble popping inside me', 'like a butterfly flapping its wings in slow motion', 'a fuzzy indistinct feeling, as if a piece of cotton wool was being pulled into different shapes', 'a tiny tumbling feeling, like an eel falling over a waterfall'.

The old term 'quickening', which was used to describe the time when a baby was first felt to move in the womb, meant coming alive, and it may well seem to you that your baby has come alive when you feel it moving for the first time. It can be a very exciting time, and many women become fond of their babies and attribute a personality to them thanks to their strange antics in the womb.

As the baby grows and the movements become stronger, you will be able to tell the difference between one kick and an entire repositioning, and you may recognise times of day when your baby is more active ... particularly if they are times when you are trying to rest. You may notice that your baby seems to move only when you are stationary. This may be simply that you are not aware of the baby moving when you yourself are on the go or it may be that your movements lull the baby, and it only wakes and moves when you are still.

Alarming though it may seem, in later pregnancy, when the baby is bigger, it is possible to distinguish the parts of the body that are suddenly jabbing out: a hand, a heel or a knee. You may also know when your baby is moving position so that it is facing up or down, or lying across you.

CASE STUDY: *'It always gives me a flutter of pleasure when I feel my baby kicking. I'm sometimes surprised how vigorous it is (said in week 30), but I always imagine this little thing curled up inside and making its little protests about the living quarters!'*

CASE STUDY: *'Well, of course, people had told me that you could tell when they had hiccups, but I thought that was a load of twaddle. Then one day I was trying to relax in the bath and my tummy started this regular sort of twitching, causing little ripples of water every time.*

There really was only one thing it could have been, the baby had hiccups.'

Some women feel little or no foetal movement throughout their pregnancy, but this need not be a sign that there is anything wrong with the baby. If you are worried because you have not felt any foetal movement at all, speak to your doctor or midwife. They should be able to reassure you that the baby is alive and well by listening to its heartbeat and relaying the sound to you with a Doppler device.

Babies tend gradually to move less in the last few weeks of pregnancy because there is less room to move, and they are settling into a position for delivery. If you notice a sudden decrease in the amount your baby is moving or if the movements have stopped altogether, contact your doctor or midwife immediately. It could mean that something has happened to your baby. You may be asked to keep a record of when your baby kicks (a kick chart) to check that it is all right.

Week 21

You are now over half way through your pregnancy, but it probably still feels as if it is a very long time before you will have your baby.

The Foetus

The foetus has been growing inside you for 19 weeks, and it now has a crown-rump measurement of about 17.5cm (7in). It is putting on around 50g (2oz) every week at this point, and now weighs about 300g (just under 11oz). The limbs are beginning to look sturdier as the muscles develop, and fat deposits build up slowly, gradually making the skin appear less wrinkled.

The placenta is now a large and very complex organ, fuelling the baby's dramatic growth.

What is Happening to the Foetus

The internal organs of the foetus continue to mature all through the second half of your pregnancy. The bones are also developing, containing more and more ossified (hard and bony) cells. The placenta has grown and developed remarkably since the foetus first implanted in the uterine wall some 18 weeks ago. It has a huge network of blood vessels filtering nutrients from the mother's bloodstream into the foetus, and removing waste products from the foetus's bloodstream to be excreted by the mother. The umbilical cord, which acts as the service route from the placenta to the foetus and allows the foetus to move around within the uterus, is now about 1cm (½in) in diameter.

How you Feel

You are likely to be feeling physically well in the middle weeks of your pregnancy, and you may feel as if you are 'on the home straight'. You might be making plans for the birth and for the things you need to buy for the baby, or you may feel that it is all a very long way away still.

Dressing with a Bump

By the twenty-first week of pregnancy, when you are nearly five months pregnant, you are likely to have a fair sized bump, and the top of the uterus will have risen above your navel, so that you can no longer wear clothes that fit around you waist. Your breasts will probably have grown enough to make bras and tops tight and uncomfortable too.

If you have loose fitting tops, and skirts, dresses or leggings with elasticated or drawstring waists, you may well be able to go through your pregnancy without buying new clothes. It is not always easy to look smart for work or a special occasion in these sort of clothes though. You may also find that, if you do use the few things that fit over and over again, you get bored with them.

If you can afford it, then, you might find that you take pleasure in choosing garments specially for your bump. There is no need for them to be specific maternity clothes in a style that you would not otherwise wear, just looser fitting clothes that are comfortable and that suit you. It is worth bearing in mind that the weight gained in pregnancy rarely drops off in a matter of weeks, so these clothes might be useful to you for a number of months.

When you first begin to have a tummy you will probably want to disguise it and carry on wearing your normal clothes for as long as you can. It is possible to buy button extenders from haberdashers which will give you an extra couple of inches on the waistband of a skirt or pair of trousers, although, of course, the zip will not do up all the way so you will need to conceal the top of the zip. A long jacket or cardigan will also help to hide the bump.

As your tummy gets bigger there will be less point in trying to conceal it, but you may want to draw attention away from it. This is traditionally achieved by choosing clothes that have particular detail near the face, such as a wide collar; you could just as easily use a top with a contrast colour near your face, or wear a scarf to lead the eye upwards.

If you have any special occasions to dress for in the last few weeks of your pregnancy, it is just as well to start planning a little in advance. Many outlets – from chain stores to designers' private shops – now sell maternity clothes. There are also agencies which specialise in maternity wear for hire or to buy second hand.

Underwear

It is important that any clothes you buy especially for your pregnancy make you feel good and confident about the way you look, but the most important consideration is that they should be comfortable. This applies to your underwear as well: make sure that your bra fits comfortably around your chest, and does not restrict your breasts. When your bras get too small, have a proper fitting for new ones to ensure that you get the right size, because your chest measurement can change during pregnancy as well as your cup size.

You may find that you need to buy new knickers for your pregnancy too, especially if you put on weight on your buttocks. Even if you do not, your knickers may constantly feel as if they are falling down, and you may find that you need skimpier ones that do not contend with your bump at all, or much larger ones that come up to your waist over it. The same under-or-over question may arise with tights: ordinary tights will probably be uncomfortable over your tummy towards the end of your pregnancy, and could slip down if you put the waistband under it. It is possible to buy maternity tights with a wider waistband to accommodate your bump.

Footwear

Your feet may swell a little when you are pregnant and they will probably ache if you stand for too long in the later weeks. Try to go barefoot when you are at home, and to wear trainers or sandals when you do not have to dress up; if you need to have smart footwear, avoid high heels which will put extra pressure on your feet and could cause you to lose your balance.

Vaginal Discharge

Some women notice an increase in vaginal discharge during pregnancy. This is normal; so long as the discharge is clear or whitish and is not accompanied by soreness, itching or an unpleasant smell, then it need not be cause for concern. If you have a lot of discharge use a panty liner, but do not use a tampon. Do not be tempted to wash yourself too vigorously with soaps and vaginal deodorants, the chemicals in them could upset the delicate balance in the vaginal mucus and could cause irritation and discomfort.

If the discharge is discoloured or contains spots of blood, speak to your doctor or midwife. This could mean that your cervix is eroding, and you may have developed a small ulcer on the cervix.

Thrush

Some women are more susceptible to thrush during pregnancy. Thrush is caused by a yeast-type of fungal infection and is typified by itchiness in and around the vagina, and a thick whitish yellow discharge that may have an unpleasant smell. Thrush is extremely common and may be very uncomfortable. It can be treated successfully with antifungal creams and pessaries, although it can recur.

CASE STUDY: *'I think the whole thing is mega-exciting but my bottom has been uncomfortable. Well, what I mean is I have had thrush, and I just didn't expect something like that. It's been demoralising.'*

Week 22

By the end of the twenty-second week of pregnancy you are actually five months pregnant, in another five months you should have a two-week old baby.

The Foetus

At the five month stage the foetus's crown-rump measurement is about 18.5cm (7½in), this is about half the crown-rump length of a full term baby. It has put on another 50g (2oz), and now weighs about 350g (12oz). The feet and hands are still maturing: the fingernails and toenails have grown so that they come almost to the end of the fingers and toes, and the muscles in the fingers and toes are growing stronger so that your baby can now wriggle its toes and grip with its hand.

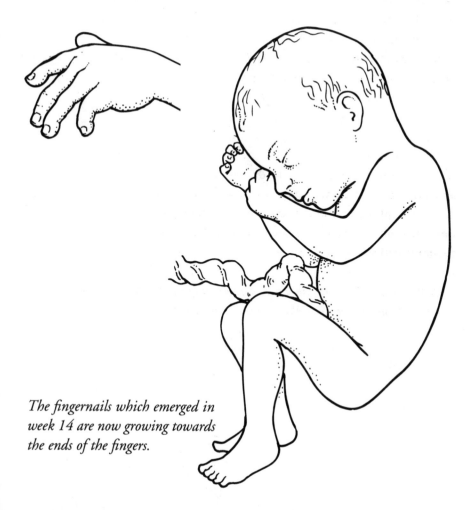

The fingernails which emerged in week 14 are now growing towards the ends of the fingers.

What is Happening to the Foetus

The foetus's skin, which was initially a fragile layer just one cell thick, is developing rapidly at this stage. It has divided into two layers, the epidermis on the outside and the dermis underneath. These layers now begin to specialise to perform their different functions. The epidermis will be the protective outer layer of the skin and the dermis develops a tiny network of blood vessels and nerve endings which make the skin sensitive to the touch. At about this stage, glands in the foetus's skin begin to secrete a white greasy substance called vernix which forms a barrier between the foetus's skin and the amniotic fluid.

How you Feel

Most women find that the middle months of their pregnancy are relatively happy and easy ones, they have shaken off the morning sickness of the early months and they are not yet tired and unwieldy as they may be in the later months. If you do not feel happy or well, try to talk about your feelings with your partner or a close friend. If you are in any doubt about your health during your pregnancy get in touch with your doctor or midwife.

Understanding the Structure of Hospital Staff

By now you will have had a number of antenatal check-ups as well as your scan, and you almost certainly know where you will be having your baby. If you have your check-ups in a hospital or if you have been to hospital for a scan or to see the maternity ward you may be a little bewildered by the number of different people that you see. You may wonder who is in charge and how the staff is structured. Members of staff will usually introduce themselves to you, but if you are ever in any doubt about who you are seeing and why, always ask.

Consultant: Every pregnant woman is referred by her own doctor to a consultant obstetrician who oversees the progress of her whole pregnancy. Consultant obstetricians are qualified specialists in pregnancy and childbirth, and they have a team of staff working with them. You might see your consultant at your booking appointment or at a later antenatal check-up, or during your labour and delivery. If your pregnancy, labour and delivery progress well, there may be no need for you to see your consultant at all.

Midwives: A midwife is qualified to manage normal pregnancy, labour and delivery. You will see a midwife for most of your antenatal visits (unless you have elected to see your family doctor) and a midwife will attend you in labour and for the delivery of your baby if everything goes smoothly. A midwife is qualified to deal with a number of complications, and can perform episiotomies (a surgical cut to the perineum to allow the baby's head to pass) and to stitch tears or episiotomies. Midwives will continue to care for you after your baby is born. Some of the midwives you see may be sister midwives, and are more senior. There will, for example, be a sister in charge of antenatal care, a labour-ward sister and a sister for each postnatal ward. Each sister has a staff of midwives qualified to care for you at every stage.

If there are any complications during your pregnancy your midwife will consult with a doctor or ask you to see a doctor at the clinic. If problems arise during labour your midwife will liaise closely with the medical staff.

Doctors: Registrars and Senior House Officers are doctors with different levels of training. A Senior House Officer is a junior doctor who is beginning to train in obstetrics. He is sufficiently qualified to attend you for minor complications such as forceps deliveries; and, like your midwife, he or she can perform episiotomies and suture (stitch) an episiotomy or a tear.

A Registrar is a more highly qualified and experienced doctor, second in seniority to the consultant. There will always be one or several registrars resident in a hospital, and they can be called upon 24 hours a day (whereas consultants tend to work more regular hours) to attend to a woman in labour or to manage a delivery if serious problems arise or are anticipated.

You may also be seen by medical students (student doctors) when you are in hospital, and you might be asked if they can attend the delivery of your baby, or even perform the delivery if everything is progressing normally. You should always be asked your permission for a student of any kind (doctor, midwife or nurse) to be present at any stage in your pregnancy, labour and delivery; and they should always be accompanied by a fully trained health professional.

Health care assistants: In addition to the midwives who handle your check-ups and care for you in labour and in the postnatal ward, you may meet health care assistants or auxiliary nurses. They will help the midwives care for you and your baby. The care they give will be supervised directly or indirectly by a midwife.

Week 23

By now it will be becoming obvious, even to people who do not know you, that you are pregnant.

The Foetus

The foetus is now putting on weight more quickly, it has gained about 100g (3½oz) in the last week and now weighs around 450g (just under 1lb). The average baby weighs nearly eight times this much at birth, so it still has a long way to go. The crown-rump measurement is about 19.5cm (just under 8in). The foetus's face is now much more defined, with an obvious browline, growing eyebrows, and well formed features. The eyelids remain closed over the eyes but they are finer now and the eyelashes longer.

What is Happening to the Foetus

Incredible though it may seem, a baby born in only the twenty-third week of pregnancy can survive with an enormous amount of specialised care. Obviously, such early deliveries are rare, and the percentage that survive only small, but this is an indication of how developed your foetus's organs are at this stage.

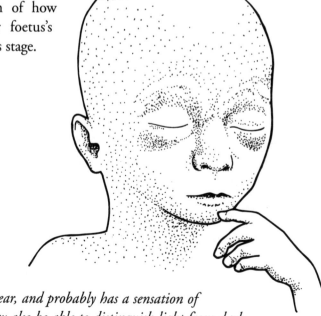

The foetus can hear, and probably has a sensation of taste-smell; it may also be able to distinguish light from dark even though its eyes are still closed.

How you Feel

You should by now be feeling your baby kicking regularly, and you may have started to notice that the baby has a pattern of resting and moving. As the baby makes more and more movements and establishes its own waking and sleeping pattern, independent of yours, you will come to see it more as a person and less a part of you. A few women feel a little afraid of the autonomy of their baby, as if they have somehow lost control of their own bodies; there is nothing unusual or wrong about feeling like this. Most women find that these signs of individuality make them more excited about meeting their baby at birth.

Feelings of Excitement and Fear

It is common for women to have mixed emotions during their pregnancy: on the one hand they are excited about having a baby and all the joy that a child can bring to their lives, on the other they are afraid of the changes that this implies, afraid of the labour and delivery, and afraid that there may be something wrong with their baby.

All of these feelings are quite normal, and you may find that you tend to swing between excitement and fear more and more as your pregnancy progresses. You can share your feelings of excitement with those around you, talking about the baby and your plans for the future. You should tell them about your fears too; talking about your anxieties will help you to face them and possibly to dismiss them altogether.

It is very common for first-time mothers to fear labour and delivery and to feel that they may not be able to cope. You have to remember that women have been having babies for millions of years, and that the labour does not go on indefinitely. Furthermore, there is not really a question of not being able to cope: it is not like climbing a mountain, you cannot stop half-way up – however you think you are coping, you will have a baby at the end of it.

It is also very common for parents to worry that their baby might be handicapped or still-born. These are very real and very normal concerns, and there is nothing wrong with contemplating these eventualities so long as you do not brood on them. If you have any tangible reasons to worry about the health of your baby you should arrange to see your doctor.

SEEING OTHER MOTHERS AND BABIES

Whatever your feelings about your pregnancy you might find that the people you most want to discuss them with are other mothers and pregnant women. Some women seem to take a malicious pleasure in discussing the horrors of appallingly long labours and traumatic deliveries but most women will be happy to talk to you sympathetically, telling you about their experiences and reassuring and advising you. Your antenatal clinic is an obvious place to meet other pregnant women and to talk about how you feel physically and psychologically. When you start antenatal classes you will have plenty of opportunities to meet other women at the same stage of pregnancy as yourself.

You may want to see other people's babies just to see what they are like: many women have hardly ever seen a very new baby when their own first baby is born. You need not be alarmed if you have no feelings for other people's babies, and no desire to hold them. This does not mean that you will not be a good mother or that you will not want your own baby. The instincts and hormones that make you want to cherish your own baby may be very specifically triggered by the process of labour and delivery and the sound of your own baby's cry. If you do know someone who has a very young baby while you are pregnant, you might ask if you can spend some time with them just to talk about what problems they are having to deal with, and to gain some experience of handling a new-born baby.

CASE STUDY: *'I was so excited about the whole pregnancy and I think it got a bit boring for my friends and family. The only people who really understood were other pregnant women. I had one friend in particular who was just a few weeks behind me, and we would speak almost every day. When we got to the stage of buying little things for the nursery and little clothes we would go round and show them off to each other.'*

Week 24

It is five months since your egg was fertilised and your foetus is now considered viable in English law. The baby has a slim but realistic chance of survival if it is born now, and it is illegal to perform an abortion after the twenty-fourth week unless there are very special medical reasons such as gross abnormality in the foetus or a threat to the mother's life.

The Foetus

At 24 weeks the foetus weighs about 550g (just over the 1lb mark). It measures about 20.5cm (just over 8in) from crown to rump. The proportions of your baby are still changing and the head is now much more in proportion with the body. The baby is now quite well covered in the greasy vernix mentioned in week 22, and the skin is beginning to appear less wrinkled as fat stores are gradually laid down and fill it out.

Greasy vernix begins to cover the foetus's body to protect its skin from the amniotic fluid.

How you Look

The top of your uterus, the fundus should now be about 4cm (1½in) above your navel, giving you a recognisably pregnant tummy. You will probably have put on at least 4.5kg (10lb) by the twenty-fourth week, although this varies from one woman to another. The weight will partly be accounted for by your bump and partly by enlargement of the breasts and fat stores laid down over the body.

Women carry their babies in different ways and these differences may start showing as early as the sixth month when your bump becomes more obvious. Some women carry high so that the bump appears higher up in their abdomen earlier than usual in the pregnancy, others carry low so that they appear to have a big 'belly' for all but the eighth month when the uterus reaches up into the upper abdomen (in the ninth month the baby often 'descends' to make a lower-looking bump).

Preparing a Nursery / What You Really Need

For obvious reasons, manufacturers and retailers of baby equipment are keen to persuade pregnant mothers that they will need an enormous amount of new equipment to accommodate their babies, and make caring for them as easy as possible. You really need very few new things in the first few weeks, and you can get other things as and when you need them.

Cots, Mattresses, Bumpers and Bedding

A baby obviously needs somewhere to sleep. In the early days you may have the baby in bed with you, especially if you are breast-feeding. A tiny baby can sleep in a carry-cot, moses basket, crib or even a drawer! Sooner or later you will need a cot which can see your baby through from birth to about three years.

There has been a great deal of publicity about the links between cot deaths and certain kinds of cot mattress. Do not use a second-hand mattress, and when you buy a new one, ask the assistant about cot deaths to check whether the mattress meets current safety regulations.

A new baby cannot move enough to warrant having a bumper round the cot, but once the baby is strong enough to roll over or push himself up towards the bars, you may decide to have a bumper round the cot to keep the baby warm and comfortable (it must be very securely attached to avoid any risk of suffocation). You will need a certain amount of cot bedding, and you should have enough sets to allow for your baby to be sick or to have a leaking nappy more often than your washing machine can keep up with. If you are buying fitted sheets, make sure that you measure your mattress beforehand.

Changing Tables and Changing Mats

There are some tremendously user-friendly changing tables on the market, but they are not cheap and you may find that it is just as easy to change your baby's nappy on top of a piece of furniture such as a chest of drawers. If you do not have a changing table, make sure that you arrange the room so that all the things you will need while you are changing your baby's nappy (cotton wool, lotion, wipes, clean nappies) are close at hand, because you should never leave your baby alone on a high surface.

A changing mat is a cheap and very useful piece of equipment. It not only provides an ideal place to change your baby's nappy while protecting the furniture beneath from unintentional spills, it is also a useful playmat for a very young baby. A changing mat covered with a towel and put on the floor is a perfect place for a baby that is not yet sitting or rolling to kick about with no clothes on. It is important to remember not to leave your baby alone, even if you think he is quite safe on the floor; and, if you have cats or dogs, shut them in another room before letting your baby lie on the floor.

Baby Baths and Bath Accessories

Baby baths may be convenient and useful for a few weeks, but they are certainly not essential items. A tiny baby can be bathed in a basin, and as he grows bigger you can bath him in the bath filled with a few inches of water (there are a number of security devices available to make your baby safer in the bath, but you should never leave a baby alone in a bath). Probably the best way to bath a baby is to have a bath with him yourself; he is safe in your arms and benefits from the skin to skin contact.

Feeding Chair

Again there is no need to buy a chair specially for feeding, but it is much more comfortable to feed on a chair with short legs. You could design your own feeding chair by cutting the legs off an existing chair.

Heat and Light

Your baby's room should ideally be kept at a constant temperature of about 20°C (70°F), so make sure that the room your baby is to live in has an adequate heating system. Remember that it is just as dangerous to overheat a baby as to keep it too cold. There is an increased risk of cot death for babies kept in very warm rooms.

It might be worth investing in a night-light or a low-wattage bulb to keep the baby's room as dark as possible for night feeds.

Miscellaneous Items

While you are researching the things that you need for your baby's nursery you should also think about other essential items that you will need for your baby such as a car seat and a pram or pushchair. If you are expecting twins you may need help and advice about how to manage your two babies and what equipment you will need for them. The addresses of organisations who can give you specialised advice on caring for twins appear at the end of the book.

Week 25

You are now well in to the second trimester of your pregnancy, and you may notice that you start putting weight on more quickly now as the baby has another period of rapid growth.

The Foetus

In the twenty-fifth week of your pregnancy the foetus measures about 21.5cm (8½in) from crown to rump. It has put on an incredible 130g (4½oz) in the last week and now weighs about 680g (1½lb). It is looking more and more like a miniature version of a new-born baby and the skin is less wrinkled now as the fat stores build up.

As the foetus continues to grow and becomes more cramped it adopts a more flexed position.

How you Feel

You may begin to feel that this pregnancy is going on for ever: you are in week 25 but there are still 15 weeks to go, and that is more than three months. You will be surprised how quickly the time does go, however: you are coming to the end of the middle months and you need to look after yourself well, eating properly, taking regular exercise and getting plenty of rest.

Booking a Place on Antenatal Classes

Many hospitals and local surgeries offer antenatal or parentcraft classes to help prepare women (on their own or with their partner) for labour, delivery and parenthood. These classes are free and they are usually given as a course of about six two-hour sessions once a week, and women are encouraged to start going to classes when they around the thirtieth week of their pregnancy (if you are expecting twins, you will probably be advised to begin attending classes a couple of weeks earlier because twin pregnancies are, on average, two or three weeks shorter than single baby pregnancies). In week 25 it is worth finding out about antenatal classes in your area, and booking a place on a course of classes.

If this is your first pregnancy you will benefit enormously from attending antenatal classes. Although the subjects covered will vary from one hospital to another, most courses will cover the following key topics:

Relaxation techniques and exercises during pregnancy
Recognising the onset of labour
When to go to hospital
What to do if your waters break
How established labour is defined
All forms of pain relief in labour
Breathing techniques in labour
What is happening to your body when you are in labour
How the baby is born (models may be used to demonstrate this)
Forms of assisted delivery such as forceps
Delivery of the placenta
Suturing (stitches)
What tests are performed on the new-born

Care of the new-born
Feeding your baby
Changes to your body after delivery (bleeding, care of stitches etc.)
Exercises to do after having a baby
Taking your baby home

Classes are usually held by a midwife, and she may be accompanied by a physiotherapist or other relevant health professional. The classes are well structured because there is a lot of material to cover but the atmosphere is usually friendly and informal, and women are encouraged to ask questions.

If you attend antenatal classes you will have plenty of opportunities to discuss any anxieties you have and to ask questions about labour, delivery and care of the new-born. You will also meet other women who are at the same stage in their pregnancies and who may well end up in hospital at the same time as you.

CASE STUDY: *'I'm going to the classes with Christine Hill [at Queen Charlotte's Hospital]. She's amazing and very thorough. I really feel prepared for it.'*

CASE STUDY: *'I was a bit shy about going to the classes at first, but hearing other people asking questions, I realised that we were all worried about the same sort of things. We were all in the same boat, you know, so there wasn't much to be shy about really.'*

Stretch Marks

Stretch marks are scar-like patterns that may appear on your skin where it has been stretched beyond the limits of its elasticity when you gain weight. They commonly appear on the tummy, thighs, buttocks and breasts. They usually consist of series of parallel lines or ridges which can be anything from silvery white to – in the worst cases – dark red or purple. However dark and obvious they are when you are at your heaviest they will fade gradually as you loose weight again, and the skin eases back.

Stretch marks are often associated specifically with pregnancy although they can be caused by any significant weight gain. Not all women will get stretch marks as a result of pregnancy, but those who put on a substantial amount of weight are more likely to.

It is not easy to predict whether you will be prone to stretch marks. The elasticity of the skin is to some extent linked to your age and the oiliness of your skin, but there is no guarantee that if you are young and have an oily skin you will not have stretch marks. Neither is there any evidence that oils and lotions applied to threatened areas can significantly reduce stretch marks.

If you are getting stretch marks and you are worried that they are unsightly, keep an eye on your weight gain. It is worth remembering that they do not hurt, they will do no harm to you or your baby, and they will fade.

Week 26

If you are planning to start your maternity leave on the earliest possible date, that is in the twenty-ninth week of pregnancy, you should have written to your employer by the end of this week.

The Foetus

The foetus is growing at an incredible rate, its crown-rump length is increasing by about 1cm (just under ½in)every week; it now measures about 22.5cm (9in). It is putting on weight even more quickly, gaining about 120g (4oz) in the last week so that it now weighs about 900g (2lb). As the weight gain continues, the limbs become fuller looking and the foetus begins to get little creases at the elbows.

The foetus begins to fill out gradually as tiny fat deposits are laid down.

How you Feel

The very fact that you could be applying for maternity leave to start in three weeks time will make you realise that time is marching on, and it really will not be that long before you have a baby. If you have not done so already, you may feel that you are ready to start work on a nursery and to do some shopping for your baby.

Adapting to Your Bump

Having a growing tummy not only affects what you wear but many other aspects of your life. You may find that you feel 'front-heavy', and are more inclined to trip up or fall forwards, for example going upstairs. This will be particularly noticeable if you wear high-heeled shoes as they throw your weight forward. You should avoid wearing high heels as your bump gets bigger because they put an extra strain on your back. Problems of balance can be overcome by making sure that you adopt the correct posture, with your 'tail' tilted under you rather than sticking out behind, counterbalancing the bump and exaggerating the curve of your spine.

> CASE STUDY: *'No, I didn't have problems of balance while I was pregnant, because I did yoga so I knew about balance. And, anyway, you adapt gradually, but after the baby was born, I did find I sometimes felt off-balance because the weight I had been compensating for suddenly wasn't there any more.'*

Some women find that driving becomes difficult or uncomfortable in the last weeks of their pregnancy. If you find that it becomes difficult to drive, you should drive as little as possible or much more slowly; it is dangerous for your reactions and movements to be impeded when you are driving.

Towards the end of your pregnancy it may be difficult to pull on socks, do up boots and shoes or even shave your legs! You may also find that you can no longer reach the bottom of a supermarket trolley; most large supermarkets offer shallower trolleys that should be easier for you to use.

> CASE STUDY: *'I had this huge tummy and I really couldn't reach my legs to shave them. I had to ask my husband to do them for me ... which probably contributed to the fact that he no longer saw me as a sex goddess!'*

Week 27

At the beginning of week 27 you are six months pregnant, two-thirds of the way through your pregnancy. You are now entering the third trimester.

The Foetus

At the six-month stage the foetus is growing very quickly; its crown-rump length is now about 23.5cm (just over 9in). It has put on another 100g (3½oz) this week and now weighs 1kg (2lb 3oz) – the same weight as a standard size bag of sugar or flour. Something very exciting happens to the foetus by about the twenty-seventh week: the eyelids are no longer fused together and it opens its eyes. The baby's irises are usually blue at this stage; the colour of the baby's irises at birth depends on his ethnic origins. Most white babies have blue eyes at birth whatever their eye colour turns out to be

What is Happening to the Foetus

Not only have your baby's eyes opened at about this time, but the retina of the eye – the 'screen' that receives images at the back of the eye to be transmitted to the brain – has developed sufficiently to receive information about light and dark. Your baby can probably see the difference between darkness and light. As the eyelids open for the first time, the muscles around the lids develop more quickly and the baby can open and close its eyelids.

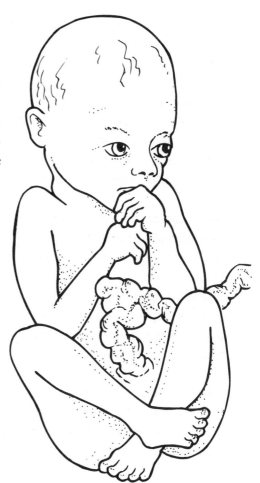

At around 27 weeks the foetus opens its eyes and can see the difference between light and dark filtering through the mother's abdominal wall.

How you Feel

If you are getting impatient about the length of your pregnancy, you may feel that once you have reached the six-month mark the end is at least in sight. You will probably be starting antenatal classes quite soon, and that will give you an opportunity to meet other women at the same stage of pregnancy.

Changing Emotions

The hormones in your blood-stream can continue to upset your system throughout your pregnancy, and this may not always manifest itself with physical symptoms. You may find that the your pregnancy changes the way you feel about yourself and how you respond to things.

Self-image

Progesterone has a relaxing effect, and this may contribute to a feeling of wellbeing and happiness. Your pregnancy might also make you feel important, and may boost your self-image: some women find that they feel increasingly confident as their pregnancy becomes more obvious in the latter months. But others say that, as they come into the third trimester, their self-image feels more fragile. You are likely to become tired more easily, you will certainly be looking bigger, which some women find difficult to handle, and you may be having doubts about how you will cope with labour and the delivery. There is nothing unusual about you if your self-image takes an occasional dent in pregnancy, but it is not something you should brood over. If you are feeling down, try to talk to your partner or a friend about your feelings. It is worth remembering that most changes to your looks in pregnancy will reverse once you have had your baby.

Mood Swings

You may also find that you become moody and switch from being happy to being short-tempered more easily in the latter stages of your pregnancy. This can be attributed to hormones, to tiredness and to the physical and psychological stresses of pregnancy. Again, there is nothing wrong or unusual about this, but try to talk with those around you who may suffer as a result of your mood swings, especially if you feel they are expecting too much of you and, therefore, adding to the demands on you.

High Emotions

Many women find that they are far more emotional when they are pregnant, rather as they may be just before a period. You may notice that you are more easily moved by films, television programmes, even news stories. Your emotions may rise more quickly and be more intense; a feeling of fear, anger or sorrow may suddenly be overwhelming and cause you to cry.

CASE STUDY: *'You do get more emotional:* Eastenders *set me off the other day! It was a particularly moving episode, but it wouldn't normally have made me cry.'*

Week 28

In the twenty-eighth week of pregnancy you again enter a new phase: from now on your antenatal visits will probably be more frequent, perhaps once a fortnight until the thirty-sixth week, when you will probably have a check-up once a week until your baby is born. (The pattern of antenatal visiting varies from one hospital to another, and your antenatal check-ups may be more frequent if there are any complications in your pregnancy.)

The Foetus

The foetus's crown-rump measurement is now about 24.5cm (just over 9½in) and it has again put on about 100g (3½oz) in a week; it weighs 1.1kg (1lb 6oz). Now that the head is more in proportion with the body as it continues to fill out the foetus looks more and more like a miniature baby. It is now well covered in the greasy vernix that usually disappears by the time the baby is born, except in creases in the skin.

The foetus curls up as space becomes more limited.

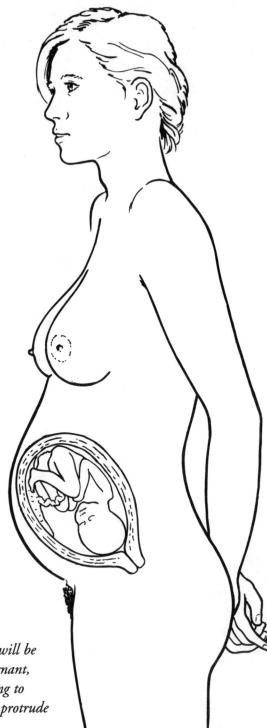

By now most women will be looking obviously pregnant, the uterus is continuing to grow upwards and to protrude outwards.

What is Happening to the Foetus

The lungs of the foetus develop fully much later than the other organs because there is no need for them to perform their function of extracting oxygen from the air until your baby is born and breathing. For many weeks the lungs remain solid and very premature babies need a lot of help breathing because the lungs are stiff. By the twenty-eighth week the lungs have developed considerably, and your baby would be capable of breathing if it was born now.

How you Look

There are very few women who can disguise even a first pregnancy by the time they have reached the six-month stage. The top of the uterus is now well up above your navel and probably protrudes very obviously by now. It now contains not only a baby with a head to toe length of about 39cm (over 15½in), but also a well developed placenta and about 750ml (1¼ pints) of amniotic fluid. The linea negra, the dark line from your pubic hair up to your navel is fairly pronounced at this stage, unless you have very fair skin. Your navel itself may be darker, and might be changing shape as your skin stretches over the growing uterus.

Your breasts have almost certainly grown at least one cup size by now (and perhaps much more), and they may have some blood vessels showing just under the skin. The nipples are darker than usual; they tend to become darker so that they are easier for the baby to see when he is rooting for a feed. Towards the end of a pregnancy it is not unusual to have leaks of colostrum (the first milk).

Back Pain

Backache is one of the most widely recognised painful side-effects of pregnancy. The hormone progesterone causes your ligaments and joints to slacken to facilitate the passage of the baby through the pelvic girdle for delivery, and this slackening makes the joints weaker and more susceptible to strain and pain. This is aggravated later in pregnancy by the changes to your balance and the demands made on your joints by your growing tummy.

A small minority of women suffer backache all the way through their pregnancy whereas others are affected only in the latter weeks. If you have problems with back pain ask your midwife whether there is an obstetric physiotherapist attached to your hospital; he or she will be able to give you specialised advice on posture and back care. You may want to contact the Association of Chartered physiotherapists in Women' s Health (their address appears at the end of the book).

Minimising the Chances of Suffering from Backache

Sitting and standing: Make sure that you stand and sit correctly. Stand erect with your 'tail' tucked in rather than allowing your spine to curve, throwing your tummy forwards and your bottom back. Sit well back in a chair, with your back straight, preferably with a small stool under your feet and with your legs uncrossed. Do not stand or sit for too long at a time; if you have a job that involves a lot of standing (such as shop work) or sitting (such as office work) let your employer know that you need to have more frequent breaks.

> CASE STUDY: *'I don't have too much trouble with backache but then I am much more aware of my posture. By the end of the day it is difficult to sit comfortably – and I try and be aware of how I sit.'*

Lifting: It is surprising how many back injuries are caused by incorrect lifting, and when you are pregnant your back is even more prone to injury and pain if you do not lift things correctly. Avoid lifting very heavy things altogether, and avoid bending over something to lift something out (for example, taking a heavy bag or box of shopping out of a supermarket trolley). Put your feet squarely on the ground, keep your back straight and bend your knees to come down to the level of the thing (or child!) that you are lifting. Then, still keeping your back straight, use the straightening of your knees to lift the object off the ground. Use the reverse process for putting things down on the ground.

Lifting does not only mean picking things up off the ground, be careful when you put things onto or take things off shelves above chin level. You may find that you arch your back backwards and this too can cause pain or even damage to your back.

Exercise and relaxation: One way of preventing back pain is to make sure that you take regular exercise (though not strenuous exercise which puts too much strain on your joints) and practice relaxation techniques to avoid tension in your joints. You may learn exercises and relaxation techniques in your antenatal classes, or you could speak to your midwife or see whether there is a qualified yoga instructor in your area.

Moderate weight gain: One of the causes of back pain in pregnancy is the considerable extra weight that you carry in pregnancy. If you keep an eye on your weight, you are less likely to put unnecessary strain on your back (by the twenty-eighth week the average weight gain is about 9.7kg or 20lb). Remember that you should not try to loose weight when you are pregnant.

Footwear: Avoid high-heeled shoes which throw your weight forward and exaggerate the curve of your back. Completely flat shoes are not always the answer either, because they give the foot no support while restricting its natural movement. If you buy flat shoes, check that they have a raised area on the inside of the insole to support your instep; if not, most large chemist shops sell raised insoles separately.

Your bed: Make sure that you have a firm mattress that will give your back plenty of support. If you wake with aches or pains in your back or neck it could be that your mattress is too soft or that you have too high a pillow. It is very important that your back is well rested, so try changing your mattress or putting a wide board under your mattress, and experiment with different thicknesses of pillow.

Pain Relief

No preventative measures can guarantee that you will not suffer back pain. You may be tempted to use analgesics for the pain. You should not use them in the first trimester because they might contain ingredients which could compromise the normal development of the foetus. If you have serious back pain later in pregnancy talk to your doctor or pharmacist about safe kinds of pain relief. Here are some other steps you could take to alleviate the pain when it strikes.

Try lying on a hard floor and bending your knees so that the small of your back is pushed into the floor. Make a conscious effort to push it down for a count of five, then release it. Repeat this several times. Lying or sitting and practising breathing exercises may also help relax the back and lessen the pain.

Sitting with a warm hot-water bottle in the small of your back sometimes helps. Make sure that the bottle is neither so hot that it feels uncomfortable or so full that it exaggerates the curve of the small of your back. Some people find that the cooling effect of a bag of frozen peas wrapped in a fine towel is more soothing than the warmth of a hot-water bottle (the peas can be re-frozen and used for this purpose again and again … but should not then be used for cooking!). You may find that using a hot-water bottle and frozen peas alternately has a soothing effect, stimulating the circulation but minimising inflammation.

CASE STUDY: *'I found that my back got tired at the end of the day, a persistent ache in the small of my back, and I got into a ritual of coming home, making myself a cup of tea and filling a hot-water bottle, and relaxing with the hot-water bottle in the small of my back … bliss!'*

Week 29

This is the earliest date that you can start your maternity leave. Very few women decide to leave work this early, but you may be getting tired and looking forward to leaving work.

The Foetus

In the twenty-ninth week of pregnancy the foetus's crown-rump measurement is about 25.5cm (10in) and it weighs about 1.25kg (2lb 11oz). It will probably weigh nearly three times this much when it is born, so it will virtually triple its weight in the next eleven weeks. The foetus usually has quite a growth of head hair by now, although this varies enormously: some babies are born with only sparse and very fine fair hair, others are born with a great deal of black hair as much as 5cm (2in) long. The colour of a baby's hair at birth is not a reliable guide as to the child's eventual hair colour.

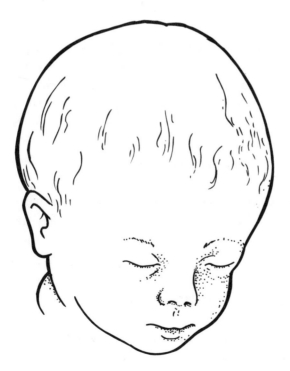

The foetus may well have quite a growth of head hair by now.

What is Happening to the Foetus

By this stage in the pregnancy virtually all the foetus's organs are fully developed; in the next ten weeks the organs – especially the lungs – will continue to mature in preparation for life outside the womb.

How you Feel

Now that you are well in to the third trimester of pregnancy, you may begin to experience some of the discomforts associated with the latter weeks. You may well get tired more easily, have backache and other aches and pains, tired feet, breathlessness, a frequent need to pass urine and difficulty sleeping. Make sure that you get as much rest as you need.

Dreams and Nightmares in Pregnancy

It is not uncommon for women to say that they have – or remember – more dreams when they are pregnant, particularly in the latter weeks. They may well be dreaming more, and the fact that they remember their dreams is probably related to the fact that women wake more often in the night in late pregnancy.

Dreams are the mind's way of addressing concerns and problems. They are healthy and natural however bizarre they may seem. You may dream that you are no longer pregnant, that you are playing with your baby, that you go out somewhere and forget your baby, even that your baby can walk and talk when it is born. It is quite normal to dream about your baby and the birth; dreams may be like practising for motherhood or for playing out fears and anxieties about the delivery or your competence as a mother, for example.

You may remember more of your dreams but find that none of them has anything to do with the baby. Some women find that they have dreams of a sexual nature which can be pleasant or unpleasant and which may not involve their usual partner. These dreams are probably partly triggered by the increase in hormonal activity, but they may also be an expression of anxieties about diminished attractiveness during pregnancy.

CASE STUDY: *'I've heard that you can have erotic dreams in pregnancy but its just my luck never to have had anything like that. I never had dreams with the first two but they were planned pregnancies, you know, intended. This one was a complete accident, and I think that must be why I'm worrying about it subconsciously. I have endless dreams about the delivery, every possible complication and going into labour in the most ridiculous situations.'*

CARPAL TUNNEL SYNDROME

Carpal tunnel syndrome is a condition that can cause tremendous weakness and pain in one or both wrists. It can affect people at any time but is more common in the latter weeks of pregnancy; if you do suffer from carpal tunnel syndrome during pregnancy, it should clear up once you have had your baby.

Carpal tunnel syndrome is caused by fluid retention in the wrist joint: the excess fluid builds up in an area called the carpal tunnel – a band of tissue which protects the carpal nerves that serve the hand and fingers – until eventually it begins to squeeze the nerves, causing a tingling feeling in the fingers. There may be some loss of sensation so that you find difficulty in picking things up and holding on to them, typing, writing, doing up buttons or anything else that requires dexterity. In the most severe cases, carpal tunnel syndrome can be extremely painful.

If you suffer from carpal tunnel syndrome, speak to you doctor or midwife. You may be offered mild analgesics to control the pain, and you will probably be given advice on how to minimise fluid retention (see the feature on fluid retention, **Swelling of Fingers, Wrists and Ankles** in **Week 31**), and you may be referred to a physiotherapist who can show you some simple exercises to alleviate the pain and help to dispel the excess fluid.

Week 30

You are now three quarters of the way through your 40-week pregnancy. It may still feel as if you have a long way to go or it may seem as if time is suddenly running out.

The Foetus

The foetus is still adding an incredible 1cm (just under ½in) a week to its crown-rump length which now measures about 26.5cm (10½in). If your baby were born now, his overall length would be about 38cm (17in). The foetus is putting on weight very quickly at this stage and now weighs 1.4kg (3lb). It has laid down considerable fat stores now, and has more or less reached the proportions of a full-term baby.

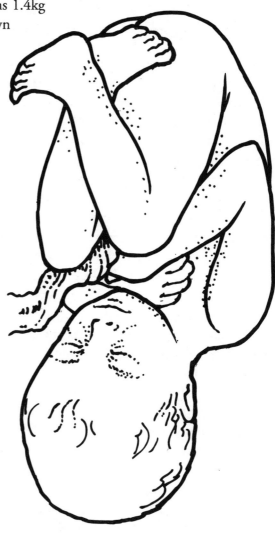

The foetus can no longer move around so freely, and begins to settle in a well flexed position.

How you Feel

As you become increasingly obviously pregnant, you may notice that complete strangers respond to you differently: they may start conversations with you spontaneously, asking when the baby is due and whether it is your first baby. They might offer to help you with things or give up their seat for you on public transport. Some women enjoy these unsolicited attentions, others find it an invasion of their privacy, as if their bump turns them into public property. It is worth remembering that, thanks to a primeval urge to further the species, we are all programmed to protect pregnant women and the very young; people's inquisitiveness and concern about your pregnancy are merely a latter-day expression of that protective instinct.

Exercise in the Third Trimester

As you get bigger and your joints become more relaxed in the latter stages of pregnancy, it becomes more difficult to take exercise without discomfort. On the other hand, it is good for you and if you continue to take some form of exercise right through your pregnancy it may even make your labour and delivery easier. Physical fitness is no guarantee of a quick and easy labour, but it will at least give you the stamina and confidence to tackle labour. Exercise is also important because it can help you to relax, and being relaxed will help you to cope with labour too.

If you already take regular exercise but find that it is causing discomfort or pain, try to adapt your routine to suit your changing limitations. Rather than running, try walking uphill which puts less pressure on the joints of the leg. Cycling (on a real bike or an exercise machine) works the major muscle groups without putting your weight on your legs at all. Swimming is an excellent form of exercise at any time, but it is especially useful in late pregnancy, because it works all the muscle groups in a medium that gives you a sense of weightlessness. If you go to a gym or leisure centre talk to the staff about the amount of exercise you are taking and the equipment you are using. It is safe to continue to use weights and weight machines, but moderate the weights you use and always make sure that you are in the correct position to use the equipment safely: the slackening of ligaments in pregnancy means that you are more prone to sprains and strains.

If you have not been taking regular exercise, now is certainly not the time to launch into a demanding fitness regime, but it is still not too late to start taking exercise! You could work on your aerobic fitness by walking or swimming, and build up muscle tone by doing specific muscle exercises (either by joining a local gym or yoga class, or by asking your midwife about exercises recommended in pregnancy). You will probably be taught some relaxation exercises in your antenatal classes.

CASE STUDY: *'I suppose I am a bit of a fitness freak: I went running and did aerobics until I was seven months when my back started complaining to the management! Then I stopped the running and did step classes instead of aerobics, because that was less pounding on my back and legs. In the last month I just went swimming three times a week, right up to the day before I had her. I had a long labour, nearly 24 hours, but I coped very well, and only had a bit of gas and air right at the end. I definitely think being fit made a big difference, not just because I felt up to it physically, but mentally as well.'*

STRESS INCONTINENCE / PELVIC FLOOR EXERCISES

One kind of exercise that is recommended throughout pregnancy is the strengthening of the muscles of the pelvic floor. These muscles form a figure-of-eight configuration under your pelvis, and support your uterus, bowel and bladder; subconsciously you use them for example to control the flow of urine from your bladder.

Towards the end of your pregnancy you are not only likely to need to pass urine more frequently, you may also find that you suffer from what is called stress incontinence. As the pelvic floor muscles relax under the effects of progesterone, they can allow small amounts of urine to pass when they are put under sudden pressure, for example when you cough, sneeze, laugh or even just bend over. This can be embarrassing and, if you do not work on the pelvic floor muscles, it might continue long after you have had your baby.

Exercises for the pelvic floor muscles are explained in the chapter **Preparing for Pregnancy**. Physiotherapists recommend starting to do pelvic floor exercises even before conceiving, but it is never too late to start. If you have a problem with stress incontinence ask your midwife whether there is an obstetric physiotherapist attached to your hospital to give you specialised advice about pelvic floor exercises.

Week 31

You are now seven months pregnant and you may well be starting antenatal classes this week, so you will have a chance to meet other women at the same stage in their pregnancy as you.

The Foetus

At the seven-month stage the foetus measures about 27.5cm (11in) from crown to rump, and its overall length would be about 40cm (18in). It continues to put on weight at a rate of around 200g (7oz) a week, and now weighs about 1.6kg (3lb 8oz). The foetus is now nearly four-fifths the length but still under half the average weight of a full-term baby; this gives you some idea just how much filling out the baby does in the last two months of your pregnancy. The foetus is likely to be moving fairly vigorously and regularly by now, and you may have recognised a pattern of sleeping and waking. You may also be confident enough to feel your abdomen and find out how your baby is lying.

How you Feel

When you start your antenatal classes you may feel apprehensive about exactly what the classes are going to entail and how much you will learn from them. Most women who attend classes, especially for a first pregnancy, say that they are invaluable and enjoyable too. You will probably just enjoy meeting other women at the same stage as you who have many of the same concerns, anxieties and discomforts. You may well find yourself saying 'Oh, so it's not just me!'

Swelling of Fingers, Wrists and Ankles

In your antenatal check-ups you will be asked whether you have noticed any swelling of your fingers, wrists and ankles. You may notice that rings and shoes feel tight and uncomfortable. This is partly because you are putting on weight but it is also a sign of increased fluid retention, known as oedema.

It is normal to have a certain amount of fluid retention in pregnancy, especially in the latter weeks, and a small amount of puffiness should not be cause for concern although it may be uncomfortable. The swelling usually gets worse if you stand or sit for any length of time; if so, avoid

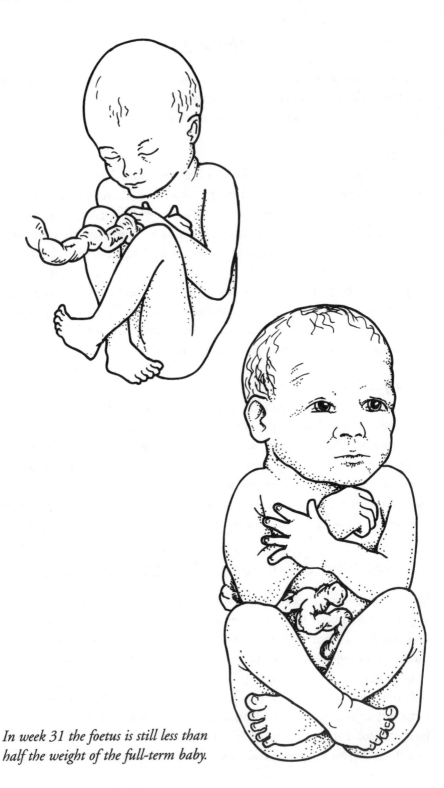

In week 31 the foetus is still less than half the weight of the full-term baby.

standing, and sit with your feet slightly raised. At the end of the day sit with your feet well up and even sleep with your feet on a pillow so that your circulation has the best chance of clearing the excess fluid. When you are resting try gently exercising your wrists and ankles, turning the hands and feet through 360° clockwise, then anticlockwise; this will improve the circulation and the draining of fluid from your joints.

Do not be tempted to drink less fluid to stop the build-up of fluid, drinking plenty of fluids actually helps to flush out the swelling. Moderating the amount of salt you consume might help too, because salt in the diet causes fluid retention.

The reason that health professionals like to keep an eye on fluid retention is that it is one of the key symptoms of a dangerous condition called pre-eclampsia. If you notice that you have suddenly put on weight or that your hands, feet and face are very puffy, you should contact your doctor or midwife and they can test for other symptoms (such as raised blood pressure and protein in the urine). If pre-eclampsia is not diagnosed, the blood pressure can rise to dangerously high levels, threatening the survival of the foetus and even of the mother herself; but properly treated with bed-rest and medical care, the condition can be controlled and the baby can be born safely. The swelling and puffiness caused by pre-eclampsia goes down shortly after delivery.

Aching Legs and Varicose Veins

Many women find that towards the end of their pregnancy their legs ache, especially if they stand for any length of time. It seems obvious that their legs will ache because they are carrying extra weight, but these aches should not be dismissed and ignored: they may be a sign that blood circulation in the legs is somehow compromised and this could cause varicose veins.

When the baby begins to fill the abdomen towards the end of the pregnancy it can put pressure on the veins which carry blood back out of the legs. The arteries continue to pump blood into the leg and the blood vessels of the leg can become swollen (it is also possible to have varicose veins in the vulva and the rectum). This causes a dull ache and may make the skin feel tingly or itchy if the blood vessel is close to the surface. As the condition progresses, the veins can be seen to be engorged and they are usually a dark purple colour. Varicose veins are unsightly and can be very uncomfortable. In some cases they are irreversible, they will not go back down after the end of the pregnancy, so it is a case of prevention rather than cure.

If there is a history of varicose veins in your family, you will be more susceptible to them so you should make a point of taking these precautionary measures: avoid sitting or standing for long periods, and try to sit with your feet raised to help your circulation; try to moderate your weight gain in pregnancy so that there is less pressure on your legs; make sure that you take regular exercise to improve your circulation; and avoid wearing tight clothes, especially elastic topped socks, knee-high tights or hold-up stockings which will restrict the flow of blood in your legs.

You may find that wearing support tights will help to make your legs more comfortable and to improve the circulation in your legs. Support tights should be put on first thing in the morning when there is no swelling in your legs and the circulation is at its best because you have been lying horizontally. They will help your circulation, minimise swelling and literally help support your legs so that you should notice less aching.

Week 32

It is now only eight weeks until your baby is due, and only four weeks until week 36 when most hospitals ask pregnant women to prepare their bag for hospital in case they go into labour pre-term.

The Foetus

The 30-week old foetus has a crown-rump measurement of about 28.5cm (just over 11in), and its overall length is about 42cm (nearly 19in) – its overall length has increased 2cm (1 inch) in the last week. It has put on another 200g (7oz), and now weighs about 1.8kg (4lb). The foetus is filling out and the placenta is also quite a large organ now; your uterus has

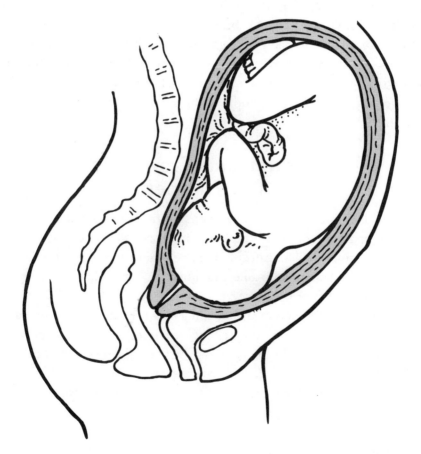

The foetus is now snugly enveloped by the uterus, and the amount of amniotic fluid begins to diminish.

nearly taken up all the available space in your abdomen, and the foetus has less freedom of movement. At about this stage in the pregnancy many foetuses adopt the characteristic legs crossed, head-down position. You may notice that the foetus makes fewer large movements now, but continues to make jabbing, kicking movements.

How you Look

In the thirty-second week of pregnancy the top of the uterus is probably about 12cm (5in) above your navel. Your tummy may well look as if it comes out straight underneath your breasts, and it is indeed about as high as it will get over the next few weeks (as the baby settles in the head-down position, and later when the head engages, your bump appears to drop); you are at the ship-in-full-sail stage. Your tummy protrudes outwards as well as upwards, and you navel is likely to be flattening out as the skin is stretched over your expanding abdomen.

Your breasts will probably have grown considerably by this stage in the pregnancy, and the nipples are often larger and darker. You may also have noticed that you have filled out on your legs, buttocks, arms and face. The average weight gain by the middle of the seventh month of pregnancy is just under 10kg (20lb).

Nutrition and Cravings in the Third Trimester

With any luck you will have no nausea in the third trimester, but you may find that you can eat only a little at a time because your uterus is pushing up on your stomach. This can also cause heartburn and indigestion which means that you have to keep an eye on how much and what you eat in the last few weeks of your pregnancy.

The principles of good nutrition and a balanced diet remain the same in the third trimester, but you are now sustaining quite a large growing and moving foetus inside you: you may be needing an extra 500 calories a day (this is equivalent to five bananas or five slices or unbuttered bread). You may find that it is easier now to have four or even five light meals a day instead of three larger ones. This will make it easier for your cramped digestive system to cope, therefore reducing the risk of indigestion. Eat your meals slowly and chew the food well. Try to avoid very spicy or fatty foods which could increase the likelihood of heartburn.

Cravings

Food cravings are among the most highly publicised symptoms of pregnancy, but many women have no food cravings at all. A number of women find that in the early weeks of pregnancy, while they are adapting to the surge of hormones, their appetite and palate alters and they crave particular foods. These are not generally regarded as true cravings but as distortions of the appetite attributed to the hormonal changes taking place. True cravings in the latter stages of pregnancy may be a direct response to a need for a particular nutrient.

You may find that you have irresistible urges to eat something, even if it is something that you do not normally like or even something that is not normally considered edible (such as coal or baking powder); this extreme condition of craving substances that are not normally regarded as foods is known as pica. The very fact that cravings can be for such obscure ingredients strengthens the argument that the body is responding to a need; although we are not aware of it, our sense of smell may be sufficiently developed to identify the lacking nutrient in the craved foodstuff. The fact that many women crave citrus fruits would seem to indicate a need for vitamin C; women who crave ice cream may not be exploiting the myth in order to have something they have always loved, they may genuinely need calcium and carbohydrates.

Women are usually encouraged to satisfy their cravings, but to do so in moderation especially if they crave foods such as ice cream or sweets which have a high calorie content but little nutritional value. Pica is not as common now as it appears to have been in the past – and this is attributed to the fact that women's diets are generally more nutritious and balanced now – but if you do crave non-foodstuffs, you should discuss it with your doctor or a nutritionist. They may be able to establish that you have a vitamin or mineral deficiency, and to prescribe you a supplement ... which is more convenient and hygienic than surreptitiously nibbling handfuls of soil!

CASE STUDY: *'I really wanted fruity things, funnily enough fruits themselves weren't strong enough, concentrated enough. Fruit pastilles, fruit gums and raw jelly were what I really wanted. Once or twice I did literally have to drive up to the service-station late at night to get some fruit gums, and I'd never really liked them before.'*

CASE STUDY: *'No, I haven't had any cravings, except I do drink a lot of cranberry and blackcurrant juice, and I never have before.*

Week 33

You may only have a few weeks left before you leave work, and you are probably looking forward to having some time to yourself to prepare for the arrival of your baby.

The Foetus

In the thirty-third week of pregnancy, seven months since the egg was first fertilised, the foetus has a crown-rump measurement of about 29.5cm (nearly 12in), and the overall length is about 43cm (17in). Its weight has reached the 2kg mark (4lb 6oz), and it is nearly two-thirds of the average weight of a full-term baby. Babies born at this stage in pregnancy still have immature lungs and they do not have enough fat to maintain body warmth by themselves, but they have a very good chance of survival with special care. The face of the foetus at 33 weeks still looks thinner than a full-term baby, with puffy-looking eyelids and a prominent upper lip.

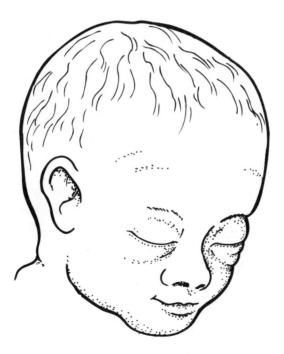

The foetus has puffy eyelids, probably to protect the eyes from constant exposure to amniotic fluid.

How you Feel

You are probably beginning to get excited about the arrival of your baby, it seems more real now that it is less than two months away, but you may also be having very real concerns about coping with pain in labour. Talk to the instructor at your antenatal classes: she will be able to tell you about coping strategies and the advantages and disadvantages of different kinds of pain-relief for labour. It's also worth talking to other pregnant women and to women who have had children themselves to build up a more complete picture. Remember, no two pregnancies and labours are alike, so do not let yourself be terrified by other people's horror stories or lulled into a false sense of security by women who say that having a baby is as easy as shelling peas!

Your Breasts in the Third Trimester

Your breasts will probably have grown considerably by the end of the seventh month, although a small minority of women notice very little change in breast size until their milk comes in, some three days after their baby is born. The size of your breasts bears no relation to your ability to breastfeed: breast size is related to fat stores in the breast and not to the size of the milk-producing structures.

Your nipples will probably be larger and darker than usual: this is to make them easier for the baby to identify when he is rooting to suckle. Your nipples may also have a slightly waxy texture; glands in the nipple secrete tiny quantities of oils to protect the nipple from cracking when your baby suckles. The best way to prepare your breasts for breastfeeding is not to toughen them up, as some books advise (even recommending chafing with a toothbrush!) but to let this natural process take its course: do not use soap on your breasts, because it might dry out the oils, dry them well after a bath or shower and use a rich body lotion or oil on them.

You may have a fizzing, tingling sensation in your nipples and you may even notice that you have some leaking from the breasts. This is caused by the first milk, colostrum, which is already being produced in preparation for your baby's arrival. This should not be cause for concern although it might be inconvenient: if you find that the leaks make marks on your clothes, buy some breast pads (they are likely to be useful when you are feeding anyway) to absorb the colostrum leaked.

The blood vessels on your breast may be much more prominent in the latter stages of pregnancy, especially if your breasts have become much larger. Although they may seem unsightly, these blood vessels are playing a vital role, supplying blood and nutrients to the milk ducts that will produce milk for your baby. They will gradually disappear as your breasts become smaller when you eventually stop breastfeeding.

Nursing Bras

If you are planning to breastfeed even for a short time it is worth investing in nursing bras. You may well have had to change your bras once already during your pregnancy, but it is not really worth investing in a nursing bra until about the seventh month when your breasts are more likely to be nearer their final size. Nursing bras are designed to support your breasts adequately – with wide straps over the shoulders and to the back – and to afford quick access to the nipple for feeds. They usually have zipped cups or front sections of the cups that un-hook from the shoulder strap. Lighter, sleeping nursing bras are also available: they will give your enlarged breasts some support while you sleep, but will not hinder you when you get up to feed your baby in the night.

Make sure that you have a proper fitting when you buy a nursing bra, and think about how the bra works in relation to the clothes you are likely to be wearing (different fastenings are more suitable for front opening clothes such as blouses, and clothes that may be lifted over the breast to feed, such as jumpers).

Week 34

You have probably been to your first two or three antenatal classes by now, and you will know more about what happens to your body in labour and during delivery. You are ready to start making more informed decisions about how you would like to have your baby.

The Foetus

In week 34 your foetus's crown-rump measurement is about 31cm (just over 12in) and its overall measurement is about 44cm (17½in). It has put on an impressive 250g (nearly 9oz) in the last week and it now weighs about 2.25kg (5lb). The lanugo (fine hairs) and greasy vernix that have covered the foetus's body for many weeks now begin to disappear, although many babies are born with traces of vernix still in folds of skin, and others still have a considerable covering of lanugo.

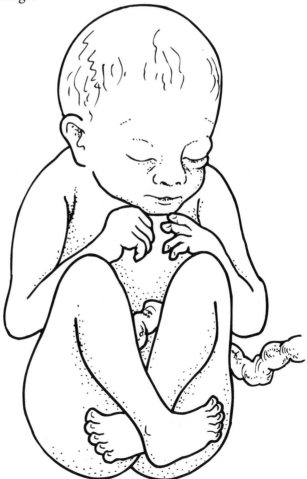

The vernix begins to disappear from the foetus's skin.

How you Feel

You may well be beginning to feel a little fed up with your pregnancy, and you should not feel guilty about this. Many women find that at various stages in their pregnancy they feel resentful or just bored: nine months is a long time, especially if you have had discomfort or other symptoms which have restricted your lifestyle. Women who have already had children will tell you that you will have even less freedom once the baby is born. This is largely true, although it may be difficult to appreciate from where you are standing, and you should try to make the most of the last few weeks to ensure that you are physically and psychologically prepared for labour, birth and motherhood. It is increasingly important to strike the right balance between activity, rest and relaxation.

Your Birth Plan

At some stage in your antenatal check-ups or classes you may be asked if you would like to draw up a birth plan. A birth plan is a written record of the way that you would like your labour, delivery and postpartum care to proceed in an ideal world. There is actually no need to have a birth plan unless there are some things that you feel particularly strongly about, but it does help to focus your thoughts on labour and delivery, and it gives you the opportunity to discuss certain aspects of labour that you may be worrying about. It is important to stress that birth plans should not be seen as cast in concrete: complications can arise, and labour can go on beyond a woman's endurance, so it is unrealistic – and will only cause disappointment and feelings of inadequacy – if you believe that you must adhere to your birth plan at all costs.

Some hospitals provide a birth plan form for you to fill in, or you could create one yourself. You will only be ready to devise a birth plan once you have had most of your antenatal classes, discussed labour and delivery with your doctor or midwife, possibly read the chapters of this book that cover labour and delivery, and talked about the plan with your partner or the person you have chosen to attend you in labour. Only when you have a full understanding of the options open to you will you be able to start drawing up the birth plan.

Your birth plan may cover the following information:

• Who your birthing partner is and whether you would like them to be with you the whole time, even if you have to have an emergency Caesarean section.

• What equipment you would like to use in labour and delivery (for example bean bags, birthing stools, birthing pools), and whether this equipment is available in the hospital or will be brought by you.

• Whether or not you have foetal heart monitoring throughout labour (this can seriously limit how much you move around while you are in labour).

• What sort of pain relief you would or would not like to have in labour (different hospitals offer different drugs, and not all hospitals can provide epidurals at any time of day or in an emergency).

• What position you might adopt for the birth.

• How you feel about being given an episiotomy.

• Whether you want your baby delivered straight onto your tummy.

• How you are planning to feed your baby (this is important because, if you want to breastfeed, the baby should be put to the breast shortly after delivery when the rooting and sucking reflexes are at their strongest).

Some women feel that there is little point in drawing up a birth plan because they cannot imagine what labour and birth are going to be like. Others have strong feelings about wanting as little or as much pain relief as possible. You may feel that, if you have a plan, you have a starting point, something to refer to and for your partner to refer to when you can no longer make decisions for yourself. The main purpose of the birth plan is that it gives you a reason to consider and discuss the options that may be open to you.

CASE STUDY: *'I didn't really have a birth plan, but I read a lot about labour and delivery before I had my baby. I knew what I wanted, and that was as little pain relief and monitoring as I could get away with. My labour went on quite a long time, so I didn't get away without the monitoring because they wanted to check that the baby wasn't in distress, but the pain relief bit worked ... well almost, just half an hour of gas and air wasn't bad going!'*

CASE STUDY: *'I haven't drawn up a birth plan – I know what I'd like but it's probably unrealistic till I know what it's like. Ideally, I'd like an epidural as soon as possible.'*

BRAXTON HICKS CONTRACTIONS

As part of your body's preparation for labour and delivery, your uterus actually undergoes regular painless contractions from the early weeks of pregnancy. These are known as Braxton Hicks contractions.

Some women never feel Braxton Hicks contractions, others – especially in second and subsequent pregnancies when they appear to be stronger – are aware of them by the middle of the pregnancy. Most find that they notice them in the latter weeks as the contractions become stronger.

When you have a Braxton Hicks contraction, the uterus contracts, making the abdomen feel rigid to the touch. You might feel a little bit of discomfort but there should be no pain. If you feel pain in conjunction with contractions, contact your doctor or midwife: you may well be going into labour.

Week 35

You are now eight months pregnant and the arrival of your baby is probably beginning to seem very real and imminent.

The Foetus

When you are eight months pregnant the crown-rump measurement of the foetus is about 32.5cm (13in), and its overall length is about 45cm (just over 18in). It has again put on 250g (nearly 9oz) in a week and now weighs about 2.5kg (5lb 8oz). It is very nearly the length of the full-term baby, but it still needs to fill out with fat stores under the skin. With only five weeks of pregnancy left, your baby only has to grow a little more and for the lungs to mature fully before it is ready to be born. A baby born in the thirty-fifth week has an extremely high chance of surviving, and may not even need any special care.

How you Feel

By this stage in your pregnancy you are likely to be thinking of your baby as an individual rather than a part of yourself. As the birth draws nearer your perception of yourself and the baby will gradually change, you are not one unit but two separate beings, and when your baby is born he will have a life of his own, although he will, of course, be totally dependant on you.

Some women have a feeling of impatience towards the end of their pregnancy, not just for the pregnancy to be over but to meet their baby, to see who this baby is going to be. Others are apprehensive, not only about the labour and the birth but about how they will feel towards the baby. Talking to other pregnant women and women who have already had their babies will help you to realise that, whatever you are feeling and thinking, there are plenty of other women who share these feelings and thoughts.

The Size and Height of your Bump

Towards the end of your pregnancy the size, shape and height of your bump may be quite a talking point, and you may feel as if your body is no longer your own: it has been taken over by an alien and is a source of entertainment and speculation for those around you. People will try to guess 'how far gone' you are, will tell you that you are carrying very high

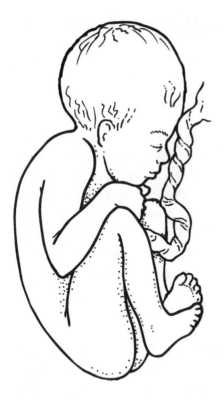

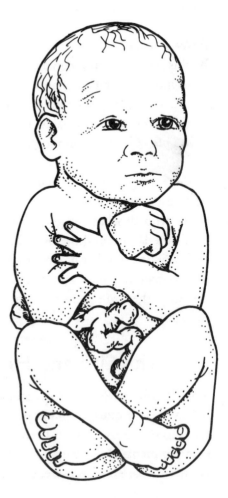

Just five weeks before the due date the arms and legs of the foetus are still much thinner than those of a full-term baby.

or very low, that the position of your bump and the distribution of your weight implies that you are carrying a boy or a girl; they may even tell you to your face that you are huge or 'very neat'.

While the size and height of your bump might be entertaining to those around you it could become a serious inconvenience to you. If your tummy is very large you may find that driving becomes difficult or uncomfortable in the last weeks of pregnancy. It may be difficult to pull on socks, do up boots and shoes or even shave your legs! And you may no longer be able to reach the bottom of a supermarket trolley.

Most of these practical problems are surmountable, but there may also be a number of physical inconveniences:

Heavy, Aching Tummy

Some women find that the bump feels uncomfortably heavy, especially towards the end of the day and when they have been standing for any length of time. This heavy feeling, particularly if it is accompanied by aching, might indicate that you are straining the ligaments that support the uterus within the abdomen. Try to avoid standing for long periods, heavy lifting and stretching. It may help to wear a special support belt under the bump to take some of the strain off your back and abdominal muscles and ligaments. If you have a lot of discomfort and would like to use a support belt, an obstetric physiotherapist would be able to give you specialised advice.

Itchy Skin

It is also very common for women to complain of itchiness on their tummy as the skin stretches to accommodate the growing uterus. If your skin becomes dry and itchy, use only a light soap or cream soap when you wash, make sure that you dry the skin well, and moisturise it with lotion or oil.

If you have excessive itching and if the itching is not only on the skin of your tummy, it is important that you speak to your doctor or midwife. Recent research carried out by Queen Charlotte's Hospital has shown that a malfunction of the liver known as obstetric cholestasis causes a build-up of bile salts in the mother's bloodstream which can produce terrible itching. Severe obstetric cholestasis can result in the death of the foetus: it is believed that the bile salts transferred to the foetus through the placenta may fatally damage the foetus, although the exact cause of death is not known. Obstetric cholestasis could be responsible for a significant proportion of stillbirths (perhaps as many as one in five, according to one estimate).

The itching caused by obstetric cholestasis usually begins in the last trimester of pregnancy, and it may be particularly bad on the hands and feet. It can be so intense that sufferers scratch themselves raw. If you have this sort of itching you can be given a blood test to see whether you have obstetric cholestasis; once the condition is diagnosed, close monitoring of the foetus's wellbeing is essential. It may be deemed safer to deliver the baby early than to allow the pregnancy to go to term.

Rib Pain and Breathlessness

If you are carrying your baby very high you could have pains in your ribs as they are forced to expand. You may also find that you are short of breath because your lungs are no longer able to expand downwards. If you do get short of breath, sit down and breathe steadily, consciously pushing your lungs out and up. Obstetric physiotherapists may be able to give you advice about posture and breathing exercises to alleviate rib pain.

Heartburn

Another problem aggravated by a high baby is heartburn. Heartburn is caused when stomach acid is regurgitated into the bottom of the oesophagus (the tube that carries food from your throat to your stomach), causing a burning sensation as the oesophagus becomes inflamed. It can be very painful and may be accompanied by sicking up of unpleasant, bitter stomach juices into the mouth. The valve at the top of the stomach is looser during pregnancy because of the relaxing effects of the hormone progesterone, and a high baby can literally squeeze the juices out of the stomach.

It is quite safe to use antacid indigestion treatments to neutralise the acids; ask your doctor or pharmacists which would be most suitable. Avoiding very greasy and spicy foods can also help. If you suffer from heartburn at night, make sure that you have your last meal two or three hours before you go to bed, and try sleeping slightly propped up so that gravity works against the backflow of acids.

Most of the problems associated with a high baby should improve in the last month when the baby tends to descend and may engage its head in the pelvis ready for delivery.

Frequent Urinating

If the baby is very low, you are more likely to be troubled by a frequent need to pass water as pressure on your bladder means that it has a smaller capacity, and the valve (which is relaxed by the effects of progesterone) signals that you need to urinate more often.

Sciatic Pain

You may also suffer from sciatic pain: this is a very distinctive pain which can range from a dull ache to an excruciating flash in the lower back and buttocks, running all the way down one or both legs. This happens when your uterus squeezes the sciatic nerve which runs down your leg. If you suffer from sciatica, try applying a warm hot-water bottle to your buttocks or legs when you are sitting down, and make sure that you rest your legs as often as possible. If the pain is very severe, and it can be quite incapacitating, talk to your doctor about exercises that may be able to ease it, and about safe forms of pain relief.

Week 36

Most hospitals ask pregnant women to prepare their bag for hospital in the thirty-sixth week in case they go into labour pre-term. From now on you will probably have antenatal check-ups once a week until your baby is born.

The Foetus

In the thirty-sixth week of pregnancy, when the foetus has only four more weeks of growing, it is very close to its final full-term length. The crown-rump measurement is now about 33.5cm (just over 13in) and the overall measurement is about 46cm (just over 18in). The weight is still going on at an impressive 250g (nearly 9oz) a week, and the foetus now weighs 2.75kg (6lb). Most babies will have assumed a head-down position by now and, if this is your first baby, its head may well descend into your pelvic girdle (engage) in the thirty-sixth week.

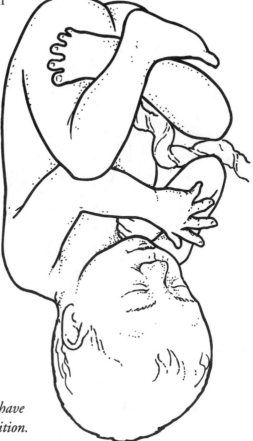

By week 36 most foetuses will have settled into the head-down position.

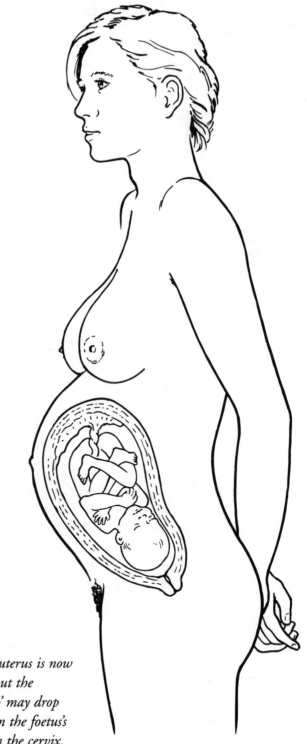

The top of the uterus is now very high up, but the mother's 'bump' may drop noticeably when the foetus's head engages in the cervix.

How you Look

If your baby has descended, particularly if the head has engaged, you will look quite a different shape now from ship-in-full-sail of of the last few weeks. Your bump has visibly dropped, and there may be a gap now between your breasts and the top of your tummy, even though the height of the fundus does actually continue to rise about 1cm (just under ½in) a week until the end of your pregnancy.

You will probably feel very big by now or, especially if this is your first baby, you might still be quite neat. Women tend to want to remain as small as possible during pregnancy but to have huge bouncing babies; the two are not mutually exclusive, but it is an unrealistic ideal for everyone. Pregnancy is not a competition; if you feel cumbersome, remember that in about four weeks' time you will have a baby to show for it.

You may have some swelling from fluid retention and you may well look flushed and feel hot as the extra blood steams around your circulatory system, and your metabolic rate is raised.

Your Hospital Bag

If you are having your baby in hospital you should have your bag ready in the thirty-sixth week of pregnancy. Some hospitals will provide you with a list of the things that you will need. These will include:

For your Labour

- Something to wear in labour (you may wear a hospital gown or you might prefer a favourite nightie or an old shirt of your partner's). You might also need some warm socks, women often say that their feet feel cold in labour.

- Books, magazines, personal stereo (anything that might help you to relax and to pass the time if your labour is slow to progress).

- Some favourite drinks or snacks (for you or your partner). Some hospitals discourage eating during labour, others let the woman follow her own instincts, and you certainly should drink if you are thirsty in labour. It may be possible to get snacks and drinks from a vending machine in the hospital, but you may prefer to take something with you.

- Coins or phone cards to announce the news!

For your Hospital Stay

- 2 nighties (front opening if you are going to breastfeed).

- 2 bras or nursing bras.

- 6 pairs of pants (old ones or buy cheap ones or disposables; you will lose a lot of blood in the days after your baby is born, and you will probably throw these pants away).

- Dressing gown and slippers (make sure that the slippers can be slipped on because you may find bending over difficult in the first few days after having your baby).

- Sanitary towels (not just a handful of panty pads, but a big pack of large, super-absorbent towels).

- Your toothbrush, toothpaste, flannel, soap, hairbrush, shampoo.

- 2 towels (if they are not provided by the hospital).

For the Baby

Some hospitals provide nappies and nighties for babies during your stay in hospital. Check what your hospital's policy is. You might need:

- New-born size nappies.

- 3 or 4 nighties or babygrows.

- 2 or 3 vests.

- A shawl, jacket or blanket.

For Going Home

Pack your going-home clothes in advance but do not take them to hospital with you unless you are on a Domino Scheme and planning to come out of hospital shortly after your baby's arrival. You will need:

- Loose-fitting clothes, underwear and outdoor shoes for yourself.

- A babygrow, cardigan or shawl and bonnet for the baby.

- A car seat for the baby (you may not be allowed to leave the hospital until you can satisfy the staff that the baby will be travelling in a car seat).

The Lie of Your Baby

By this stage in your pregnancy, you may be very aware of the lie of your baby, the position that it has assumed inside you. You might be able to tell where its head and bottom are at any time. The doctor or midwife who

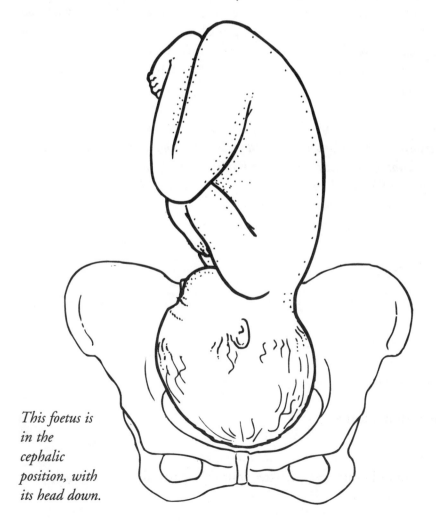

This foetus is in the cephalic position, with its head down.

does your check-ups will pay special attention to the lie of your baby now, because it can effect how easy your labour and delivery will be.

The most common position for the baby is to be head-down, tightly curled with arms and legs crossed, and turned so that it is facing your back. This is also the best position it can be in, with the head as the presenting part putting pressure on your cervix. If the baby is facing your front, you may have a slower labour and you may suffer from backache.

If the baby is in a breech position and remains in the breech position when you go into labour you may have to have a Caesarean section. There are a number of different breech positions, some of which can be delivered normally without harm to the mother or baby.

If there is any doubt about the lie of your baby at this stage, you will be closely monitored in case you need to be admitted to hospital or to have a Caesarean section. In the great majority of cases, the baby is head down by week 36 and the head will probably have engaged if this is a first pregnancy. Most women are aware that their baby's head has engaged: they notice that the bump is lower and they may feel a slight aching in their pelvis.

CASE STUDY: *'I carried my baby very low for the whole pregnancy so I thought I probably wouldn't notice when he dropped and engaged. But, don't you believe it, it suddenly felt as if he was between my knees and my hips felt like a pair of nut-crackers. I was actually conscious of the shape of his head cradled in my pelvis.'*

Week 37

As your due date approaches you need to check that everything is ready for the arrival of your baby and that you have made arrangements for any other dependants. If you have other children, an elderly relative, even a pet, you need to make sure that they will be looked after at least for the time that you will be in hospital.

The Foetus

With just three weeks to go, the foetus's crown-rump measurement is now about 34.5cm (just over 13½in) and the overall measurement is 47cm (18½in). It is still filling out and building up vital fat stores; it has now reached the 3kg mark (6lb 8oz). Babies need fat stores to insulate them and to nourish them in the first few days of life while their bodies adapt to digesting milk rather than the nutrients supplied by the placenta (most babies lose weight in their first three days, and begin to put weight on once your milk has come in). The foetus's face is filling out too, the nose is becoming smoother and more rounded, the cheeks fuller, and the neck is thicker. The eyelids still look puffy but they can open and close easily and are complete with eyelashes.

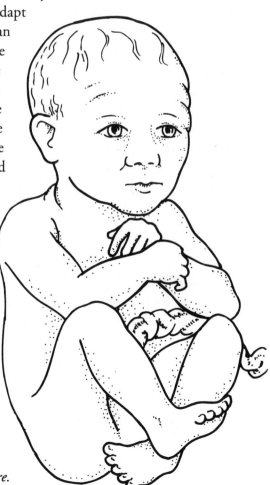

Although the foetus still needs to lay down more fat stores at this stage, it is not unusual for babies that are born in the thirty-seventh week to need little or no specialised care.

How you Feel

Time may suddenly be running out for you. You may be rushing around making arrangements for your dog to be fed and walked while you are in hospital, and stocking your freezer with oven-ready meals for the weeks ahead when you will be learning how to be a mother. You may still be at work, and you are probably feeling tired and a little fed-up with the pregnancy. Try to rest whenever you can, and rest your legs even when you are doing something: sit down to do the ironing or to prepare a meal if possible. It is important not to exhaust yourself before your baby arrives; not only have you got the labour and delivery to cope with, but you will then have a baby to look after ... and it may be months before you have an undisturbed night's sleep.

YOUR RELATIONSHIP AND SEX IN THE THIRD TRIMESTER

Many couples find that by the third trimester of pregnancy they no longer make love very often. The woman may be tired and quite cumbersome, and both partners may find that they have less appetite for sex. Some women continue to have a high libido throughout their pregnancy, but they may find that they need to be more imaginative about positions for sex as their bump gets larger.

Whether or not you are making love in the last months of your pregnancy, your relationship with your partner is very important at this stage. Your body is coping with tremendous demands and you are approaching a turning point in your lives: you need support from each other. When you are both tired or anxious about the baby or financial changes that the new arrival implies, it is likely that you will be irritable with each other, but try to be tolerant and try to discuss your anxieties. Many couples find that the shared excitement of the imminent arrival of a baby brings them closer.

CASE STUDY: *'He's been fantastic. I'm now going through a phase when I'm irritated by him (said in week 34). I think it's mutual. I don't go on about the pregnancy the whole time, but it's always there, and we both have the odd day when we're tetchy.'*

CASE STUDY: *'You get closer as it gets nearer, he's been brilliant.'*

Visiting the Unit

If you are having your baby in hospital, you may have had a brief visit to the maternity unit when you first started your antenatal check-ups, but most women do not see the maternity unit until a visit is arranged during the course of their antenatal classes.

However prettily the postnatal wards are decorated and however charming the hospital staff are, there is no escaping the fact that a maternity unity contains a great deal of equipment. As many women hardly set foot in a hospital except to have a baby, the equipment can appear very daunting. It is important to remember that having a baby is a very natural and usually safe process: the unit is bound to be stark and uncluttered in order to keep it a clean and safe environment for new-born babies and newly delivered mothers, both of whom are very susceptible to infection. The equipment is there to monitor the progress of mother and baby in labour and to assist delivery if necessary.

Your visit to the maternity unit is an opportunity for you to familiarise yourself with a place where you might spend some of the most intense hours of your life. Ask the staff what the various pieces of equipment are, how they work, and when and why they may be used.

CASE STUDY: *'I have seen the unit, and it all seems very real to me now. It did look very clinical and there seemed to be a lot of apparatus around, but then I suppose that should be reassuring not off-putting.'*

Week 38

Many women leave work at about this stage in the pregnancy, allowing themselves a fortnight to prepare for the arrival of their baby. If this is the case with you, make sure that part of that preparation is to rest and look after yourself.

The Foetus

In the thirty-eighth week of your pregnancy, 36 weeks since your egg was first fertilised, the foetus is still growing steadily. The crown-rump measurement is now about 35.5cm (14in) and the overall length is about 48cm (19in). The weight gain is slowing down slightly; in the last week it has gained about 150g (5oz) and it now weighs about 3.15kg (6lb 13oz). The foetus's fingernails and toenails have hardened and they reach the end of the fingers and toes. It is possible for a woman's vagina and thighs to be scratched by her baby's fingernails and toenails during delivery.

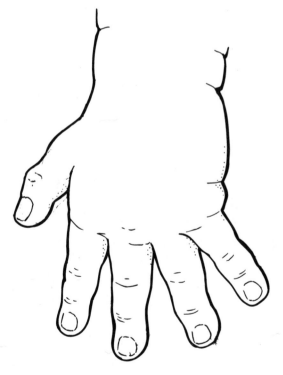

The finger nails have nearly reached the ends of the fingers and they are now quite hard and sharp.

How you Feel

Your baby is very nearly ready to be born, in fact it is considered normal for a baby to be born up to three weeks before full-term. If your baby were born now there is every chance that he would need no special care at all and could be treated like a full-term baby. You may well feel that it is high time that your baby arrived: you have been pregnant for nearly nine months and you may be getting very tired and uncomfortable at this stage.

It is not uncommon for women to feel bored and fed up in the last few weeks of pregnancy, you may even have feelings of resentment for your partner or the baby because your life no longer seems to be your own. There is nothing wrong with feeling like this, and it does not mean that you will not be a good mother. On the other hand, you may be very excited about the arrival of your baby, or apprehensive about labour and delivery. If you have any real fears about the labour discuss them with your partner and with your doctor or midwife.

The Internal Furnace

Towards the end of your pregnancy you may notice that you feel hot the whole time. This is because your metabolic rate has speeded up to cope with the demands of pregnancy: you are consuming and burning about 500 calories more a day, you have more blood circulating in your body and your circulation is probably working more efficiently than usual.

If the last three months of your pregnancy coincide with the coldest winter months, this hot feeling could be an advantage, but at any other time of year it can cause you considerable discomfort. You may find that you sweat very easily, that you feel flushed and even light-headed, and that it is difficult to find clothes that are comfortable.

It is quite normal for you to feel warm or even hot, and you will find that loose-fitting cotton clothes and mesh fabrics that breathe will be more comfortable and stay cooler. If you feel feverishly hot or if you suddenly feel cold, you could have a temperature. Take your temperature and if you have a fever contact your doctor.

CASE STUDY: *'I normally feel the cold very easily and my fingers and toes go white because my circulation is so bad, but being pregnant has made a huge difference (said in December in week 36). My husband has noticed it almost more than me because he no longer gets icy toes tucked between his legs to warm up in bed!'*

Week 39

You should have everything ready for your baby's arrival by now because very few babies actually arrive on their due date, and there is no way of knowing whether yours will choose to come just before, just after, or bang on.

The Foetus

The foetus is now fairly cramped in the uterus and there is less amniotic fluid than a few weeks ago. It is close to its full-term length and weight, with a crown-rump measurement of 36.5cm (14½in), an overall measurement of 49cm (nearly 19½in), and weighing about 3.3kg (7lb 5oz).

The uterus is moulded round the foetus now so that it can no longer move freely, but it can still make jabbing movements with its arms and legs.

How you Feel

You will almost certainly have left work by the end of this week and you will probably have finished your course of antenatal classes and visited the maternity unit where your baby will be born. You may well be swinging between feelings of excitement about the arrival of your baby and apprehension or even fear about the preceding labour and birth.

Difficulties Sleeping

It seems unfair that just when a woman's body is being stretched to its limits by the latter stages of her pregnancy, there should be so many things that can stop her from having a good night's sleep. Many women find that towards the end of their pregnancy they wake several times in the night, and this can be for a number of reasons:

Needing to empty your bladder in the night: You may well be woken more than once in the night to empty your bladder, especially once the baby has dropped and puts more pressure on your bladder. It is not a good idea to cut down your fluid intake, but try to avoid drinking in the last hour before you go to bed, and you may be woken less frequently by your bladder.

Waking every time you turn over: Many women find that as they get bigger they wake every time they turn over in their sleep because the bump gets in the way of their manoeuvring. So long as you do not have trouble getting back to sleep this is merely an inconvenience.

> CASE STUDY: *'By the end I had the turning circle of an oil-tanker, and just turning over in bed was difficult. I might wake two or three times in the night to turn over. Some nights were good. Some were bad.'*

Waking because you are uncomfortable: You may be woken simply because your sleeping position is uncomfortable, and it is worth experimenting with different sleeping positions and strategically placed pillows to find a position that is comfortable and gives your tummy some support. Many women find that lying on their side and having a pillow supporting the bump is comfortable; it is also an easy position to change over when you turn over in the night. If you find that there is not really room for you, your bump, your pillows and your partner in bed, it is worth talking to him about one of you moving to another bed. He should understand that you are not rejecting him, but trying to find the best position to sleep.

Waking because you are hot: As you come towards the end of your pregnancy your raised metabolic rate makes you feel hot, and you wake in the night because you are hot. Make sure that you do not have too many bedcovers or night clothes on. Use cotton sheets or duvet covers; they are cooler than synthetic ones, and don't tuck them in around you.

Having trouble getting to sleep: In the latter weeks of pregnancy it is not unusual for women to have difficulty getting to sleep in the first place or getting back to sleep when they have woken. If you find that you cannot get to sleep because your mind is racing and you are worrying about things, try to work out whether you really need to be concerned about these things and discuss them with your partner or midwife. It might help to get into a regular routine, winding down for a good hour before bedtime, so that your body recognises the pattern leading up to sleep.

Sometimes you may feel very tired and your mind may be blank but you could still find it difficult to get to sleep. This is because your metabolism is still fuelling the growing baby even when you are trying to sleep, and your body may find it difficult to switch off. It is important that you rest even if you are not sleeping, so try not to get agitated and worry about how much or how little sleep you are getting. Use the time to rest physically, and read a book or listen to some music to take your mind off the thought of getting to sleep. Do not use sleeping pills, even herbal ones, without consulting your doctor or pharmacist.

CASE STUDY: *'I have trouble getting to sleep, and I seem to wake at 4 o'clock – I'm woken either by the bump or because I need to go to the loo – and I'm awake for two hours. Still, I suppose I'm going to have to get used to it when the baby comes.'*

Week 40

This will very probably be the last week of your pregnancy, although a proportion of babies – especially first babies – are born after the 40-week term.

The Foetus

After 38 weeks growing inside you the foetus is now ready to be born. The average full-term crown-rump measurement is about 37.5cm (15in) and the overall measurement is about 50cm (just under 20in). The average weight of a full-term baby is about 3.4kg (7lb 8oz). The baby's head may now be fully engaged and your cervix may even have started to efface, to thin out in preparation for dilating to allow your baby to be born.

At 40 weeks the baby's head (or other presenting part) is usually engaged in the pelvis, although in second and subsequent pregnancies, the presenting part may not engage until labour has begun.

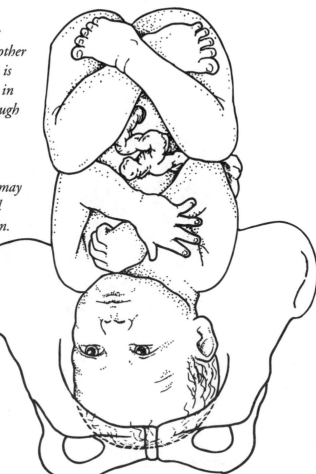

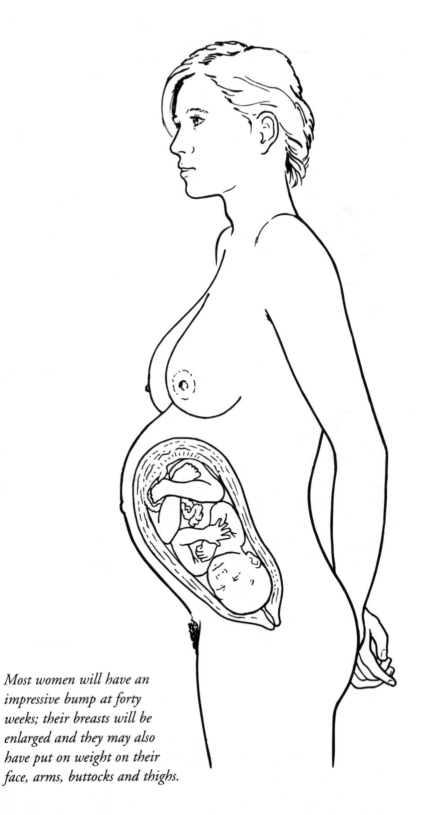

*Most women will have an
impressive bump at forty
weeks; their breasts will be
enlarged and they may also
have put on weight on their
face, arms, buttocks and thighs.*

How you Look

The foetus has grown several centimetres in length and has filled out considerably since week 36, so your tummy is likely to be protruding noticeably more. Many women find that the rate at which they put on weight slows down in the last weeks of pregnancy, but your body may have laid down some fat stores in preparation for lactation, so your outline could be more rounded than four weeks ago. In most cases, the bump has descended and the foetus's head (or presenting part) will almost certainly have engaged by now if this is your first pregnancy.

Feeling Afraid / Feeling Prepared

You may well be worrying about the labour and delivery, about whether or not you will recognise the onset of labour, and how you will cope with your contractions. It is natural and normal for a woman to feel apprehensive or even afraid of labour and childbirth, especially when she is expecting her first baby.

Women who feel prepared for the arrival of their baby – who have made all the necessary preparations and arrangements at home, have attended antenatal classes and perhaps have read books such as this one about pregnancy and childbirth – may be no less apprehensive about what lies in store, but they feel able to face it with greater confidence. One of the aspects of childbirth that women find frightening is the feeling of loss of control; if you understand what is happening to your body and know what options are open to you, you are more likely to feel as if you are in control of the situation and to have a more positive experience.

If there is anything that you are genuinely concerned about or if you have any questions that you would like to have cleared up before you go into labour, talk to your doctor or midwife.

CASE STUDY: *'Actually, I have just blanked out the labour and I worry about bringing the baby home. It think that's my way of dealing with it.' (said in week 37)*

CASE STUDY: *'Yes, I did worry about labour, but towards the end I thought less about being pregnant and going through labour and more and more about the baby. It was like a natural progression, and the end – i.e. the baby – sort of justified the means, however terrible they were going to be.'*

Week 41

You may not still be 'here' in week 41, you could well have had your baby at this stage, but more babies – especially first babies – are born late than early, and fewer than 10% of babies actually arrive on their due date.

The Foetus

If your pregnancy goes into a forty-first week this could either mean that your dates were wrong or that you will be having your baby post-term or late. If your dates were a little inaccurate, the baby will still be growing normally and will be reaching the size and appearance of the full-term baby illustrated in week 40. If you are now overdue, the foetus can undergo a number of changes and some of them are actually harmful to the foetus (that is why many hospitals will not allow a woman to go more than two weeks beyond term).

Towards the end of the pregnancy, the greasy vernix which protected your baby's skin from the amniotic fluid has all but disappeared. If the skin is exposed to amniotic fluid for several days it begins to absorb it, and it may become puffy and bloated with fluid. This is especially noticeable at the joints, particularly the fingers.

How you Feel

Most women cannot help feeling fed-up if they go overdue with a pregnancy. Even if you feel relieved to have escaped the ordeal of labour and delivery so far, you know that it cannot be postponed indefinitely. You are probably eager not to be pregnant any more, to get the birth over with and to have your baby. It is especially difficult if you have friends who were due at about the same time as you and who have already had their babies. You will begin to wonder when it will ever be your turn.

You should try to make the most of these extra days to make sure that you are absolutely ready for your baby's arrival, and to get plenty of rest. Keep your feet up as often as possible, because you are increasingly prone to oedema as your pregnancy goes beyond term.

KEEPING BUSY

Even though you have now passed your due date, you could still have over a week to wait before your baby is born. More than 60% of babies are born after their estimated date of delivery (EDD), and it is considered normal for a baby to be born up to the forty-second week of pregnancy (although hospitals have different policies about exactly how many days to wait after the EDD before inducing labour artificially).

It is tempting to assume that your baby will arrive on time, and you may have left the pages of your diary blank after the magic date in anticipation of this arrival. If and when you enter the forty-first week of your pregnancy you may find that you become bored and unnecessarily anxious if you have nothing to do, especially if you normally work full-time and are used to being busy all day.

You are likely to tire more easily by this stage in your pregnancy, so it is unwise to plan a hectic schedule of activities, but make sure that you have one or two outings or visits to look forward to in the days after your baby is due.

CASE STUDY: *'I was so persuaded that the baby was going to be early, but he was actually nearly two weeks late. After the first week I was climbing up the walls and I started arranging to see friends and go to the cinema. Then it was brilliant ringing people and saying, "sorry, I can't come over but will you come and visit me in hospital instead"!'*

Week 42

It is considered normal for a baby to be born as late as the forty-second week of pregnancy: about 10% of all babies (a much higher percentage of first babies) are born in week 42; a much smaller proportion of babies are not born until the forty-third week, although you will almost certainly be given a date for an induction if you do not seem to be going into labour spontaneously towards the end of your forty-second week.

The Foetus

Unless your dates were a full two-weeks out, your baby will now be post-term. Some babies continue to grow and to put on weight after term, so that some post-mature babies can be very large, especially if they are bloated with amniotic fluid as described in week 41. This itself can pose a problem, particularly if the baby's head circumference continues to grow: the mother becomes less likely to be able to deliver the baby herself; forceps deliveries and Caesarean sections are more common with very overdue babies.

On the other hand, the foetus can actually lose weight if it goes overdue. Once your due date has been reached and your placenta has reached its optimum performance, its condition and efficiency can begin to deteriorate. The post-mature placenta may not be nourishing the foetus efficiently (in a very small minority of cases the supply of oxygen to the baby could be compromised) and some overdue babies appear long and thin, and are very hungry on arrival.

In some women, the production of amniotic fluid decreases after the due date, making the uterus a less safe and comfortable environment for the foetus. If there is very little amniotic fluid present the baby may be born with delicate and even sore or cracked skin.

How you Feel

You will almost certainly be fed up with your pregnancy if you go into a forty-second week, and you may be finding it very difficult to sleep or to settle to anything because you know that it cannot be long now until you have your baby. You may well be having frequent Braxton Hicks contractions or even periods of false labour when you have regular and quite painful contractions for as long as a couple of hours, but they then stop.

Many women begin to worry that there will be something wrong with their baby if they go very overdue. Try not to worry about this: firstly your dates may be wrong so that you are not actually overdue at all, secondly you will be closely monitored. You will continue to have check-ups right up until your baby is born, and you may be asked to come in for check-ups more frequently after your due-date so that you can be monitored more carefully. Your doctor or midwife will keep a close eye on your health and the wellbeing of your baby (by monitoring its heartbeat). If there is any evidence of foetal distress they will probably induce labour or, in extreme cases, give you an emergency Caesarean section. It is important that you ring your doctor or midwife immediately if you have any vaginal bleeding; this could indicate that your placenta is beginning to detach from the uterine wall. If this happens, the placenta may no longer be able to maintain an adequate supply of nutrients and oxygen to the foetus.

Encouraging the Onset of Labour

There are a number of quite safe ways of trying to encourage the onset of labour that you can use yourself at home. However keen you may be to have your baby, you may not like the idea of being artificially induced, and these methods might help to kick-start your labour.

Newborn babies: If you have a friend who has just had a baby – and of whom you may be horribly envious at the moment! – she and her baby could actually be very useful to you. Just holding a newborn baby and hearing it cry can cause your womb to make a series of contractions, and this can sometimes be enough to jump-start labour.

If you cradle a newborn baby near your breasts, especially if the baby tries to root on you, you may be able to feel a tingling feeling in your breasts as they respond to this stimulation. The production and flow of milk are directly linked to contractions in the uterus (when you feed your own baby, the sucking of the baby triggers contractions in your uterus to help it shrink back down to its pre-pregnancy size and position). Stimulating your nipples with the presence of a newborn baby could provoke contractions and the onset of labour.

Nipple stimulation: You can, of course, stimulate your nipples at home, either by yourself or with your partner. It is, anyway, a good idea to keep the skin of your breasts and nipples well moisturised with lotion or oil to keep it supple as it stretches to accommodate your growing breasts. You may find that it is very pleasurable to smooth lotion into your nipples. Stimulating them like this can also induce labour.

Intercourse: If your partner helps you with the nipple stimulation described above, this could well lead to intercourse (even if you both thought you had completely forgotten about sex at this stage in the pregnancy). You may have to be inventive about positions for love-making if you are very big, but the contractions of the cervix that you experience during intercourse (especially if you reach orgasm) are a mild, painless variant on the contractions of labour. Substances called prostaglandins which are present in semen have the effect of inducing the effacement and dilation of the cervix. Some couples swear by love-making as a way of inducing labour.

Raspberry leaf tea: A herbal tea made from raspberry leaves is known to cause uterine contractions in some women, and it may encourage your uterus to go into labour. (It is dangerous to drink raspberry leaf tea in the first few weeks of pregnancy when you are at the greatest risk of losing the tiny foetus.)

Chapter 3

Illness During Pregnancy

However well your pregnancy is progressing, the likelihood of your going through an entire nine months without suffering at least a cold is very slim. Some women notice that they feel very well when they are pregnant, and they may even notice that their resistance to common ailments such as colds is improved. Others find that their physical resources and resistance are depleted by the demands of the pregnancy (your immune system is slightly suppressed in the early weeks of pregnancy so that your body does not reject the baby, which is – after all – a foreign body).

One of the best ways of dealing with illness in pregnancy is to try and avoid it in the first place by keeping fit and well. Avoid contact with people you know to be ill wherever possible (don't visit a friend whose child has the flu, or your aunt who has bronchitis); keep yourself well fed with a good diet and plenty of fluids; make sure your home is hygienic; prepare foods carefully and cook them thoroughly; and take regular exercise. Finally, ensure that you get sleep, rest and relaxation, and that you are not subjected to too much stress. These last are crucial: exhaustion and stress are linked to suppressed immune responses.

Many women are concerned about the effects of illness on their growing baby. There are two things to be concerned about here: the effects of the illness itself and the effects of the medication to treat the illness.

The majority of minor ailments such as coughs and colds cause the foetus no harm at all, whereas some of the over-the-counter drugs we usually take to cure them or to control the symptoms may be harmful to the foetus, especially if they are taken in the first three months of pregnancy. A number of more serious viral infections such as measles and German measles can be harmful to the foetus, and so can chronic conditions such as diabetes and asthma.

Effects of Common Illnesses on the Foetus
(listed alphabetically)

Coughs, colds and sore throats: Ordinary sore throats, coughs and colds that involve no fever, although they may be very unpleasant and may lay you low for as much as a week, will not actually harm your baby. Make sure that you get enough sleep or rest, that you eat well (even if you have little or no appetite) and that you drink plenty of fluids.

Cystitis: Cystitis and other infections of the urinary tract are common in pregnancy and they do no harm to the foetus, but they must be treated to avoid their progress to kidney infection. If you experience pain or a burning sensation when you urinate and / or if you feel as if you need to urinate all the time, you may have cystitis. Contact your doctor and make sure that he knows that you are pregnant before he prescribes any medication. Most urinary tract infections can be cleared up with a course of antibiotics – your doctor will prescribe you one that is safe to use when you are pregnant. You should not be tempted to try and go without the medication or to stop using it as soon as the symptoms clear up. Take the whole course of medication or the infection could come back and might even work its way up to your kidneys. Kidney infections can be very painful and can take a long time to clear up.

Food poisoning: If you have violent symptoms similar to those experienced with a tummy bug (see below), and if other people who shared a meal with you have all or some of the same symptoms you could be suffering from food poisoning. Some forms of food poisoning are powerful or possibly life-threatening, and they can pose a threat for the foetus. Even if it is not particularly virulent, food poisoning can drag on for longer than a simple gastro-enteritis virus, and this can weaken and dehydrate you. If you think you are suffering from food poisoning, get in touch with your doctor.

Influenza: The fever associated with influenza (flu) can be harmful to the foetus. A significant rise in body temperature sustained for more than a day may cause abnormalities in the developing foetus in the early weeks of pregnancy and can cause miscarriage. In the latter weeks it can lead to more serious illness and can even cause you to go into labour pre-term. Do not be tempted to take any medication to control your symptoms without consulting your doctor. Get in touch with your doctor if your temperature rises above 102°F for half a day or more.

Thrush: Thrush is caused by a yeast-type of fungal infection and is typified by itchiness in and around the vagina, and a thick whitish yellow discharge that may have an unpleasant smell. Some women find that they are more susceptible to thrush during pregnancy. It is extremely common and can be very uncomfortable, but it will do the foetus no harm. It should be treated for your own comfort if nothing else, and can be treated successfully with antifungal creams and pessaries which are harmless to the foetus. Unfortunately, even if it clears up completely it can recur.

Tummy bugs: The microscopic viruses that cause gastro-enteritis (upset tummies with diarrhoea, vomiting and abdominal cramps) are very unlikely to harm your baby. You may find that you are unable to eat or to 'hold anything down' for a day or so, and this too should do the foetus no harm; it may not be advisable to force yourself to eat, because food can aggravate and prolong the condition. It is very important that you drink enough fluids when you have gastro-enteritis, otherwise you will become dehydrated. Your doctor may be able to prescribe you a special powder to mix with your drinks to replace the vitamins and minerals that are leached out of your body when you have diarrhoea and vomiting. Contact your doctor if you cannot keep water down, or if you have any fever with your other symptoms.

Effects of Common 'Childhood Diseases' on the Foetus
(listed alphabetically)

Most of the so-called childhood diseases (which can usually be contracted at any age) are now fairly rare in Britain because babies and young children are systematically inoculated against them. It is still possible for a pregnant woman to contract them, especially if she did not contract them or was not immunised against them as a child, and if she works in an environment that brings her into contact with children. It is not generally thought to be possible for the foetus to contract or be affected by any of these diseases if the mother is immune to them.

Chicken pox: If you contract chicken pox in the first trimester of your pregnancy there is a very small risk of birth defects in your baby and also a risk of miscarriage. In addition, i you contract it at the very end of your pregnancy – within days of delivery – there is a fairly high risk that your baby will be infected. As with measles, chicken pox can be a very serious illness in the newborn infant. As well as the attendant risks to the foetus and the baby, you yourself may be struck fairly hard by the disease, and it can lead to a number of complications, including a related form of pneumonia.

Measles: Measles contracted by a woman during her pregnancy is not known to have any effects on the foetus, although the mother herself may be particularly ill with it. If the mother is infected at the end of her pregnancy or while she is breastfeeding there is a very high chance that she will pass on the disease to her baby, and the baby may become very ill with it. If you suspect that you or your newborn baby has measles let your doctor know; he may prescribe gammaglobulin to help you and / or the baby cope with the disease, and to minimise the symptoms.

Mumps: If you are exposed to mumps and you are not immune to it, it can pose a threat to your baby. One effect that mumps can have is to induce contractions of the uterus: in the very early stages of pregnancy this could cause a miscarriage, and in the latter months it could make you go into labour pre-term.

Rubella: If you are not immune to rubella (German measles) and you contract it during the first few months of your pregnancy it can have a very damaging effect on your unborn child: it may cause blindness, deafness, brain damage and heart defects. Women who are planning a pregnancy are advised to have their immunity checked, but if your pregnancy was unplanned or if you were unaware of the dangers of rubella, it is not too late to have your immunity checked to put your mind at rest.

If you have had German measles or were immunised at school, you will still be immune; it is very rare to lose your immunity, but if you are in any doubt it is worth going ahead with the test. A simple blood test will assess whether or not you are immune. If you discover that you are not immune to rubella when you are already pregnant, your doctor may recommend that you have tests regularly to check that you have not contracted German measles. As with all 'childhood illnesses', rubella is becoming increasingly rare in Britain as babies are now usually immunised at 13 months; but you should be aware that there may still be a risk of catching rubella if you travel abroad.

Medication in Pregnancy

In the first three months of pregnancy the cells that make up the foetus begin to differentiate into the limbs and skeleton, the vital organs and the nervous system of your unborn child. While these crucial changes are taking place the foetus is most sensitive to the chemical changes in the mother's bloodstream caused by medication and other drugs. Some medicines can produce malformations in the foetus if they are taken at this stage in the pregnancy, and some can continue to have harmful effects even in the second and third trimester of your pregnancy.

If you are ill and you need some sort of medication to cure the illness or to control your symptoms, you should always tell your doctor or pharmacist that you are pregnant before asking them to suggest any medication for you. Even when they have prescribed or recommended some form of medication, always read labels carefully before taking them.

Remember that it is always dangerous to stock-pile old medicines and to prescribe them for yourself when you suffer similar symptoms again. This is especially true when you are pregnant – particularly because stock-piled medicines are rarely stored neatly with all the necessary notes and leaflets about contra-indications. When you first know that you are pregnant, you should clear out your medicine cabinet just in case there is something there that you might be tempted to use and that could harm your baby.

There are some conditions which may themselves be more harmful to your own health and your foetus's development than the medications used to control them (for example, if you are asthmatic it may be more harmful to deprive your foetus of oxygen than to give it oxygen with the help of steroids). If your doctor tells you to use a medication – even for what seems to you to be a minor complaint – do not ignore his advice or secretly throw the medication away. If you are afraid that it could be harmful to your foetus discuss this with him, and take his advice.

If you are tempted to take medication just to curb the unpleasant symptoms of a common complaint such as a cold, ask your pharmacist to recommend a safe alternative to the pain-killers and decongestants you might usually use.

Effects of Common Medicines on the Foetus
(listed alphabetically)

What is known about the effects of various medicines on the foetus changes all the time, and new drugs are brought onto the market every day. The following is to give you an idea of the risks associated with common medicines.

Antibiotics: Antibiotics are used in the treatment of infections and there are a number that are known to be safe in pregnancy. So long as your doctor knows that you are pregnant when he prescribes antibiotics he should choose one that will pose no risk to the foetus.

Anti-depressants: Most anti-depressants are regarded as dangerous to the foetus: they can cause malformations. If you were on anti-depressants when you became pregnant, discuss your course of action with your doctor. If you suffer from depression during your pregnancy, talk to your doctor before taking any kind of treatment. He may call on the help of a psychiatrist or community psychiatric nurse to offer you counselling. If they decide that you would benefit from anti-depressants they will prescribe one that is regarded as being safe to use in pregnancy.

Antihistamines: Used for treating allergic conditions such as hay fever and allergic reactions such as skin irritations. They can cause drowsiness and may cause malformations in the foetus if taken in the early weeks of pregnancy. They are usually considered safe after the fourth month.

Aspirin: Aspirin is one of the most common analgesics (used to relieve pain); it is also valued for its blood-thinning properties for the treatment of a number of circulatory disorders. It is safe to use aspirin in low doses during pregnancy, and it may be used to help prevent miscarriage in some cases. In high doses, however, the blood-thinning effects of aspirin may compromise the correct development of the baby's blood-clotting mechanism, and may even cause the mother to bleed excessively during delivery. There is an increased risk of abnormality in the foetus if analgesics are taken in conjunction with alcohol.

Codeine: Codeine is a powerful analgesic often used for headaches, toothache or backache. It is present in a number of brand-name pain-killers. It can be addictive, and this means that if it is taken during pregnancy the foetus can become addicted, and the baby will suffer withdrawal symptoms after delivery. It has also been associated with certain malformations of the face such as cleft palates. There is an increased risk of abnormality in the foetus if analgesics are taken in conjunction with alcohol.

Contraceptive pill: If you became pregnant while you were using the contraceptive pill and continued to take the pill for the first weeks of your pregnancy, there is a small risk of growth defects in the foetus. Stop taking the contraceptive pill as soon as you realise you are pregnant and speak to your doctor about the particular risks associated with the brand that you were using. He may advise that you have an early ultrasound scan to assess whether the foetus has been affected.

Decongestants: Decongestants are used in cold cures, treatments for sinusitis and cough medicines to relieve mucus congestion in the nose, sinuses and lungs respectively. Some decongestants may impair the development and function of the foetal heart, even after the early weeks of pregnancy. Make sure that your doctor or pharmacist knows that you are pregnant before recommending a decongestant.

Diuretics: If you suffer from oedema (fluid retention) during your pregnancy you may be tempted to use diuretics to dispel the excess fluid. Diuretics may cause problems with the correct formation of the foetal blood cells and circulatory system. It may also be dangerous to mask the symptom of oedema as it can act as an indicator of serious conditions that can affect you in pregnancy. Check with your doctor or pharmacist whether it is safe to use diuretics.

Paracetamol: This very common analgesic can be taken in tablet form, and it is also present in a number of cold and flu cures, and brand-name pain-killers. Although paracetamol has been associated with an increased risk of kidney and liver malformations if used in the early weeks of pregnancy, it is generally regarded as the safest analgesic to use during pregnancy. Certainly in the second and third trimesters it is unlikely to harm the foetus. There is an increased risk of abnormality in the foetus if analgesics are taken in conjunction with alcohol.

Steroids: Steroids are used in some of the stronger treatments for hay fever and allergic forms of asthma and eczema. There is a small risk of malformation of the foetus if they are used in early pregnancy and, because they are chemically similar to male sex-hormones, they may compromise the normal development of the sexual organs of a female foetus if taken in large quantities. If your doctor advises you to continue using steroids during your pregnancy, you should take his advice: in certain cases the benefits of the drug outweigh the risks to the foetus.

Travel-sickness pills: Many travel sickness pills (and other anti-nausea drugs that you may be tempted to use to combat morning sickness) contain antihistamines and other ingredients which may cause malformations in the foetus if they are used in the early weeks of pregnancy. Some women notice that they are more prone to travel-sickness during pregnancy. If you do suffer from travel-sickness or other nausea, try to overcome the nausea using the suggestions made in the feature on **Morning Sickness** in **Week 6** of the **Your Pregnancy Week by Week** section.

Alternative Therapies and Medicines During Pregnancy
(listed alphabetically)

Many people recognise the real or perceived risks of using conventional medicines even when a pregnancy is not implicated, and they turn to alternative therapies and remedies to treat a variety of conditions. The risks to the foetus posed by conventional medicines are well researched and documented (some of them are listed above), but pregnant women should do some research before turning to alternative remedies to treat their symptoms. The effects of alternative therapies and remedies on the unborn child have not always been thoroughly studied or published, and it is certainly never safe to assume that – because something is ancient, traditional or alternative – it will not harm your unborn child.

The following descriptions of a number of alternative therapies are only intended as an introduction. If you are considering using an alternative therapy to relieve symptoms of any kind during your pregnancy, you should read more specialised material on the subject or contact an organisation that specialises in that therapy (you may find some useful addresses and telephone numbers at the back of the book). The practitioners of some or all of these alternative therapies may be unwilling to treat a woman in the first trimester of pregnancy; this does not necessarily imply that the treatment poses any threat to the foetus, the practitioners are merely protecting themselves from being blamed for the miscarriages that might occur during that period anyway.

Acupressure: Acupressure works on the same principles as acupuncture (see below) except that here, instead of inserting a needle, a firm and sustained pressure is applied to the relevant point on the body. Once you have learned the acupressure points you can apply the pressure yourself or even buy special bands to apply pressure more permanently to the acupressure point. As with acupuncture, acupressure can be used quite safely during pregnancy, and may even be helpful in the treatment of morning sickness. If you have acupressure treatment or use acupressure on yourself, make sure that the person treating you is aware of the acupressure points that may not be safe to use during pregnancy.

Acupuncture: The theories on which acupuncture is based were developed in China more than 5000 years ago. Chinese doctors developed these theories by observing patients and their symptoms: they concluded that every kind of illness was caused by an imbalance of forces in the body (the female force *yin* and the male force *yang*) which interrupted the flow of energy (*qi*) between the organs of the body along routes called meridians. By inserting a very fine needle into a recognised point along the interrupted meridian, the flow of energy and the Yin – Yang balance could be restored.

Although many people recoil from the idea of 'having needles stuck in' them, most people who have acupuncture treatment experience little or no pain, and have an immediate feeling of wellbeing after their treatment. This feeling is probably related to the release of endorphins (natural pain-killers, which respond to the puncturing of the skin) and not to a miraculous cure. The mechanics of how acupuncture actually works cannot be satisfactorily explained by conventional medicine, but this does not make it a less effective form of therapy.

Acupuncture can be practised safely on a pregnant woman by an experienced practitioner. It has even been used successfully in the treatment of morning sickness and other complaints brought on by the pregnancy itself. The British Acupuncture Council recognises that acupuncture can be a very helpful therapy in pregnancy but warns that there are certain acupuncture points on a pregnant woman that should not be used. It is, therefore, very important to ensure that your practitioner is fully qualified, has experience of treating pregnant women and knows that you are pregnant.

Aromatherapy: The modern use of aromatherapy was launched by a French chemist called Gattefosse, although there is documentation of Egyptian, Chinese and Indian civilisations using plant oils and unguents up to 4000 years ago. The theory of aromatherapy is that the powerful oils (essential oils) obtained from plant sources can have a variety of beneficial effects on the body. These changes are produced physiologically because the oils activate certain enzymes and hormones, and psychologically as the individual responds to the smell of the oil. The oils are not used to treat conditions but symptoms, for example an 'invigorating' oil could be used to overcome tiredness that may have been caused by physical or emotional strain.

The oils should never be ingested or applied to the skin neat but can be used in a number of ways. A few drops of essential oil can be added to a bath (this works best if the oil is first mixed with a spoonful of milk so that it is diffused throughout the bath water); or to a 'base' oil such as sweet almond oil which can then be used to massage the essential oil into the skin. Essential oils can also be used more topically, for example for a headache, if a few drops are added to a hot or cold compress. Finally, they can be used to give a therapeutic ambience to a room if a few drops are put into a bowl of water on a radiator.

It is tempting to assume that these oils derived from plant sources are absolutely harmless, but there are a number of essential oils that should not be used at all during pregnancy and others that should not be used for at least the first trimester. Aromatherapy can be a useful therapy for the stresses and strains of pregnancy and can even be used in the treatment of morning sickness (oils of ginger, mints and citrus fruits are said to be particularly beneficial).

If you already have a collection of essential oils at home, speak to an experienced aromatherapist about which ones are safe to use during pregnancy. If you are thinking about using aromatherapy during your pregnancy in order to avoid using conventional treatments for minor complaints, contact a trained aromatherapist or read the labels carefully before buying any oils from a health shop.

Chiropractic: Chiropractic is a system of treatment in which manipulation of the body, especially the spine, is used to correct mechanical dysfunctions of the joints which can be the underlying cause of pain, discomfort or even disease. The philosophy behind chiropractic is that the body is capable of healing itself; when – through accident or lifestyle – a joint or vertebra becomes slightly misaligned, chiropractic manipulation can restore normal alignment and allow self-healing.

Chiropractic is a safe, drug-free treatment; after medicine and dentistry, it is the third largest primary health care profession in the western world. It can be used to treat a range of complaints including back pain, sciatica, tension headaches, migraine and neck, shoulder and arm pains. Many of these sorts of joint and muscular pains and disorders may be brought on by pregnancy, and it is safe to have chiropractic treatment during pregnancy. If you are prone to backache or other aches and pains, it may be worth speaking to a chiropractor even before conception to see whether the problem can be corrected before it is aggravated by the muscle-relaxing effects of progesterone. A chiropractor will also be able to give you more general advice on posture, diet and other aspects of your lifestyle.

If you are interested in having chiropractic treatment during pregnancy it is important that you find a practitioner who has experience of treating pregnant women, and you should let him or her know that you are pregnant before having treatment. The British Chiropractic Association (whose address appears at the end of the book) may be able to provide you with a list of registered chiropractors in your area.

Herbal medicine: The use of herbs in medicine has been documented for nearly 5000 years and is still widespread to this day. Many conventional Western medicines are based on herb and spice extracts, and traditional herbal medicine is enjoying renewed popularity in the Western world.

Herbal medications are usually taken in the form of infusions or decoctions (teas made from various parts of the plant), although they can also be made into ointments or pastes. Traditionally, the entire plant is used and herbal medications are, therefore, not as potent or potentially dangerous as the essential oils used in aromatherapy. Most herbal remedies can be taken quite safely during pregnancy, but there are a number of herbs that are contra-indicated. If you are interested in trying herbal remedies during your pregnancy to avoid using mainstream drugs, you should try contacting a medical herbalist who will not only tell you which herbs are safe for you to use, but may prepare combinations of herbs specifically to treat your symptoms.

Homeopathy: Homeopathy is a relatively new therapy, devised just over 200 years ago by Samuel Hahnemann in Germany. The word homeopathy means 'treating with the same', and the principle of homeopathy is to treat an illness with a minute dose of a medication which – in larger doses – would produce the same symptoms as the illness. The well-documented success of homeopathic treatment has not been satisfactorily explained scientifically, but this should not detract from its validity as an alternative therapy.

The drugs used in homeopathy may be plant or mineral extracts, or combinations of the two. They are used in such tiny doses that they pose no threat to the foetus. Homeopathy is, therefore, a very useful alternative to mainstream drugs during pregnancy, and it has been used successfully in the treatment of morning sickness.

In order to benefit from homeopathic treatment you need to pay very special attention to your symptoms, because the treatments are designed to match symptoms not to cure specific conditions. If you are interested in having homeopathic treatment during your pregnancy, it would be worth contacting a registered homeopath who can get to know you and will know how to match your particular symptoms with a treatment.

Hypnotherapy: Hypnosis has been used in the treatment of a variety of physical and psychological conditions since 1842, and it was especially popular in the late nineteenth century. The hypnotist puts the subject into a state of deep relaxation and – traditionally – cured them of their complaint by telling them or suggesting to them that they would no longer suffer from it. The British Hypnotherapy Association is at pains to point out that it no longer endorses or recommends the use of suggestion in hypnotherapy, but that the state of relaxation should be used to explore the subject's underlying psychological reasons for having a complaint, by helping the subject to remember and to bring problems to the surface.

Hypnotherapy can be used quite safely during pregnancy, because it is non-invasive and uses no drugs. There is no danger that you will be controlled by your hypnotist or made to do anything against your will. Hypnotherapy can be used to give you a 'psychological spring clean' before your baby is born, possibly making your experience of labour and birth easier and more relaxed, and reducing your chances of suffering from postnatal depression (which may be triggered by long-standing underlying psychological problems).

There are a great many hypnotherapists who advertise their services and make impressive claims about what they can do for their subjects. If you are thinking of contacting a hypnotherapist, it is worth asking the British Hypnotherapy Association for the name of a registered practitioner in your area rather than responding to an advertisement (their address appears at the end of the book).

Osteopathy: Osteopathy is a system of healing in which the bones and muscles are manipulated and / or massaged to correct the equilibrium of the musculo-skeletal system. It is useful in the treatment of aches and pains in all parts of the body, postural problems and even digestive disorders; it might be helpful in the treatment of backache during pregnancy. Osteopathy poses no threat to the unborn child, but you should let your osteopath know that you are pregnant so that manipulations that involve pressing on the lower abdomen can be avoided.

Reflexology: Reflexology is a non-invasive treatment which aims to help the body balance itself and improve its own flow of energy by the application of controlled pressure to recognised points on the feet. There is no satisfactory scientific explanation for the theory that the major organs are affected by pressure on specific points of the foot, but reflexology should not be ignored as it is an effective drug-free form of therapy.

Reflexology is considered safe during pregnancy, and research has shown that it can be a relaxing, complementary way of dealing with some problems associated with pregnancy such as high blood pressure and heartburn. It can also be used successfully to relax women in labour. Before having reflexology treatment you should ensure that your practitioner is fully trained and registered, has experience of treating pregnant subjects, and knows that you are pregnant.

Stress and Pregnancy

We all experience moments of stress in our lives, and a certain amount of stress is stimulating and even beneficial, although the amount of stress that a person finds beneficial rather than destructive varies considerably from one individual to another. When we are presented with a stressful situation – whether it is a physical stress such as the need to run for a bus suddenly, or a psychological one such as an astronomical telephone bill – our bodies always respond in the same way. The hormone adrenaline is released into the bloodstream: it speeds up the heart rate, making us more alert and ready for rapid physical activity.

For most animals, stressful situations demand a physical response – fight or flight – and physical activity exploits the special state of alertness created by the adrenaline, and disperses the adrenaline itself. Most of our sources of stress in an industrialised country (that telephone bill for example) do not require physical action, so that the adrenaline is not exploited or dispersed. The heart rate and blood pressure remain artificially elevated by the effects of adrenaline and may not have a chance to recover before the next stressful stimulus pushes them up again.

Some people thrive on the stress associated with high-powered jobs and decision-making, but we all have a threshold beyond which our bodies find it difficult to cope with stressful stimuli. Even a succession of small problems can have a dramatic cumulative effect, causing a build-up of stress responses. If the body is constantly reacting to stressful stimuli, the person becomes nervous and jumpy, possibly argumentative and unable to concentrate. They may lose their appetite, suffer constipation or diarrhoea, and have difficulty sleeping. The body's resistance to infection will be lowered, making them more susceptible to coughs, colds and other contagious illnesses.

Prolonged stress is detrimental to health at any time, but it can be especially damaging in pregnancy. Pregnant women are anyway susceptible to sleeping difficulties, lack of appetite and reduced immune responses; they will be doubling the physical and psychological demands on themselves if these problems are compounded by stress. Stress in pregnancy is associated with low birth-weight babies, with an increased incidence of depression during pregnancy and with postnatal depression.

There are three ways of dealing with stress: avoiding the stressful stimuli in the first place, looking after your health (so that your body is best equipped to cope with stressful situations and its own response to them), and countering the stress response when it occurs.

Avoiding Stress

This certainly sounds obvious but it might also seem impossible; if your job or financial status causes stress you may feel you cannot avoid stress. It is important to remember that stressful stimuli have a cumulative effect: you may set standards for yourself, or try to do too many things in too little time as well as having a demanding job or financial worries. On days when you feel particularly over-wrought, make a list of everything that you have done and see whether they were all essential. Rewrite a prioritised list, so that next time you do only the things that really matter. Try to think of things on your lists that could be delegated to other people, and do not take on new commitments. Then write a list of the things that have caused you anxiety. Think them through or talk about them with someone else – you may find that by talking about them they lose some of their 'stress-value'.

Looking After your Health

If you are fit and well you are far more likely to cope well with the effects of even sustained stress. Part of your stress response is psychological, and you should not lose sight of the old adage: a sound mind in a sound body. Make sure that you have a well-balanced diet, that you get plenty of sleep and exercise, and avoid smoking (see the guidelines for a healthy lifestyle in the chapter **Preparing for Pregnancy**).

Countering the Stress Response

There are a number of ways of dealing with your pent-up energy when your body responds to a stressful situation. One of the most effective is to take some exercise; you may not be in a position or in a physical state to run a mile, but you might be able to run up a few flights of stairs or just walk briskly around the garden a few times. The physical demands and the regular breathing induced by even slight exercise will diffuse much of the tension.

Breathing is a key to the release of tension. Even if you cannot take exercise you can concentrate on taking deep breaths to help you relax (take slow deep breaths on a count of ten, then release on a count of ten; or breathe in, hold for a count of ten and breathe out). Singing is another excellent way of releasing tension and controlling your breathing. It is also something that you can do almost anywhere, self-consciousness permitting: if your drive to work is very stressful, turn the music up and sing!

If you feel angry or have pent-up feelings of resentment or fear, it might help to take your feelings out on an inanimate object such as a pillow or something satisfyingly firm such as the back of an armchair. Your adrenaline is preparing you for a 'fight' response, but society tells you that that would be inappropriate behaviour. The longer you go on controlling your feelings, the more strain you are putting on yourself, and it is perfectly healthy to release aggressive tension by punching an inanimate object. Taking a deep breath and screaming or shouting at the top of your voice is also a very refreshing release, although it is not always easy to find a sufficiently open or private place to do this without attracting attention!

Use any techniques at your disposal to relax yourself – breathing exercises, warm baths, massage – because this will help you to sleep, and sleep is vital if you are to cope with stress successfully.

Depression and Pregnancy

If you are suffering from depression – especially if you are taking anti-depressants – when you become pregnant it is important that you let your doctor know, because he may want to change your treatment. The effects of anti-depressants on the foetus are not well documented, and few anti-depressants are considered safe in pregnancy. All but the most extreme cases of depression can be treated very satisfactorily with counselling from a psychiatric nurse or a psychiatrist.

A small percentage of women become depressed during pregnancy. In some cases this is the result of factors that would have led to depression even if there had not been a pregnancy; in others, the pregnancy itself can be a contributory factor. The additional physical and psychological stresses of pregnancy can bring on periods of mild or even moderate depression, especially in women with financial, domestic or health problems, or those prone to mood swings, pre-menstrual syndrome or mental illness.

Depression is typified by feelings of emptiness, flatness and futility, which may be accompanied by permanent tiredness, sleeping difficulties, lack of appetite (or excessive appetite), an inability to make decisions, and indifference to normal interests. Depression rarely just 'goes away': if it is left untreated it can become far more serious, ultimately threatening the victim's own health and safety, and – in the case of a pregnant woman – that of her baby.

It is important to remember that there should be no stigma attached to depression: it is caused by a chemical imbalance affecting our moods, rather as diabetes is caused by a chemical imbalance that affects our ability to metabolise sugars. Talking to your doctor about depression, and understanding what it is, can be important steps on the road to recovery. If you think that you are suffering from depression, or have had any of the symptoms listed above continuously for more than a week, it would be worth talking to your partner and to your doctor.

Chronic Conditions During Pregnancy
(listed alphabetically)

If you suffer from a chronic condition and are now pregnant or are planning a pregnancy, the chances are that you will already have discussed with your doctor the implications of your condition and the necessary medication on your pregnancy. The following paragraphs give only an outline of the effects and limitations of the most common chronic conditions on pregnancy.

Anorexia and bulimia: The anorexic and the bulimic, if they conceive at all, go into pregnancy at a great disadvantage because their bodies are not correctly nourished: the anorexic is very undernourished and is unlikely to be able to supply the foetus with the full compliment of vitamins and mineral; the bulimic leaches her body of vital nutrients by inducing vomiting or diarrhoea, and could also harm the foetus by using laxatives and diuretics. The long-term health of both mother and baby are threatened.

One of the problems with eating disorders is that the sufferer is often very secretive about and ashamed of their condition. If you suffer from anorexia or bulimia and you are pregnant or are planning a pregnancy, try to use your pregnancy as the motivation to seek help from your doctor or a support group. These are not physical disorders, they have their roots in psychological problems, and you need to address these problems for your physical and psychological wellbeing if you are to carry a baby and become a parent.

Asthma: Mild asthma may not pose problems during pregnancy, but in about 30% of sufferers, asthma can be aggravated by pregnancy, especially in the latter months when women are prone to breathlessness (it can also remain stable or be improved). Bad asthma can have more serious implications for the foetus.

If you are asthmatic you very probably know the allergens or circumstances that trigger your attacks. However, during your pregnancy you should be especially vigilant about avoiding these triggers and about your general health so that you are not prone to coughs, colds and influenza. Your doctor will tell you which drugs are safe to use and in what doses as preventatives and to overcome attacks. Do not be tempted to skip medication to spare your baby from the effects of the drugs: the lack of oxygen is more potentially damaging than the drugs. If you should suffer from an attack and the drugs that you have been prescribed cannot control it, contact your own doctor or your local hospital immediately for further assistance.

Diabetes: You may have had diabetes for years when you become pregnant or you may develop it during pregnancy; in either case, diabetes can threaten the health of mother and baby if it is not detected or properly monitored and treated. You will have to do a lot of self-monitoring in order to keep your diabetes under control and to maintain a steady blood sugar level, but if you do you will have no higher risk than a non-diabetic of having any other complications during your pregnancy.

It is important that you listen to and follow the instructions given to you by your obstetrician and / or your doctor. You will certainly be given detailed instructions about what and how often to eat (to keep your blood sugar levels steady) and to keep a close eye on your weight gain (excessive weight gain is associated with diabetes in pregnancy and can lead to further complications). You will be encouraged to take regular light exercise to boost your metabolism, and to get plenty of rest so as not to sap your energy. You will have to monitor your blood sugar levels and take medication regularly throughout the day.

If you do not follow these instructions and maintain stable blood sugar levels, your own health and that of your baby may be threatened. The most common problems with poorly controlled diabetes are that the placenta begins to fail towards the end of the pregnancy, depriving the foetus of nutrients and oxygen, and that the foetus grows very large, making a normal vaginal delivery impossible.

Epilepsy: Epileptic seizures may have a damaging effect on the foetus, as may some of the drugs used in the treatment of epilepsy. If you suffer from epilepsy it is advisable to speak to your doctor when you are planning a pregnancy so that he can plan a drug strategy for you, at least for the first trimester of the pregnancy when the foetus is most vulnerable to the effects of drugs. If your pregnancy was not planned you should let your doctor know immediately that you are pregnant so that he can adjust your medication. He may offer to carry out tests on the foetus to see whether it has been adversely affected by drugs.

Epileptic women are usually monitored more closely during pregnancy and may be prescribed a number of vitamins that are deficient in epileptics or leached out by the medication they take. If you find that the frequency and severity of seizures or the effectiveness of your medication changes during your pregnancy, let your doctor know immediately so that he can review the drugs and dosages that he is giving you.

Heart disease and coronary artery disease: In all but the extreme cases of heart disease and coronary artery disease (CAD) a woman and her baby should be able to cope with pregnancy and childbirth, but they will need careful monitoring.

Pregnancy makes enormous demands on the heart and coronary artery: not only does the heart grow and have to work much harder, pumping more blood around the body more quickly, its 'workspace' is also restricted as the uterus pushes up towards the chest. Women with heart disease and CAD have traditionally been advised not to become pregnant and to terminate accidental pregnancies because of the risk to their own and the babies' lives. If you have heart disease or CAD and you are pregnant or planning a pregnancy you should speak to your doctor immediately about your own condition, how serious it is and how it would be affected by pregnancy.

Pregnant women with heart disease and CAD will be advised to moderate their weight gain, to take only very light exercise and to avoid stress which makes further demands on the heart. They may need to spend much of their pregnancy resting, and they may be advised to have a Caesarean section to avoid the exertion of delivery.

Hypertension: Chronic hypertension (high blood pressure) in pregnancy can pose a threat to the mother and the baby especially because in some cases pregnancy causes a raising of blood pressure anyway. If you suffer from hypertension – especially if you control it with medication – and you are pregnant or are planning a pregnancy it is important that you contact your doctor immediately so that he can adjust your medication and dosage in the light of this.

To reduce the risks to your own health and that of your baby, you and the baby will be closely monitored throughout the pregnancy. You may be asked to monitor your blood pressure regularly yourself and to be especially alert to any changes in your body (you will be particularly prone to the dangerous condition pre-eclampsia, see the chapter **When Things Go Wrong**). You will need to avoid stressful situations, to rest and relax frequently and to stick to a healthy diet, in order to give yourself the best chance of enjoying a normal pregnancy. Do not be tempted to skip your medication if you are feeling well and your blood pressure has dropped: the dangers posed by a rapid rise in blood pressure are greater than those posed by a medication prescribed by a doctor who knew you were pregnant.

If you do suffer from a chronic condition and you are pregnant or are planning a pregnancy it is very important that you discuss your individual case, your needs, diet and medication with your own doctor or specialist. It is also important that, despite the 'special needs' that may be associated with your condition, you remember that pregnancy is a normal and healthy process. It might be helpful to contact support groups and speak to other women who are having or have had the same experiences as yourself (you may find some useful addresses at the back of this book).

Chapter 4

When Things Go Wrong

There are a number of conditions or symptoms that can develop at various stages during a pregnancy and may give cause for concern. You should be alert to changes in your body and how you feel, because – in most cases – if conditions are identified and treated early enough they should not threaten the health of the mother or the baby.

I f they go undetected and untreated there are a number of conditions that can actually be fatal to both mother and baby. Potentially fatal problems only occur in a small percentage of women, but – when you consider how many thousands of women are pregnant at any one time – you cannot assume that you will not be affected.

Some of the more common problems that occur in pregnancy are explained below. They appear in alphabetical order.

Abdominal Pain

It is not unusual for women to experience abdominal pain in the last trimester of pregnancy. This may be caused by flatulence or by the strain posed on the round ligaments that support the uterus. These conditions may be uncomfortable but do not pose any threat to the mother or the foetus. If a woman has acute abdominal pain, it could, of course, be caused by an unrelated disorder such as appendicitis and it should be investigated immediately. If acute abdominal pain is felt very early in the pregnancy – perhaps even before you realise you are pregnant – you may have an ectopic pregnancy (see **Ectopic Pregnancy**, below), which can have very serious consequences.

Abnormalities Detected in the Foetus

Even if you are in good health and your pregnancy seems to be progressing normally, there are a number of abnormalities and illnesses that can affect your foetus, threatening your chances of having a normal, healthy baby. These may be chromosomal abnormalities such as Down's Syndrome or physical defects which can range from the minor hare-lip to debilitating physical abnormalities and physiological disorders.

There are extensive screening facilities available to check for abnormalities in the foetus (for explanations of the tests available and the abnormalities they may be able to detect see **Your Pregnancy Week by Week: Week 10** for the nuchal fold test; **Week 16** for alpha-fetoprotein (AFP) test, triple test, amniocentesis and chorionic villus sampling (CVS); and **Week 18** for ultrasound scan). Some hospitals carry out one or several tests routinely on all pregnant women in their care, and many hospitals offer several tests to women who are perceived to be at high risk of having a baby with abnormalities either because of their age, their blood group, their health or their family history.

Before you decide to have any tests on your unborn child, you need to think about why you are having them performed. Few of these tests are 100% reliable and some carry a small risk of causing a miscarriage. Are you having these tests to reassure yourself that the baby you are carrying is normal and, if so, are the risks worth taking? If you discover that your baby has some kind of abnormality, what action would you take? You may be faced with the decision to terminate your pregnancy, or you may use this early warning to prepare for a baby with special needs and find out as much as possible about your baby's condition.

If any test result shows that there is something wrong with the foetus, it may take you some time fully to understand the implications of this test result. If there is anything that you do not understand, or if you were too shocked to take the information in when you first received the news, speak to your doctor; he or she will explain exactly what the results mean and what courses of action are open to you. You may be offered a termination and, if this is something you want to consider, you may be under pressure to make a decision quickly before the legal limit for abortions elapses in the twenty-fourth week.

Whether you choose to continue with your pregnancy or to terminate it, you will have to come to terms with a very different picture of the future to the one you may have been imagining so far. It can be an enormous strain on your physical and psychological resources and on your relationship with your partner. It is very important that you talk about your feelings and your plans for this pregnancy with your partner, your doctor and possibly your own family and friends. Whatever you decide to do, you will need a great deal of support from them. There are also many organisations that can give you advice and support whether you choose to terminate your pregnancy or to keep your baby. Their addresses are listed at the back of this book.

CASE STUDY: *'I had all the usual tests done, but no extra ones. I was lucky though, they never came up with any problems, and I never really thought about what I would have done if anything had been wrong. In a way, I think having the test is like half admitting that you would have an abortion if there was something wrong, and I'm not sure that's a good thing.'*

Abnormalities Detected in Urine

You will be asked to take a urine sample to every check-up during your pregnancy so that your midwife can check for any abnormalities in the urine. Regular urine tests are a useful way of checking for problems that can arise during pregnancy.

The presence of sugars in your urine sample could mean that you have developed a form of diabetes known as **gestational diabetes** (see Gestational Diabetes, below). Diabetes need not pose any threat to the wellbeing of mother or baby if it is detected and controlled.

If proteins are detected in your urine, this could imply that you have an infection of the urinary tract. Your doctor will probably check whether you have any fever, and may ask whether you have a burning sensation when you pass water. Urinary tract infections need to be dealt with speedily with antibiotics (there are several antibiotics that are known to be safe, even in the first trimester of pregnancy). Left unchecked, the infections can spread to the kidneys, possibly causing long-term damage, or even into the vagina, coming perilously close to the cervix and the uterus.

Protein in the urine is also one of the symptoms of pre-eclampsia (see **Pre-eclampsia**, below). If you have signs of protein in your urine, and any of the other symptoms of pre-eclampsia, your doctor will take immediate action to treat the problem.

Baby's Size

One of the most obvious ways of assessing whether a foetus is developing normally is to check that it is growing at the optimum rate by comparing its size to the expected size of the foetus at the same stage in the pregnancy. The size of the foetus can be measured approximately by measuring the height of the fundus (the distance from your pelvic bone to the top of the uterus, this distance grows by about 1cm [½in] a week as the uterus pushes upwards in the abdomen); and by abdominal palpation to feel the actual size of the foetus (after about week 20). An accurate reading of the foetus's size can be obtained during an ultrasound scan.

If your baby is found to be smaller or larger than expected this could mean that your dates are not accurate. Further measurements taken using an ultrasound scan will probably be able to assess the exact age of the pregnancy and you may be given a revised due date. If your baby is smaller or larger than expected but its stage of development implies that your dates are correct, the foetus is said to be small-for-dates or large-for-dates respectively. Neither of these are necessarily cause for concern, but they could be an indication of more serious problems and – especially in the case of large-for-dates babies – they could mean that you may need a Caesarean section.

If you attend all your antenatal clinics, your doctor or midwife will soon pick up on the fact if you have a small- or large-for-dates baby. They will implement further tests and they may ask you questions about your lifestyle to assess why the baby is not growing at the expected rate. It may then be possible to take action to help the foetus to grow at a more normal rate.

Small-for-dates Babies

A baby may grow more slowly than expected for a number of reasons connected with the mother's lifestyle and general state of health: if the mother is very underweight, fails to gain weight in pregnancy or takes excessive exercise; if she smokes, drinks excessively or abuses drugs; if she has an on-going or chronic illness, or becomes ill during her pregnancy; or if she is under great psychological stress. Complications of pregnancy such as repeated vaginal bleeding and placenta praevia also increase the likelihood of having a small-for-dates baby.

When the mother's lifestyle is implicated it is possible to improve the foetus's growth rate if the mother has the will and the will-power to make the changes. If you know that you are carrying a small-for-dates baby think carefully about the tips for a healthy lifestyle given in the chapter **Preparing for Pregnancy**: it is never too late to start living healthily. Your baby is pre-programmed to thrive as best it can in the womb: if you make a dramatic turn around now, so could the foetus, possibly catching up completely with its own expected weight.

If the problem is related to illness or a complication in pregnancy, good nutrition and as much rest as possible (complete bed-rest in some cases) coupled with safe treatment for specific conditions where appropriate, are the best way of improving foetal growth. The mother's energies will not be sapped by her own activities and can be channelled into growing a healthy baby.

You and the foetus will be monitored more closely if you are carrying a small-for-dates baby. If the foetus continues to be very small or shows signs of stress after the twenty-eighth week of pregnancy (when its chances of survival in a special care baby unit are good), the baby may be delivered by inducing labour or by Caesarean section. If you go to term and are known to be carrying a very small-for-dates baby, you may be advised to have your baby in a hospital with a special care baby unit, where babies with even very low birth weights have a good chance of survival.

Large-for-dates Babies

One of the commonest incidences of large-for-dates babies is in mothers who have diabetes: the excesses of blood sugar passing through the placenta are turned into fat stores under the baby's skin. Women who are themselves overweight are also more likely to have large-for-dates babies.

The most important implication with a large-for-date baby is that the mother will be unlikely to have the baby vaginally because of the disproportion between the size of the baby's head and the mother's pelvis. If a baby is growing very large, the mother may be induced or given a Caesarean section pre-term in order to avoid further complications and unnecessary strain on the mother's body. (Although the baby will appear fully-grown, it may not be fully developed and it is likely to need the special care given to any pre-term baby). If the baby is allowed to go to term it is very likely that a Caesarean section will be necessary.

Full-term, large babies born to healthy mothers should not need any special care (although they may have proportionately larger appetites!); those born to diabetic mothers may need special care similar to the care given to pre-term babies.

Blood Pressure Problems

Your blood pressure should be taken every time that you have a check-up throughout your pregnancy, not only because it is a good indication of your general state of health and how your heart is coping with the demands of pregnancy, but because changes in blood pressure can be indicators of more serious problems, which will require treatment.

As your pregnancy progresses you actually produce more blood and your metabolic rate is raised so that the blood is pumped around your body at a faster rate than usual. By the end of the pregnancy your heart may be working 30 to 50% harder than it was in your pre-pregnancy state. Blood is pumped from your heart through your arteries, and the walls of the arteries offer resistance to the flow of blood. This resistance may be raised or lowered during pregnancy by the effects of pregnancy hormones on the lining of the arteries. If the resistance is very high, your blood pressure reading will be high, and your heart will have to work even harder to pump the blood around your body.

Understanding your Blood Pressure Readings

On your notes, your blood pressure readings will appear as a high figure – say 125 – over a lower one, say 80. The high figure (the systolic level) is the reading taken when your heart muscle contracts, pumping blood out; the lower figure (the diastolic level) is taken when the heart muscle is resting between beats. The higher figure may be raised when you are taking exercise or if you are dealing with a stressful situation, and an occasional reading of up to about 140 need not be cause for concern. The lower figure remains steadier and a rise in this figure is, therefore, a more important indication of possible problems.

High Blood Pressure (Hypertension)

If the lower figure of your blood pressure rises to 90 or more (and the higher figure is then likely to be 135 or over) your blood pressure will be considered high. It is not good for you or the baby for your blood pressure to remain high, and it could lead to other complications. One of the problems with hypertension is that the individual may not feel any different until the blood pressure is dangerously high; without regular monitoring, hypertension could go undetected until it has become a serious threat to both mother and baby.

Moderately high blood pressure in early pregnancy may not be very serious and might well be controlled without using any medication (see **Controlling your Blood Pressure**, below). A very high reading in early pregnancy could indicate that you have diabetes or that your kidneys are not performing efficiently. It might jeopardise the normal development and growth of your baby. You would be given further tests to establish what effects the raised blood pressure was having on you and the baby; you might be given medication to lower your blood pressure and bed rest might be recommended.

In the latter half of pregnancy, especially after 28 weeks, high blood pressure can be an indicator of the life-threatening condition pre-eclampsia, which requires immediate treatment (see **Pre-eclampsia**, below).

Controlling your Blood Pressure

High blood pressure is a common problem even for people who are not pregnant, and can be caused by a number of factors, the most common being stress and a diet high in saturated fats and salt. The hormonal changes to a woman's arteries during pregnancy may add to these pre-existing factors to increase her chances of suffering from hypertension.

If you are keen to avoid using medication to control your blood pressure during pregnancy you should make sure that you are adhering to the guidelines for a healthy lifestyle outlined in the chapter **Preparing for Pregnancy**. Pay special attention to your diet, cutting down on salt and salty foods, and avoiding foods that contain animal fats, such as fatty meats, butter and lard. Keep an eye on your weight gain, and take regular gentle exercise; strenuous exercise can aggravate blood pressure problems, but gentle exercise is useful as a form of relaxation.

Relaxation and rest are crucial to controlling blood pressure. The one counters the effects of stress which is a primary cause of high blood pressure; and the other gives your body a chance to recover from the physical demands of pregnancy and stress. For ways of dealing with stress see the section on **Stress** in the chapter **Illness During Pregnancy**.

If your blood pressure cannot be controlled by adjusting your lifestyle, your doctor will prescribe medication to control it. However loath you may be to take medication, especially in the first trimester of your pregnancy, you should not be tempted to ignore your doctor's advice. Sustained hypertension poses more threats to you and your baby than medication prescribed by a doctor who knows that you are pregnant.

Low Blood Pressure

It is not uncommon for a woman's blood pressure to drop during pregnancy, and it may drop further after about the twentieth week when the placenta begins to take on some of the work of pumping blood to the foetus, reducing the workload of the mother's heart. Although a low blood pressure is considered healthy and is usually a good sign, it can occasionally drop so low (to 80/50 or even lower) that the mother begins to feel faint. Some of the symptoms associated with periods of low blood pressure are: feeling floppy, absent or faint; actually fainting; a fluttering heart and trembling fingers and limbs (these last two indicate an accelerated heart-rate which is symptomatic of low blood pressure). If you do feel faint, try to get to a source of fresh air, but most importantly sit down so that you cannot fall and hurt yourself. Try to keep your head low, between your knees if necessary, if you feel very giddy. If you faint or feel faint repeatedly you may be anaemic or you may have low blood sugar levels: you should contact your doctor so that he can check on the underlying causes and treat you accordingly.

Ectopic Pregnancy

'Ectopic' means in an abnormal position, and an ectopic pregnancy occurs when the fertilised egg implants itself anywhere other than the lining of the uterus. If the sperm travel right out of the fallopian tube towards the ovary and fertilisation takes place in the abdominal cavity, there is a chance that the fertilised egg will implant itself in the external surface of the uterus, fallopian tube, ovary or other abdominal organs. In these rare cases the foetus usually becomes detached and is lost in the abdominal cavity (although it is possible to sustain an entire pregnancy outside the uterus).

The most common form of ectopic pregnancy is called a tubal pregnancy because the fertilised egg implants itself in the lining of the fallopian tube rather than completing its journey to the uterus. It is in these incidents that the woman may experience severe abdominal pain, which may be accompanied by vaginal bleeding and fever. By about the sixth week of the pregnancy the foetus will have grown so much that it may rupture the wall of the fallopian tube, possibly damaging it permanently and irreparably, and causing infection which can damage the nearby ovary.

Ectopic pregnancies are difficult to detect before they have caused this sort of damage because there are few obvious symptoms (if you are known to be at risk of having an ectopic pregnancy – perhaps because you have had one already – it is possible to monitor hormone levels in your urine: levels of human chorionic gonadotrophin do not rise so quickly in ectopic pregnancies). If you have abdominal pain you should contact your doctor and discuss it with him because the implications not only to this pregnancy but to your future fertility are serious. If your doctor thinks that you have an ectopic pregnancy he may arrange for you to have an ultrasound scan or a laparoscopy (when a tube is inserted through a tiny incision under your navel to view the fallopian tubes).

It is not possible to save a tubal pregnancy, and the damage to the tube – or to the ovary from infection – may limit your chances of conceiving in that tube again. If the tube is very damaged or infected, it will have to be removed by surgery. This would mean that any chance of conceiving in the future is limited to the other ovary and fallopian tube.

About 1% of pregnancies implant ectopically, and women who have had an ectopic pregnancy have a greatly increased chance (about13%) of having another one. This means that women who have had an ectopic pregnancy need to be especially vigilant for symptoms of ectopic implantation in subsequent pregnancies. If one fallopian tube has been damaged or removed, you may only be able to conceive in the other fallopian tube; every effort must be made to protect this second tube from damage which would threaten your chances of conceiving naturally altogether.

Fluid Retention

During your pregnancy you may notice that your fingers, wrists and ankles become puffy or swollen so that rings, watches and shoes do not fit so comfortably. This is partly because you are putting on weight but it is also a sign of increased fluid retention, known as oedema. Pregnancy hormones alter the way in which the body eliminates fluids or retains them within body tissues.

It is common to have a certain amount of fluid retention in pregnancy, especially in the latter weeks, and a small amount of puffiness should not be cause for concern although it may be uncomfortable (for ways of alleviating slight swelling see the feature on fluid retention in **Week 31** of the **Your Pregnancy Week by Week** section).

Although a small amount of fluid retention may be unsightly, and may mean you have to remove your rings with soap and leave them off until the swelling has gone down, it should do no harm to you or your baby. Do not be tempted to drink less fluid in order to stop the build up of fluid: drinking plenty of fluids actually helps to flush out the swelling. You should not use diuretics without medical advice, because some diuretics may be harmful to the foetus, especially during the first trimester.

If your fingers become so puffy that you find it difficult to use your hands normally, if your face is swollen or if you have excessive swelling at your joints, you should let your doctor know immediately. It could mean that your kidneys are not functioning normally or that you are suffering from the dangerous condition pre-eclampsia (see **Pre-eclampsia**, below).

Gestational Diabetes

It is possible for a woman who has never had diabetes to develop diabetes when she is pregnant. This is because the way in which the body controls blood sugar levels alters during pregnancy to adapt to the requirements of the foetus, and this alteration does not always calibrate the supply and demand of blood sugars perfectly.

Gestational diabetes develops in about 5% of pregnancies, usually in the second or third trimester. About 98% of women who have gestational diabetes will regain normal blood sugar control after delivery. Although this form of diabetes is known as 'gestational' because it is brought on by the pregnancy, it does not actually differ in symptoms, mechanics or effects from pre-existing diabetes.

If gestational diabetes is detected and controlled, it need not pose any threat to the mother or the baby. If it is not detected early enough it can lead to a number of complications and can do permanent damage to the mother's and the baby's health. One common problem with diabetes in pregnancy is that the excess blood sugar supplied through the placenta causes the foetus to grow very large, greatly increasing the incidence of difficult labours, assisted deliveries and Caesarean sections.

Signs of Diabetes

The most recognisable sign that you might have diabetes is not one that you can pick up on yourself, but one that is checked for at every antenatal visit: the presence of sugar in your urine. This is another good reason to attend all your check-ups and to ensure that you take a urine sample with you. If sugar is detected in your urine, it will not necessarily mean that you have developed diabetes, but it will indicate that your metabolism is struggling to adjust to different blood sugar requirements. Your doctor or midwife may ask for another urine sample a few days or a week later: if there are sugars in the next sample you will probably be given further tests for diabetes.

There are also some physical symptoms associated with diabetes: you may feel very hungry or very thirsty, and you may need to pass urine frequently and in considerable volumes (not like in early pregnancy when you want to urinate often but produce only a little urine). If the condition is more advanced you could notice a sudden weight loss and you could have periods of giddiness, overwhelming tiredness and blurred vision (if you have any of these symptoms – with the possible exception of tiredness which may be caused by the pregnancy itself – you should contact your doctor).

Treating Diabetes

The treatment for gestational diabetes is just the same as that for pre-existing diabetes: the close monitoring – by medical staff and by the individual at home – of blood sugar levels, and controlling them with diet and, possibly, medication. The difference here is that the individual concerned has never had to deal with the problem before, and will have to learn how to cope with diabetes along with all the other extra demands of pregnancy.

It is important that you listen to and follow the instructions given to you by your obstetrician and / or your doctor. You will certainly be given detailed instructions about what and how often to eat (to keep your blood sugar levels steady) and to keep a close eye on your weight gain (excessive weight gain is associated with diabetes in pregnancy and can lead to further complications). You will be encouraged to take regular light exercise to boost your metabolism, and to get plenty of rest so as not to sap your energy. You will have to monitor your blood sugar levels at home and, in more serious cases, to take medication regularly throughout the day.

You may find it a great strain dealing with the monitoring and the complicated rules about what you are and are not allowed to eat, and you will have to remind yourself that it is for the sake of your own permanent health and your baby's. You will need plenty of help and support from your partner and family, and it may help you to contact the British Diabetic Association who can put you in touch with a local support group (their address appears at the end of the book).

> CASE STUDY: *'The worst thing about the diabetes was shopping. The first few times I went shopping, it took me two hours to get round the supermarket because I had to look at my lists and look at every label and think about what I was and wasn't allowed. You have to rethink the whole way you plan your meals, but you do adapt quite quickly.'*

To add to the ordeal, even though your own blood sugar levels may return to normal soon after delivery, your baby may suffer temporarily as a result of your diabetes. Some babies of diabetic mothers grow very large with considerable fat stores. They have problems feeding and maintaining body warmth, similar to those of a premature baby (see **Premature Labour**, below), and may have difficulty controlling their own blood sugar levels.

Incompetent Cervix

A woman is said to have an incompetent cervix if her cervix slackens towards the end of pregnancy, possibly giving rise to vaginal bleeding or to premature rupture of the membranes, causing her to go into labour pre-term. It is rare for a woman to be born with an incompetent cervix, but the ability of the cervix to remain tightly closed under the pressure of pregnancy can be compromised if a woman has had a previous very difficult labour or a poorly executed abortion.

Unfortunately, an incompetent cervix may go undetected until it is too late, that is until you have had a miscarriage and the cervix was found to be incompetent. This need not mean that you will never be able to carry a baby: you can have a small 'purse-string' stitch across the cervix (this is performed under anaesthetic) to save the next pregnancy. The stitch is then removed around the thirty-sixth week of pregnancy so that labour and delivery can occur naturally.

Miscarriage (Spontaneous Abortion)

The fear of miscarriage is probably the greatest concern of pregnant women in the early weeks of their pregnancy. Around 10% of pregnancies do abort spontaneously, although this figure is open to conjecture because some miscarriages are not reported and others may happen so early on that the woman may not even know that she was pregnant. In first pregnancies the figure is much higher, perhaps as many as 30% of first pregnancies miscarry.

The commonly held belief that physical or emotional shocks cause miscarriages is not entirely accurate. Although shocks can induce miscarriage, a high proportion of miscarriages occur quite spontaneously in the first few weeks of pregnancy. Research has shown that embryos (the name given to the foetus up to the eighth week) aborted in this way often have an abnormal arrangement of chromosomes or they are not developing correctly. The mechanism by which the mother's body recognises abnormalities and rejects them – if that is what happens – is not fully understood.

Missed Abortion

In some cases of spontaneous abortion, the embryo's growth stagnates or the embryo may even die several weeks before the woman has any suspicions that her pregnancy is not progressing normally. She may have no bleeding, experience no cramping, and she may continue to feel pregnant, because the hormones in her blood stream will still be circulating as if the pregnancy was being maintained. Sometimes, missed abortions are not diagnosed until the woman goes to her booking appointment or for an ultrasound scan, and no heartbeat or image of the foetus is picked up.

If you have a missed abortion, you will probably be given an appointment for a dilation and curettage (D & C), a simple operation in which the cervix is opened up and the uterus is cleaned of any 'products of conception' such as the rudimentary placenta. The fact that your embryo may have been abnormal might be of some comfort to you, but you may be disturbed by the thought that it died some weeks ago, and you may be concerned that the same thing could happen again. Discuss your concerns with your doctor or consultant.

CASE STUDY: *'When I went for my scan they all went very quiet and I knew something was wrong. I had to wait until they'd found the consultant, and he explained that the baby had died probably two weeks previously ... my main feeling then was to get it out, I didn't like the idea that I was going round with a dead baby inside me. It was only afterwards that I felt sad about what we had lost.'*

Threatened Abortion

If you bleed at any time in the first half of your pregnancy this could be what is known as a threatened abortion. The bleeding may be light or quite heavy and could go on for a number of days; it may be accompanied by abdominal cramps. You may not lose your baby, but the bleeding is a warning signal that your pregnancy is at risk. You should contact your doctor immediately if you have any bleeding. He may recommend that you have an ultrasound scan to see how the pregnancy is progressing. In the mean time, your best chance of preserving the pregnancy is to rest as much as possible, lying flat so that your uterus benefits from an optimum blood supply.

Inevitable Abortion

If you lose a lot of blood – possibly including blood clots – and you experience abdominal cramps like powerful menstrual cramps, you will almost inevitably miscarry. The bleeding indicates that the placenta has come away from the wall of the uterus, and the site on the uterine wall is bleeding freely; and the cramps are caused by contractions of the uterus, dilating the cervix and expelling the foetus and placenta. If you have these symptoms you should call your doctor immediately; it is very unlikely that it will be possible to save the pregnancy at this stage, but you are likely to need professional care.

Depending on how many weeks you were into your pregnancy, you may be able to recognise the tiny foetus when you miscarry, and this can be very distressing. However upsetting it may be for you, you should keep the foetus and any other tissue and membranes that you lose in a clean container; by examining these, medical professionals may be able to explain why you miscarried. You could lose a lot of blood, and your doctor may recommend that you have a D & C to ensure that all the products of the pregnancy have been expelled.

CASE STUDY: *'I had intermittent bleeding from eight weeks, then I was rushed in at twelve weeks because the bleeding suddenly increased. I lost the baby and they told us afterwards that the he wasn't growing normally and he couldn't possibly have survived. I suppose that should make me feel better about it but I just keep thinking "God, I was over a quarter of the way through, and now I've got to start all over again."'*

Why Miscarriages Happen

There are a number of different reasons why women miscarry. As explained above, it could be that there were some chromosomal abnormalities in the embryo or that it was not growing normally. It could be that the levels of pregnancy hormones failed to rise quickly enough to maintain the pregnancy, or that the placenta developed too slowly to sustain the growing foetus.

Miscarriages can also occur if the woman's uterus is an abnormal shape or has uterine fibroid tumours, or if her cervix is 'incompetent' (see **Incompetent Cervix**, above). Illness and infection in the mother are associated with an increased incidence of miscarriage, as are smoking, excessive drinking, drug abuse and exposure to radiation and certain chemicals.

Coping with a Miscarriage

A miscarriage, especially a late one, can be frightening, painful and heartbreaking. You will need the support of your partner and your family to recover from it physically and emotionally.

Many women feel as if they have failed when they have a miscarriage. You may feel bereaved, inadequate, guilty, angry and depressed. You may find it difficult to come to terms with your loss, especially if you feel that other people do not understand why you are so sad. Talking about your feelings with family, close friends, your doctor or your midwife, may help you to come to terms with the loss of your baby.

Only you will know when you are ready to try to have another baby. Physically, you may be ready to conceive very soon after the miscarriage, but it may take you longer to adjust emotionally. Even if your feelings towards another pregnancy are ambivalent, remember that you may not conceive straight away, and that the pregnancy itself will give you nine months to adjust to the idea. No subsequent pregnancy will ever replace the baby that you lost; it will be a whole new beginning.

CASE STUDY: *'I couldn't really give advice about coping with it. I don't think that I did anything in particular. I did take it very hard, and I do still think about it, but all I could think of was that I still wanted a baby so we tried again almost straight away and I was pregnant again very quickly.'*

Repeated Miscarriages

Women are often very keen to know why they had a miscarriage and whether there is anything that the medical profession can do to minimise their chances of miscarrying again. Unfortunately, because miscarriages are very common – occurring in at least 10% of all pregnancies – it may simply be bad luck if a woman has more than one miscarriage, especially if they occur at different times and for different reasons. This is known as recurrent abortion, and a doctor is unlikely to be able to offer help until a woman has had several recurrent abortions. The woman herself may be able to increase her chances of maintaining her pregnancy if she adheres to the guidelines for a healthy lifestyle laid out in the chapter **Preparing for Pregnancy**.

If a woman has successive miscarriages at about the same stage in her pregnancy and for apparently the same reason, this is known as habitual abortion. After three habitual abortions a doctor may be able to run tests to discover exactly why the woman is spontaneously aborting in the hopes of safeguarding subsequent pregnancies.

Obstetric Cholestasis

If you have excessive itching during your pregnancy it is important that you speak to your doctor or midwife: you could be suffering from a condition called obstetric cholestasis. It is not uncommon for women to have some itching, especially on the skin of the tummy as it stretches over the expanding uterus, and further itching may be caused by skin rashes and by sweating, especially in the latter stages of pregnancy, but intense burning itching sensations should not be dismissed as normal.

Recent research carried out by Queen Charlotte's Hospital has shown obstetric cholestasis, which is a malfunction of the liver brought on by the pregnancy, causes a build-up of bile salts in the mother's bloodstream which can produce terrible itching. Severe obstetric cholestasis can result in the death of the foetus: it is believed that the bile salts transferred to the foetus through the placenta may fatally damage the foetus, although the exact cause of death is not known. Obstetric cholestasis could be responsible for a significant proportion of stillbirths (perhaps as many as one in five, according to one estimate).

The itching caused by obstetric cholestasis usually begins in the last trimester of pregnancy, and it may be particularly bad on the hands and feet. It can be so intense that sufferers scratch themselves raw. If you have this sort of itching you can be given a blood test to see whether you have obstetric cholestasis; once the condition is diagnosed, close monitoring of the foetus's wellbeing is essential. It may be deemed safer to deliver the baby early than to allow the pregnancy to go to term.

Placenta Praevia

If you have vaginal bleeding that is not accompanied by abdominal pain, especially if it is in the last trimester, it could be that your placenta is positioned very low in your uterus and covers some or all of the aperture of the cervix. This is known as placenta praevia and it occurs in about 1% of pregnancies; but the percentage occurrence is even lower in first pregnancies.

Normally the placenta attaches itself high up in the uterus, but it may be forced to attach itself to a site lower down because of damage to the uterine wall, either because the woman has had many previous pregnancies, has had one or several Caesarean sections, uterine fibroids or infections of the uterus.

If you have bleeding at any time in your pregnancy you should contact your doctor, and he may recommend that you have an ultrasound scan to see whether the pregnancy is progressing normally. The scan will show if the placenta is positioned low in the uterus. If your placenta is positioned over or partly over the cervix you will continue to have bleeding for the final weeks of your pregnancy. The bleeding can be heavy, and bed-rest may be advisable to minimise the loss of blood.

Women with placenta praevia are sometimes hospitalised at the very end of their pregnancy so that the loss of blood can be monitored. If the bleeding is severe and if the baby is in the breech position (which is common with placenta praevia), the woman may be advised to have a Caesarean section.

Pre-eclampsia

Pre-eclampsia (or toxaemia) is one of the most serious conditions to which pregnant women are vulnerable, and it occurs in about 7% of pregnancies. The figure is considerably higher in first pregnancies, possibly as high as 12%. This may not sound like a high percentage, but when you go for a hospital check-up or to an antenatal class, and you see ten, twenty or even thirty other pregnant women, just imagine that one in ten of those women – and one of them could be you – could suffer this potentially lethal condition. Many of the tests carried out during your antenatal visits are designed to cross-check for pre-eclampsia, so it is important that you attend your clinics and co-operate with the tests.

Pre-eclampsia is, in fact, a dangerously high blood pressure brought on by the pregnancy, usually towards the end of the pregnancy. How or why the blood pressure becomes raised is not entirely clear. It may be a side-effect of the mother's immune system responding to the presence of the baby as a foreign body: enzymes released by the immune system are known to alter the lining of the arteries, making them less flexible and, therefore, raising the blood pressure.

Treated properly, pre-eclampsia can be controlled and it need pose no threat to mother or baby. After delivery, probably within the first two days, the mother's blood pressure will return to normal. If it is not detected and treated swiftly, pre-eclampsia can threaten the mother's health permanently by causing irreparable damage to the blood vessels and by putting excessive strain on the kidneys, heart and nervous system.

It may also compromise the supply of nutrients and oxygen to the foetus, possibly retarding the growth of the foetus and causing brain damage or other abnormalities. Fortunately it is very rare for pre-eclampsia to progress this far, but in a tiny minority of cases the condition goes undetected and proceeds to eclampsia itself: the mother's blood pressure rises to the point when she may have convulsion or go into a coma. Ultimately, the mother's heart will fail to cope with the strains of the excessively high blood pressure, and both mother and baby can die.

Signs of Pre-eclampsia

There are a number of early warning signs of pre-eclampsia that a woman may notice herself at home; these are a sudden weight gain, a drop in the volume of urine even if she is drinking normally, and excessive puffiness of the fingers, wrists and ankles. All of these symptoms are caused by an excessive increase in fluid retention. If you have all or any of these symptoms, contact your doctor immediately and he can test for two other warning signs: high blood pressure and protein in your urine.

If you do not have or do not pick up on early signs your blood pressure will continue to rise and may give you headaches and stomach aches; it may also cause giddiness, blurred vision, disorientation and irritability. It is very important that you contact your doctor if you have any combination of the above symptoms.

Treating Pre-eclampsia

If pre-eclampsia is caught in the early stages, when the woman has some fluid retention and mildly raised blood pressure, she is unlikely to need drugs to control her blood pressure. Full bed-rest, usually in hospital where she and the foetus can be closely monitored, may be enough to stabilise it. If she is considered well enough to go home she will need to be especially vigilant for further symptoms, and she may be asked to attend her clinic more frequently so that medical staff can keep an eye on her blood pressure and the wellbeing of her baby. Many women with pre-eclampsia have to stay in hospital until their baby is due.

Pre-eclampsia is rare in early pregnancy and the incidence increases as the pregnancy progresses. When pre-eclampsia is detected very late in pregnancy, particularly if the cervix is beginning to ripen indicating that spontaneous labour is imminent, most hospitals will choose to induce labour and deliver the baby straight away. Both mother and baby will be spared the dangers of maternal hypertension with little risk to the baby.

In more advanced cases of pre-eclampsia the maturity of the foetus is a key factor in deciding what treatment should be given. Many hospitals will choose to induce labour if the pregnancy is in or after the thirtieth week (or even the twenty-eighth week), when the baby's chances of survival in a special care baby unit are good. The dangers of pre-eclampsia and of the drugs that may be used to control the hypertension outweigh the risks of premature delivery after 28 weeks.

A high percentage of cases of pre-eclampsia occur after the twenty-eighth week; if advanced cases occur before this time, when the baby's chances of survival would be slender, every effort is made to stabilise the mother's blood pressure and oedema with medication and bed-rest. In some cases, the condition can be stabilised and the woman may go to term – although she will almost certainly have to stay in hospital until she has been delivered – but many will be induced once the foetus is deemed mature enough.

Premature Labour

There are a number of reasons why a woman may spontaneously go into labour pre-term, some of which can be controlled to delay delivery and give the foetus a chance to mature further. In many instances pre-term delivery is inevitable and there are considerable risks to the foetus. It is, of course, possible for a woman to appear to be in labour prematurely if her dates are wrong but, if she has been attending her antenatal check-ups, it is likely that a discrepancy in dates would have been picked up on by this stage.

Why Labour may Start Prematurely

Some women go into labour pre-term without any obvious reason; it may simply be an undesirable variation on the norm. In some cases, though, it is possible to explain why a woman goes into labour pre-term: the incidence of pre-term labour is increased if the woman is carrying two or more babies; if her uterus is an abnormal shape or she has an incompetent cervix; if she has developed gestational problems such as an excess of amniotic fluid or an abnormal placenta; if she becomes seriously ill, especially if she has a fever; if her membranes rupture prematurely; if she has a considerable physical shock such as a car crash or a bad fall; or if the foetus has abnormalities or has died.

Dealing with Premature Labour

It is important for doctors and midwives to try and assess accurately why a woman has gone into labour pre-term because they will then be equipped to decide how best to proceed. If the competence of the placenta is under question the baby might be safer in a special care baby unit, and the labour may be allowed to continue at its natural rate or even accelerated. In most other cases, doctors may try to arrest the progress of labour by sedating the mother or administering specialised drugs which subdue the contractions of the uterus. This is done in an attempt to prolong the pregnancy, therefore giving the foetus a chance to mature. Once a woman has threatened to go into true labour pre-term she may have to remain in hospital on complete bed-rest until her baby is born.

Dangers to the Foetus of Going into Labour Pre-term

There are many ways in which it is dangerous for the foetus if the mother goes into labour pre-term. Firstly, the cause of the premature labour, such as an inadequate placenta, may already have given rise to abnormalities in the foetus and compromised its chances of survival. The second and most obvious danger is that the baby will simply be too small and too immature to survive whatever specialist care he is offered. Luckily, most premature labours occur after about 32 weeks when the baby does have a good chance of survival.

Premature babies have an increased incidence of physical and mental handicaps – in very premature babies these handicaps can be severe. Even if the baby has no defects before delivery, he may be so small and fragile that the delivery itself causes some damage to him. Premature babies are unable to maintain body heat; they may need to have assistance in breathing because the lungs develop only in the last weeks of the pregnancy; they are very prone to infection; and they may need to be fed intravenously because they are often not strong enough to feed for themselves (it is easier for a weak premature baby to feed from a bottle than from the breast but this does not mean that he need be denied the great advantages of drinking his mother's milk: the mother can use a breast pump to collect her milk for her baby).

With the equipment that is currently available it is possible for a baby to survive delivery at just 23 weeks, although it is likely that he will be handicapped, will need specialist treatment all his life, and that he may not live very long. The financial and emotional costs of helping premature babies to survive is enormous, and little is known about the pain threshold of the babies themselves while they undergo necessary treatment and tests. Whatever financial or ethical arguments there may be to say that nature should be allowed to take its course, most parents and most hospitals will do everything in their power to save a premature baby.

Problems in your Day-to-day Life

Not everything that can go wrong during your pregnancy is necessarily connected to the pregnancy itself. It may be that something goes wrong in your everyday life. Your relationship with your partner could suffer or break up completely, you might be faced with financial problems, trouble at work or illness in the family.

Whatever problems you have to deal with in your everyday life you should not underestimate the effects that stress and anxiety can have on your general health and the normal progression of your pregnancy (see the section on **Stress** in the chapter **Illness During Pregnancy**). Talking about problems with your partner, your employer, your doctor or midwife, possibly the Citizens' Advice Bureau or a voluntary organisation such as the Samaritans (whose address appears at the end of the book) will help you to see things in perspective and to decide what action to take.

Try not to bottle up your feelings or to take on too many new responsibilities. You may feel as if you are being selfish but, during your pregnancy, when you think of yourself you are actually thinking about two people: yourself and the baby.

Termination

If you are faced with the fact that your baby has an abnormality and you have to decide whether or not to terminate your pregnancy, it will probably be one of the most difficult decisions you have to make in your life. Whether you choose to terminate the pregnancy or to keep the baby there are likely to be times in the future when you regret your decision.

You may feel that the full responsibility for the decision to terminate lies with you, but you should share the responsibility with those who advise you, such as your doctor or midwife, and those close to you. First of all, make sure that the doctor, consultant or relevant specialist explains to you fully how and to what extent your baby's abnormalities may affect your life and the length and quality of the baby's own life. Discuss the implications with your partner, your family and – if you feel that it is appropriate – your friends. You might find it useful to talk to families who have decided to rear a child with the same abnormality, or to families who have decided to terminate a pregnancy because abnormalities were detected in the foetus (organisations who can put you in touch with other families are listed at the back of the book).

The decision becomes increasingly difficult as the pregnancy advances. In the early weeks, before the baby has started kicking, many women find that – however excited they are about their pregnancy – they do not perceive the foetus as a real person. Terminations before about 14 weeks are anyway often less traumatic for the mother because they can be performed under general anaesthetic. Just because the process may be less harrowing does not mean that you should opt for termination any more readily in the first trimester, but if you know that ultimately you will decide to have a termination you should avoid procrastinating the decision until after the 14-week watershed. If you do have an early termination you will not be able to see the foetus.

After 14 weeks, unless the foetus is especially small, a termination is likely to take the form of an induced labour. You will have to go through the whole process of labour and birth in the knowledge that you will not have a baby as reward at the end. This is especially hard after about the eighteenth week when you may well have felt the baby kicking.

Unfortunately, because many of the tests for abnormalities are not available until about the sixteenth week, and some results cannot be deemed accurate until a fortnight later, many women are faced with this very difficult decision as they approach the middle of their pregnancy, when they may have felt their baby kicking, when they believed they were 'half way' to having a baby, and when they are under pressure to make a decision before the legal limit for abortions elapses at 24 weeks.

If you decide to have a termination after the fourteenth week of pregnancy, you will be asked whether you would like to see the baby. You may find the idea repulsive or you may be afraid that you will have feelings of guilt and shame if you see the aborted foetus, but many couples find that it helps them to come to terms with their loss if they at least see the baby. Even if you do not like the idea of seeing your baby, the staff may offer to take a photograph of him, and you may find at a later date that you want to see the photograph. Some couples like to hold the baby, to name him and to arrange a small service of blessing. If you would like to arrange a religious ceremony for the baby, speak to the hospital about the legal requirements (they vary according to the age of the foetus at the time of termination).

A termination is physically and emotionally draining. Not only do you undergo surgery or labour, you also suffer the rapid withdrawal of pregnancy hormones without the stimulus of a baby to help your body with this transition. The emotional loss can be devastating: you may feel grief, exhaustion, anger, resentment and regret for weeks or months, and you may find it difficult to settle to anything. You and your partner will need a lot of support from each other, from family and friends, and possibly from your doctor, a counsellor or a local support group.

CASE STUDY: *'It was all very sudden. They told me at the scan that the baby's internal organs were not growing properly and that it would probably be stillborn or die after a few hours. It had no chance of living really, so it seemed obvious to end it all straight away. I stayed in and had the operation that night, and it was only afterwards that it started to bother me; it all happened so quickly that I hadn't had time to think about what I was doing and why. Now that I look back on it, I think we probably did make the right decision, but for a long time I felt we should have let nature take its course.'*

When to have Another Baby

If the baby you were carrying had a genetic disorder such as cystic fibrosis or muscular dystrophy you will need to talk to your doctor about the likelihood of any subsequent babies having the same condition, and about ways of limiting the risks. A number of other complaints can be linked to the mother's lifestyle and to nutritional deficiencies (a deficiency in folic acid, for example, is linked to a higher instance of nural tube defects such as spina bifida). If this was the case with you, your doctor will advise you how to alter your diet or lifestyle to minimise the chances of having another baby with the same problem.

Many foetal abnormalities are accidents of nature, and the chances of having a second pregnancy with a similar complication are extremely small. In these cases, it is up to the couple to decide when they feel ready to have another baby. No one else can tell you when the right time is, and you may even feel that the time will never seem right. Again, whatever decision you make you may find that you regret it, but as soon as you are pregnant again you will have a new focus for your attention, and you will have the nine months of the pregnancy to adjust to the idea of having another baby. A new baby will never replace the one that you lost, but he may go a long way towards easing the pain of your loss.

Vaginal Bleeding

It is not uncommon for women to have bleeding or spotting at the time of their expected period for the first month or even two or three months after conception. Although this is not necessarily a warning sign, it could indicate that the foetus is not satisfactorily implanted or is becoming detached. Spotting and bleeding can also happen at other times of the cycle; you should always contact your doctor and let him know if you have bleeding at any time in your pregnancy because it could be an indication that you are likely to miscarry. If you have repeated bleeding your doctor may want to monitor your pregnancy more closely with ultrasound scans.

If you notice that you bleed after taking exercise or after making love, your doctor will advise you not to take such strenuous exercise, and to choose a different position for love-making or to abstain from penetrative sex (at least for the first trimester when the foetus is at greatest risk of miscarriage). If bleeding is accompanied by abdominal pain and / or fever in the very early weeks of pregnancy, it could mean that you have a tubal pregnancy (see **Ectopic Pregnancy**, above) and that the tube has ruptured.

If you have excessive or prolonged bleeding in early pregnancy, and your bleeding is accompanied by abdominal cramps rather like menstrual cramps you may well be miscarrying (see **Miscarriage**, above). If you have copious bleeding towards the end of your pregnancy your placenta may have adhered low down in your uterus, over the aperture of the cervix (this known as **Placenta Praevia**, see above).

Weight Gain Problems

It is normal for a woman to gain between 7.5 and 13.5kg (17 and 30lb) during her pregnancy, although it may be acceptable for her to gain more or less than these guideline figures. The amount of weight a woman should gain in order for her and her baby to be healthy depends to some extent on her frame and her weight before the pregnancy. A woman who is underweight will need to gain more weight to nourish herself and her baby than one who has a normal weight or is overweight before the pregnancy starts.

To ensure that you gain an acceptable amount of weight in pregnancy, you should try to eat three or four regular meals a day, and you should avoid snacking on sugary foods, which are very calorific but have little nutritional value. It is especially important to have a well-balanced diet during pregnancy, providing your own metabolism and your growing baby with the full complement of nutrients, vitamins and minerals (see the section on **Nutrition** in the chapter **Preparing for Pregnancy**).

Your weight gain will be monitored once you start having antenatal check-ups, because the amount of weight you gain can have several knock-on effects. If you gain too little or too much weight this may have an adverse effect on your health and the health of your baby, and it could be a symptom of a more serious health problem.

Poor Weight Gain or Weight Loss

There are more problems associated with poor weight gain in pregnancy than with excessive weight gain, and pregnancy is definitely not a time to think about dieting and losing weight.

It is not uncommon for a woman to gain very little weight or even to lose a little weight early in pregnancy, particularly if she suffers from morning sickness. Unless you were very underweight before your pregnancy started your baby will probably suffer no ill-effects if you gain no weight in the first trimester. It will, however, take its toll on you because the baby will take the resources it needs from you so that your body's reserves will be depleted.

If your poor weight gain is caused by morning sickness, you should begin to investigate what triggers your morning sickness (see the feature on morning sickness in **Week 6** of the **Your Pregnancy Week by Week** chapter). If you do not have morning sickness and you are not gaining weight you need to think carefully about your diet and lifestyle, and whether you are making too many demands on your body. If you cannot explain your weight loss, you should arrange to speak to your doctor who may be able to give you further advice about diet or to carry out tests to investigate the problem.

If you continue to gain little or no weight as your pregnancy progresses into the second and third trimesters, your baby could begin to suffer. Your body may not be able to supply the foetus with adequate nutrients to grow at the normal rate, so that when your baby arrives he may be very small, with vitamin and mineral deficiencies and associated problems. In mothers who gain very little weight there is an increased incidence of miscarriage, of babies with physical and mental abnormalities, of long labours and of neo-natal death.

If you attend your antenatal check-ups and your ultrasound scan appointment your doctor or midwife should notice if you are not putting on adequate weight, or if your baby is not growing at the expected rate. They will investigate the causes of your poor weight gain, and give you advice about your diet. If you are advised to gain more weight it is important to remember that it is not how much you eat but what you eat that really matters: eating cakes and chocolate bars for a fortnight will certainly impress your bathroom scales but it will do nothing to improve the nutrients available for your growing baby.

Excessive Weight Gain

The old adage of 'eating for two' is a dangerous one, implying that you have a free rein to eat as much as you like during pregnancy. You may have a huge and capricious appetite, but you are certainly not feeding two fully grown adults. If you do not moderate what you eat, and you gain excessive weight you could compromise your own and your baby's health.

It is generally considered acceptable for a woman to gain up to about 13.5kg (30lb) during pregnancy – although this figure would be lower for a woman who was very overweight at the beginning of her pregnancy – and there is likely to be no cause for concern if you gain as much as 18kg (40lb). Your weight will be measured regularly at your antenatal visits, and if your doctor or midwife feels that you are putting on weight too quickly, he or she will give you advice about diet and exercise.

If you are advised that you are gaining too much weight it is important to remember that you should not try to lose weight during pregnancy, but to control further weight gain. There are some vitamins and minerals that cannot be stored in the body so you need a good balanced diet to supply them to the body daily. The quality of what you eat is far more important than the quantity.

Excessive weight gain in pregnancy can cause high blood pressure and puts unnecessary strain on the mother's heart, which will anyway be working at 130–150% its normal output by the end of the pregnancy.

The increased bodyweight makes extra demands on the joints and ligaments of the hips, legs and feet, causing numerous aches and pains, and increasing the incidence of sciatic and back pain. If you gain too much weight in pregnancy you are unlikely to be physically fit, and you may not cope so well with the demands of labour and birth. Excessive weight gain can cause complications in later pregnancy and is associated with an increased incidence of gestational diabetes (see **Gestational Diabetes**, above) and the need for Caesarean sections.

Another reason that your weight gain is closely monitored is that a rapid weight gain, especially one that is not associated with over-eating, could be a symptom of a more serious problem such as pre-eclampsia (see **Pre-eclampsia**, above).

Chapter 5

Labour and Delivery

One of the questions most commonly asked by women towards the end of their pregnancy is 'how will I know when I am in labour?' The trite answer is that labour is such a strong, painful and overwhelming experience that you cannot miss it.

In reality women's pain thresholds and their experiences of labour are so different that some will believe they are in full-blown labour when they experience their first Braxton Hicks contractions, whereas others will feel little more than 'discomfort' until the cervix is all but fully dilated.

The Build-up to Labour

Those who do not ask 'how will I know when I am in labour?' may believe what they see in films! On screen, women always seem to be catapulted dramatically into full-blown labour, the uterine equivalent of 0–60 in half a second. This only happens in a very small minority of cases; in most cases, there is a gradual build up to labour. To make it even more difficult to identify, what appears to be the onset of labour may be only Braxton Hicks contractions, prelabour or a false labour.

Braxton Hicks Contractions

As part of your body's preparation for labour and delivery, your uterus actually undergoes regular painless contractions from the early weeks of pregnancy. These are known as Braxton Hicks contractions.

Some women never feel Braxton Hicks contractions, others – especially in second and subsequent pregnancies, when they appear to be stronger – are aware of them by the middle of the pregnancy. Most find that they notice them in the latter weeks as the contractions become stronger.

When you have a Braxton Hicks contraction, the uterus contracts, making the abdomen feel rigid to the touch. You might feel a little bit of discomfort but there should be no pain, and you are likely only to feel the occasional contraction rather than a series of regular contractions. If you do feel pain in conjunction with contractions, you should not dismiss them as Braxton Hicks contractions: you may well be going into labour, and you should seek advice from your GP or midwife.

Pre-labour

In the latter stages of pregnancy, a woman's body may begin to prepare itself for labour gradually so that there is a period of transition in which changes start to take place in the body, but true labour cannot be said to have started. During the pre-labour period, which does not occur in all cases and may not be noticed in others, women may empty their bowels more frequently and they may experience some of the symptoms of the onset of true labour (see **Recognising the Onset of Labour**, below). There may be sporadic bouts of contractions or regular mild contractions spaced many minutes apart. In some cases, the cervix may be fully effaced and even partly dilated during pre-labour.

False Labour

Towards the end of pregnancy it is possible for a woman to experience what is known as a false labour once or several times; the incidence of false labour is higher in second and subsequent pregnancies. It may be very difficult to distinguish false labour from the real thing: the contractions are strong and can be very painful, and they may come regularly for several hours. The contractions do actually differ from those experienced in true labour in that they tend to be shorter and they tend to cause pain in the lower abdomen in general rather than the uterus (contractions generating in the top of the uterus are specifically associated with true labour).

False labour can be a very frustrating experience: you may have regular painful contractions for two or three hours, you may even go so far as contacting your doctor or midwife only for the contractions to stop as abruptly as they started. The only consolations of a false labour are that they do not pose any threat to the foetus, and they indicate that the real thing is probably not far behind!

CASE STUDY: *'It was very annoying, especially because I didn't really know what I was looking out for. I had three false starts before I went into labour properly. Luckily I didn't actually get around to ringing the hospital because I knew I wanted to stay at home as long as possible anyway ... All I can say is you won't be sure if it's the real thing if you're in false labour: but you'll definitely know it's the real thing when it's the real thing!'*

Recognising the Onset of Labour

There are a number of tell-tale signs that can indicate the onset of true labour. Unfortunately, no two labours are the same and some of these signs might be absent or might happen in a different order.

SIGNS OF TRUE LABOUR

A show
Spontaneous breaking of the waters
A dull ache in the lower back and / or up inside the vagina
Regular painful contractions becoming longer, stronger and more frequent

---

Show

As a woman comes to term in her pregnancy she may notice a one-off pinkish mucus discharge from her vagina. This is known as a show, and it is, in fact, the plug of mucus (usually coloured pink by blood) that has been blocking the entrance to the cervix during the pregnancy, guarding the uterus from infection. As the baby's head – or other presenting part – descends and engages in the cervix, the pelvis begins to stretch and early contractions may begin: the plug then becomes dislodged.

A show is often a sign that labour will be fairly imminent. Labour will usually follow within the next couple of days although it is possible to have a show up to two or even three weeks before delivery. There is no need to notify your doctor or midwife if you have a show, unless there is a heavy loss of blood with it.

CASE STUDY: *'We were decorating our new house and we had a pretty tight schedule before the baby was due to arrive. One day, about two weeks before I was due, I felt a tickling wet feeling in my vagina. I had a pinky yellow discharge, quite a lot of it. We went into panic mode thinking we had run out of time, but actually it was another ten days before he finally arrived.'*

Spontaneous Breaking of the Waters

The membrane enclosing the foetus and the amniotic fluid will break at some stage before your baby's head is born; this is known as the breaking of the waters or rupture of the membranes. When the membrane breaks under the pressure of your baby's head you will be able to feel the amniotic fluid running down your legs. Amniotic fluid is usually a golden yellow colour, and can easily be confused with leaks of urine due to stress incontinence: however, it has a sweeter smell than urine and you may be able to feel that it is coming from within the vagina not the tiny urethra.

In a few cases, the membrane does not break until the very last minute before the head appears, and the baby may have a cap – or caul – of membrane on his head when he is born. More commonly the waters will break during labour, and there is often a noticeable acceleration of labour after the breaking of the waters because the baby's head, no longer cushioned by the amniotic fluid, pushes more firmly on the cervix, stimulating its dilation. Another reason that labour accelerates is that substances called prostaglandins that are present in the amniotic fluid induce the effacement and dilation of the cervix.

It is not uncommon for the breaking of the waters to be the first sign that a woman is going into labour. Many women are afraid that their waters will break in a great torrent in a public place. Although there is a considerable amount of fluid to be lost, it does not usually come in a great rush. There may be an initial gush followed by slow seeping for several hours (the baby's head will have descended further, allowing the fluid to seep out only slowly).

What to do if your Waters Break

If your waters break contact your doctor or midwife. If there is evidence of blood or meconium in the fluid you may need to go to hospital straight away (see below). Once your waters have broken you may well go into labour quite quickly in which case you need to keep an eye on your contractions and speak to your doctor or midwife when you think it is time to go to the hospital (see **Timing Contractions** and **When to go to Hospital**, below). If you are having a home delivery you should let your midwife know when your waters have broken, and you should keep her abreast of your progress by telephone over the next few hours until she comes to you.

In some cases, labour does not follow quickly after the rupture of the membranes. This may be because only one of the two areas of amniotic fluid has been released and another is still cushioning the baby's head. The greater volume of amniotic fluid is in front of the baby's head (this is called the fore-waters), and there is a smaller volume behind the baby's head (the hind-waters). When the hind-waters break, labour does not always follow so promptly because the baby's head is still not applying pressure to the front of the cervix.

Once your waters have broken, the uterus and the baby are at risk of infection. You should be very careful to keep yourself clean and safe from infection: use sanitary towels instead of tampons to absorb the leaking fluid, wipe yourself from front to back when you wipe after urinating or wash, and do not be tempted to have intercourse as a way of helping labour on its way. You should check with your GP or midwife as to whether it is safe to have a bath at this stage, because there may be a risk of infection from the bath water. Finally, do not put your fingers inside your vagina to 'see what's going on'.

CASE STUDY: *'My waters broke on a Sunday morning three days before I was due. It didn't flood out but I was surprised how much of it there was. I was using those really thick old sanitary towels and I got through a whole packet in a few hours. Then the contractions started and I went into hospital mid-afternoon. She didn't make an appearance until the following afternoon, but that's another story!'*

Even if you do not go into labour spontaneously, you should let your doctor know your waters have broken: he may well ask you to go into hospital and – in order to avoid prolonging the risk of infection – it may be necessary to induce labour if it does not start spontaneously within 24 hours.

If your waters break and there is a considerable amount of blood with the amniotic fluid or if it is tinged a greenish black colour, you should contact your doctor or midwife straight away. Bleeding may indicate that your placenta is beginning to come away from the uterine wall. If this does happen, the supply of nutrients and vital oxygen to the foetus may be compromised. The greenish colour that is sometimes seen in amniotic fluid is the first stool excreted by the baby. It is called meconium and is usually not excreted until after the baby is born. The presence of meconium in the amniotic fluid could indicate that the baby is in stress or that he is very post-mature.

If you are not sure whether your waters have broken, you should anyway speak to your doctor or your midwife. They can run a couple of simple painless tests to check for amniotic fluid in your vagina.

Lower Back / Vaginal Pain

Some women are aware of a dull aching pain in their lower back, lower abdomen or their vagina before they feel actual contractions. This sort of pain may come and go throughout the last trimester, but it is especially intense when it comes as a precursor to labour. If you have this sort of pain, there is no need to contact your doctor or midwife straight away but it could be a sign that you will go into labour soon.

CASE STUDY: *'I had a lot of pain in my back for all of Monday and my husband kept saying it could be the baby. But – I feel silly saying this now, because I know better – but I thought your waters had to break before you went into labour, so I just didn't know what it was. When I finally started having proper contractions and went to the hospital I was already 7cm dilated and my waters still hadn't broken.'*

Regular Painful Contractions

The surest sign that you are in labour is if you have regular painful contractions, only in a small minority of cases (mostly with second and subsequent babies) do women feel little or no pain while their uterus is contracting. If you do start having regular painful contractions you could, of course, be having a bout of false labour (see above), but contractions in false labour tend to stay at the same intensity and then stop within a few hours.

In true labour, the contractions become longer, stronger and more frequent, and in most cases they continue this escalation uninterrupted until your baby is born. There is no need to contact your doctor or midwife when you first start having contractions unless they are very strong, lasting a minute and only three to five minutes apart (see **When to go to Hospital**, below).

What Contractions are For

The contractions of the muscles of the uterus start at the top of the uterus and radiate downwards towards the cervix and serve a number of purposes. In what is known as the first stage of labour the contractions of the uterus combined with pressure from the baby's head on your cervix force the cervix open. The muscles of the uterus are actually pulling the cervix up and out of the way: at first the cervix becomes effaced, thinning out and flattening against the baby's head. Once it is fully effaced it begins to dilate, to open up. When the cervix is fully dilated, leaving a gap of about 10cm (4in), your baby's head should be able to pass and the second stage of labour can begin.

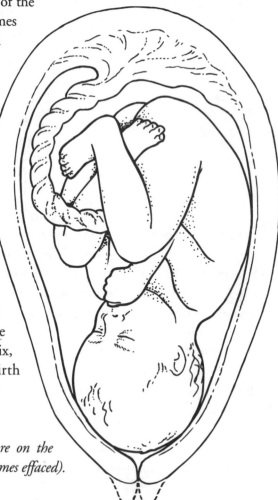

During the second stage of labour, the powerful contractions from the top of the uterus work with your pushing to push the baby through the dilated cervix, along your vagina (the birth canal) and into the world.

As the baby's head puts pressure on the cervix, the cervix thins out (becomes effaced).

The pressure of the baby's head and the powerful muscular contractions of the uterus dilate the cervix, opening it up to allow the baby's head to pass.

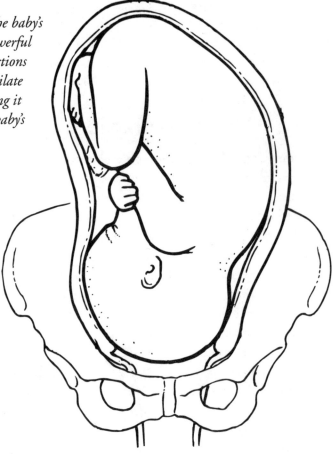

Many women are not even conscious of the third stage of labour (the delivery of the placenta) either because it has been assisted with drugs or because they are so busy getting to know their new baby. In the third stage, the contractions are considerably weaker but, by making the surface area of the uterine wall smaller they dislodge the placenta (the afterbirth) from its position on the uterine wall so that it can be delivered.

Uterine contractions do actually continue after the delivery of the afterbirth, although you may not be conscious of them. The uterus gradually contracts back to its pre-pregnancy size and position over the next few days and weeks; this process is usually faster if the mother is breastfeeding because the contractions are stimulated by the sucking of the baby. Some women experience considerable pains, known as afterpains, as the uterus contracts back.

Why Contractions Hurt

Many women ask why contractions hurt so much, and unsympathetic men may comment on the fact that animals appear to give birth without much fuss, whereas human mothers have a panoply of pain relief available. Firstly, contractions hurt because they are affecting very large muscle groups, spasms of muscle so powerful that they can efface and dilate the cervix which is normally quite firm and about 3cm (1¼in) long, and they can expel a baby through a 10cm (4in) aperture.

Secondly, contractions do hurt animals – if you have ever watched an animal giving birth you will have noticed signs of distress – but animals do not have the same means of communicating their pain as we do. They also have one great psychological advantage over humans: it is believed that most animals lack the power of imagination, of thinking 'how long will this go on, when will the next contraction be?' and so on. This means that the female animal's intelligence limits her to getting through one contraction at a time, and relaxing completely between contractions. A ewe can be seen to graze peacefully between contractions right up until her lamb is born. Women who manage to see their labour in the same way, to take one contraction at a time and make the most of the pauses in between, usually have a much better experience of labour and tend to need less pain relief or intervention.

The most significant differences between humans and animals are physiological. We are alone among mammals in walking upright on our hind legs, and this puts great demands on the cervix during pregnancy. Throughout the pregnancy, the human cervix has to be firmly closed to ensure that the baby remains safely in the uterus. It is, therefore, especially hard for the human cervix to efface and dilate during labour. Furthermore, the human baby has an especially large head in relation to the size of his mother's pelvis, and this means that the cervix has to be fully dilated before birth is possible.

Timing Contractions

Once you start having regular painful contractions you may be aware that they gradually become longer, stronger and more frequent. The length and spacing of your contractions is a good indication of how advanced your labour is. When you contact your doctor or midwife, he or she is likely to ask how frequently your contractions are coming and how long each contraction lasts.

If you attended antenatal classes you will probably have been taught how to time contractions. This is easiest if you have a watch or clock with a second hand and if someone is there to help you. To time how long each contraction is, look at your watch as you feel the first twinge of a contraction and then time it until the pain has gone away. If you time several contractions you may notice that they are of varying lengths; it is the average or most common time that matters.

To time how frequently your contractions are coming, look at your watch as you feel the first twinge of one contraction and make a note of how long it is until the first twinge of the following contraction. There will probably be less variation in the frequency of contractions than in their individual lengths, and this measurement is a key indicator of how advanced your labour is.

Most first-time labours are longer than subsequent labours, and they build up gradually over several hours. When you first start timing contractions they may well last only 20 seconds and be coming erratically about every eight to ten minutes.

Coping Strategies at Home

Labour, especially a first one, can be a long haul, and most women find that their experience of labour is improved if they stay at home for the first few hours. Here at least they can benefit from the privacy and familiarity of their own home, their own cup of tea made just as they like it, and their own bath.

So long as your contractions are erratic and spaced more than five minutes apart it is quite safe to stay at home. At this stage the contractions may or may not be painful, but they are likely to be uncomfortable and to preclude the possibility of grabbing a last minute sleep!

There are a number of ways of keeping the pain under control to prolong your stay at home before going in to hospital:

Staying on the move: Many women find that by keeping on the move, they actually feel less pain with their contractions. By moving around you are not cramping the actions of the large muscle groups in the uterus, and you ensure a good blood supply to them. You may feel like a caged lion pacing around the house, but you could also use the stairs and the garden if you have one. You may find that leaning your elbows on a table and just 'wagging' your bottom from side to side is enough movement to ease the pain.

Finding a comfortable position to rest: When you tire of moving about or if your legs are hurting with every contraction (which is not uncommon) it is very important that you find a comfortable position in which to rest. You cannot assume that curling up in your favourite chair will be right in the circumstances.

You may find that you want to rest leaning forwards, for example by kneeling in front of a bean bag and resting on it face down, or by sitting backwards astride an upright chair, resting your head and elbows on the back of the chair. These positions stretch out the back which can become very sore in labour.

Sitting on a bed in the corner of a room or on a sofa can be very comfortable: your legs can be stretched out in front of you, and you have support to the back and to one side of you. You may find that resting is even more comfortable with a warm hot-water bottle on your lower back or just under your bump.

Breathing: If you have attended antenatal classes you will have learnt about breathing techniques for labour and it is never too early to start using these techniques to help you through your contractions.

Some women automatically take in a deep breath and brace themselves when they feel a contraction coming on, not breathing again until the contraction has worn off. If you have ever been to an aerobics class or done weight training you will know that you should exhale when you make the effort and inhale when you are recovering. This is why you should let your breath out slowly when you have a contraction and breath deeply in between. As the contractions become longer and stronger you will need to be inhaling during the contractions too, but you should take a series of short shallow breaths, taking deeper breaths between contractions.

Having a bath: Having a bath in the early stages of labour can be useful in two ways, and this is thanks to the relaxing effects of the water. Because you will be more relaxed, your contractions are likely to hurt less, and some women notice that their contractions 'calm down' if they have a bath during labour. Another result of the relaxing effect of a bath can be to speed up labour: your body takes advantage of your relaxed state to get on with the business in hand, and accelerates the process.

If you do have a bath, have the water not too hot, and make sure that there is someone in the house to help you out and to act swiftly if your labour accelerates rapidly. (If your waters have broken, check with your doctor or midwife whether they consider that it is safe to have a bath at this stage; some clinicians will discourage you from having a bath once your waters have broken because of the slight risk of infection.)

CASE STUDY: *'They [the contractions] started to get uncomfortable at about midnight so I ran myself a bath ... It was just so comfortable, that I stayed there for two hours, turning into a prune and topping up with hot water. I could actually watch my tummy hardening with the contractions, but they seemed less painful, and my back didn't ache so much.'*

Massage: An effective and comforting way of easing pain in labour is back massage; this is especially helpful if the pain seems to be concentrated in the lower back (see the feature on **Backache Labour**, below). Whoever administers the massage does not need to have any sort of qualifications, just smooth, firm movements and quite a lot of staying-power! You will know which part of your back needs the attention, and you will be able to say how firm or how gentle you want the massage to be. The areas that are most commonly relieved by massage in labour are the lower back (which may be causing pain) and the shoulders (which can become tense).

TENS machine: You may be able to hire a small machine called a TENS machine from your local hospital to control the pain of your contractions right from the beginning of labour (for more background information on TENS machines see the section in the feature on **Pain Relief in Labour**, below).

TENS is most effective if it is used from the very early stages of labour, starting with a tiny current and building to a stronger one as the contractions become more powerful. Used like this, the TENS machine stimulates a steady production of endorphins.

If you would like to hire a TENS machine from your local hospital, talk to your doctor or midwife about how to use one and how to get the most out of it. Make sure that you book one well in advance of your due date in case you go into labour early.

Distract yourself: It is surprising how absolutely normal you feel even between very strong contractions towards the end of labour, so there is no reason not to feel quite normal, well and alert in between early contractions while you are still at home. Try to find something to keep you busy or at least interested in between contractions; if you drop everything and concentrate on the fact that you are going into labour the whole process will seem longer and more painful.

Even if you are on the move you can still watch television or a favourite video, or listen to music or the radio. If you are leaning on a table or sitting down you can also read a book or a magazine. How long is it since you played a simple game of snap or did a crossword? It may be a long time before you have a chance to do either again – soon you will have a tiny baby to care for – so use this opportunity to play a game and take your mind off the contractions.

Probably the most pleasing distraction for a woman in labour is to prepare her baby's nursery: making up the cot and unsealing bottles of lotion. Next time you come into that room, you will have your baby with you. You should also use this time to check that you have everything you need for your time in hospital (see the feature on **Your Hospital Bag** in **Week 36** of the **Your Pregnancy Week by Week** section), and for when you return home from hospital.

If you have older children, parents or pets who will need caring for while you are in hospital, you should use these early stages to ring the people who will be caring for them. Do not be tempted to leave these sort of arrangements until the last minute, in case your labour accelerates rapidly.

When to go to Hospital

If your waters break and labour has not started spontaneously you may be advised to go into hospital straight away (see **What to do if your Waters Break**, above). If you have any bleeding you should contact your doctor who will probably arrange for you to be taken to hospital straight away.

If you are one of the minority of women whose labours start in full-swing – that is, you are having long, powerful contractions every three or so minutes from the start – you should also go to hospital straight away. It may be that your labour will slow down in the latter stages, but if it continues at its initial rate you need to get to hospital quickly or your partner could end up having to deliver the baby at home or in the back of the car!

If your labour has built-up gradually and you have been timing contractions, it is usually recommended that you contact your doctor and / or go to hospital when your contractions are lasting about 45 seconds and are coming regularly every three to five minutes. If you are having trouble coping with the pain before you reach this stage or you have any cause for concern you can, of course, contact your doctor much sooner. Like pregnancy, labour is not competition, there should be no comparisons about how long anyone 'lasts' before going to hospital or without pain relief; every labour is different. If you do go into hospital in the very early stages, you may well be advised to go home again, but you will at least have had your mind put at rest and you will be able to ask for advice about pain relief.

Booking in

When you arrive at your maternity unit you may be taken to an examination room or straight to the labour ward for an initial examination. A midwife will check your heart rate and blood pressure, and will time your contractions with you. Your baby's heart beat will be monitored either using a Pinards (a specialised stethoscope) or using an electronic monitor (see **Electronic Foetal Monitoring**, below); often a trace of the baby's heart rate is recorded.

The midwife will probably give you an internal examination to see whether your cervix has started dilating, which would confirm that you are in established labour. You will be asked to lie down so that she can feel your cervix; it is important to try to relax and take shallow breaths when she is doing the internal, this will make it more comfortable for you, and easier for her to assess the situation quickly.

Internal examinations can be either encouraging or discouraging: you may be coping well with the pain and be told that you are already 5cm dilated, or you may already be tired and overwhelmed only to hear that your cervix has not yet started dilating.

CASE STUDY: *'I got to the hospital at 6am, my contractions had started very gradually at about seven the night before. I'd been up all night, and now they were coming every four minutes. But the midwife who booked me in said I had not started dilating which meant I was not in established labour. I was so disheartened. I think she could tell, because she said very encouragingly "but it is fully effaced". I didn't start dilating until 1 o'clock that afternoon. It was very exhausting but, having "practised" for so many hours, it was then only just over three hours before she was born.'*

When you are being booked in to the labour ward, make sure that your midwife knows about your birthplan if you have one. Remember that it is never too late to change your mind about what is on your birth plan: the drug-free labour that may have seemed a good idea at an antenatal class on a bright summer evening may not seem so realistic at 5 o'clock one autumn morning when you have already been labouring all night. If you have any anxieties or questions, now is a good time to clear them up.

Induction

There are a number of reasons why a woman's labour may be induced. In extreme cases where the mother is very ill or the baby is showing signs of distress, it may be decided that the strains of induced vaginal delivery will be too great and the woman will be offered a Caesarean section.

If your midwife or consultant says that your labour needs to be induced make sure that you understand the reasons. In most cases induction is recommended for the safety of the mother or the baby.

Reasons for Inducing Labour

The foetus is post-mature: If the woman is well past her due-date induction may be advisable. Most hospitals will give a date for induction if the dating of the pregnancy is reliable and the pregnancy goes into a forty-second week. After the due date, the placenta can begin to deteriorate, and the supply of nutrients and – more crucially – oxygen to the foetus may not be adequate.

CASE STUDY: *'I wasn't much past 40 weeks but because of my age they said that I should be induced. They gave me a pessary and things started up gradually, and I was fine because I'd decided to have a mobile epidural anyway.'*

The foetus is not thriving: Even before the due-date is reached, the placenta may begin to fail and / or the foetus may stop growing. If there is any evidence that your foetus is failing to thrive in the latter part of your pregnancy, you are likely to be induced because your baby's chances of survival will be better outside the uterus.

> CASE STUDY: *'I'm 36 weeks now but they're keeping me on complete bed-rest because the baby's growth slowed down when I got to 30 weeks. They've said they will induce me at 38 weeks.'*

If you have vaginal bleeding in the last trimester: Vaginal bleeding in late pregnancy can indicate that the placenta is no longer fully attached to the uterine wall, in which case it may no longer be supplying nutrients and oxygen to the foetus efficiently. The cause of the bleeding and the wellbeing of the foetus will be investigated and induction may be recommended.

If you have diabetes: Whether you have always had diabetes or you have only had it during your pregnancy, there is a danger that your baby will grow very large. This could cause a number of further complications and could preclude the possibility of a vaginal delivery if the pregnancy is allowed to go to term (see the sections on **Diabetes** and **Gestational Diabetes** in the chapters **Illness in Pregnancy** and **When Things Go Wrong**, respectively).

If you have high blood pressure: High blood pressure poses a number of threats to both mother and baby (see the section on **Hypertension** in the chapter **Illness in Pregnancy**), and early delivery may be appropriate.

If you have pre-eclampsia: Pre-eclampsia is pregnancy-induced high blood pressure and in its most sever form it can threaten the life of both mother and baby (see the section on **Pre-eclampsia** in the chapter **When Things Go Wrong**). If your symptoms cannot be controlled and you have passed the twenty-eighth week of your pregnancy, it may be safer for you and your baby for labour to be induced.

If you have a chronic illness: If you have a chronic illness such as heart disease the strain of the last few weeks of pregnancy may be too great for you, and labour may be induced before you reach term.

If the baby has Rhesus disease: This is now a relatively rare disease which affects second or subsequent babies with Rhesus positive blood born to mothers who have Rhesus negative blood. The disease is usually forestalled by an injection which can be given to the mother after the birth of any Rhesus positive baby (see the section on **Blood Groups** in the chapter **Preparing for Pregnancy**). If the problem is severe and the foetus is found not to be thriving because of the antibodies in the mother's blood, it may be necessary to induce labour because the baby's chances of survival will be better outside the uterus.

Spontaneous labour has stopped or stalled: Another reason for induction is that a labour which started naturally and spontaneously may have stopped altogether. Induction can help to kick-start the contractions again. Some hospitals may be over-keen to use induction in these circumstances for their own convenience, even if the woman is happy to let nature take its course. If you have been reassured that your baby is in no danger and showing no signs of distress, there is no reason why you should not let your pregnancy and labour continue at their natural pace rather than being induced.

Breaking of the waters has not been followed by spontaneous contractions: A fairly common reason for induction is if the waters have broken but labour has not started spontaneously within the desired time. Once a woman's waters have broken she and her baby are at increased risk of infection. In order to minimise this risk, most hospitals will induce labour if it has not started spontaneously within 24 hours.

Spontaneous contractions are ineffectual: In some cases, labour may start spontaneously and the contractions may become frequent and regular but the cervix may fail to dilate. Even when the cervix is not dilating, the contractions can be very painful, and this can be an exhausting and disheartening situation. A woman who remains in pre-labour for a long time and whose cervix fails to dilate, may be offered an induction to help establish true labour.

CASE STUDY: *'I had to be induced because my waters broke and then nothing happened. I was put on a drip and the contractions built up very quickly. I dilated 5cm in two hours. I managed just with breathing for the first hour then I had to move onto pethidine.'*

Methods of Induction

There are three main ways in which labour may be induced. If your midwife or consultant says that your labour needs to be induced, make sure you understand why, which method is going to be used and how it will affect you.

Prostaglandin pessaries or gel: Prostaglandins are naturally occurring hormones which promote the softening, effacement and dilation of the cervix, therefore producing mild contractions. Prostaglandins are actually present in amniotic fluid, and this is one of the reasons that labour tends to speed up after the waters have broken; they are also present in semen, which is partly why making love is a natural way of trying to induce labour.

Prostaglandin pessaries or gel, which may be referred to as dinoprostone or Prostin E2, can be applied internally directly around the cervix. They produce a gradual softening of the cervix and gently augment contractions but may not always be sufficient to induce a really recalcitrant labour. If an initial treatment is not successful or sufficiently powerful, the treatment can be repeated. If labour is not established after two or three successive treatments, another method may have to be used.

Artificial rupture of the membranes (ARM): When a woman's membranes rupture spontaneously, her labour is likely to follow of its own accord (see **Spontaneous Breaking of the Waters**, above), and the same effect can sometimes be achieved by rupturing her membranes artificially. If ARM is to be performed on you, you will be asked to lie down as if for an internal examination, and the doctor will use a small hooked instrument to enter the cervix and gently puncture the membrane surrounding the foetus and the amniotic fluid. If your cervix is already slightly dilated (either naturally or with the use of prostaglandins) and you are relaxed, this should be no more than a little uncomfortable.

Once the membrane have been ruptured, labour may follow quite quickly (as it would if the waters had broken spontaneously) or it may need further induction.

Syntocinon drip: The syntocinon drip uses a concentrated synthetic form of a substance called oxytocin, which is produced by the pituitary gland. Syntocinon induces powerful contractions, and – when given intravenously in the drip – it is a very effective method of induction. That is its strength but in many ways also its weakness because the contractions caused can be really strong and painful quite quickly so that the woman has not had a chance to 'build up to them' as she would have done had the labour progressed naturally.

In the past, syntocinon got a bad name for itself because of its dramatic effect. Today it has been 'tamed' somewhat; this is because doctors and midwives do not induce labour now unless there is a very good reason, because syntocinon is used more carefully to try and mimic a more natural augmentation of contractions.

If you have been told that you need an syntocinon drip to induce your labour make sure that you understand why and that you know about the options for pain-relief that are available. Some hospitals systematically offer an epidural (see the feature on **Pain Relief**, below) with an syntocinon drip.

Effects of Induction

The different methods used to induce labour attempt to mimic spontaneous labour as much as possible, and prostaglandins and ARM do this quite well.

The contractions induced by the syntocinon drip are usually powerful, and only a small percentage of women will cope with them without any form of pain relief. There is, therefore, a higher than average incidence of the use of pethidine and epidurals in women who are being treated with syntocinon (for the effects of pethidine and epidurals see the feature on **Pain Relief**, below).

First Stage of Labour

Once you have been booked into your labour ward and been given your internal examination, you will probably be well on in the first stage of labour. As explained in the section **What are Contractions For?**, above, in the first stage of labour your cervix is effacing and dilating to allow your baby to pass out of the uterus and into the world.

Length, Strength and Frequency of Contractions

The length and strength of your contractions will build up gradually over the first stage of labour. When you arrive at the hospital your contractions may be lasting about 40 seconds and coming every three to five minutes; they will probably be very uncomfortable but manageable. By the time you are ready for the second stage of your labour the contractions may be about a minute long and there may be only one minute breaks in between them. They will now be overwhelmingly powerful and painful, but the pain is not constant for the full minute of each contraction: it builds slowly to a peak towards the end of the contraction and then drops away more quickly.

How you will Feel

Apart from being in pain, one of the things most commonly reported by women in labour is that they feel tired. Labour can go on for a long time and almost invariably disrupts at least one night's sleep; it is also physically and emotionally draining. It is indeed very tiring, and that is another good reason for keeping physically fit and getting plenty of rest during your pregnancy.

Many women feel at least a little frightened by labour – not the fear of the unknown that you may have during your pregnancy – but a fear because you know that the labour is more powerful than you, that you have no control over it and it will not let you go. It is not uncommon to feel like a little girl again, to be restless, moody, weepy, and to want to go home.

Labour can also be an exhilarating experience; the body is working at full tilt and you will have adrenaline circulating in your blood stream making you feel alert. You will also have endorphins in your bloodstream, these are the natural painkillers that are triggered by pain, injury or strenuous activity – they are what give you a 'buzz' when you take exercise, and some women feel slightly 'high' on endorphins during labour.

Even if labour is not physically exhilarating for you, it is an exciting time. You are on the threshold of a completely new chapter in your life, from now on the dynamics of all your relationships and the structure of your whole life will change because you will soon have a baby.

CASE STUDY: *'I'd had a couple of false starts but when I finally got to Queen Charlotte's and they said I was 5cm, my husband said "oh, it's exciting!"' I knew what he meant but – much as I was looking*

*forward to seeing the baby – I had this terrible feeling of apprehension.
I had the whole labour to get through first.'*

HOW LONG DOES LABOUR LAST?

This is a question that first-time mothers ask with nervous curiosity
before they actually go into labour and then with increasing anxiety
as their labour progresses! Unfortunately, it is not a question that
anyone can answer satisfactorily. All that anyone can tell you is the
average length of labour: First labours are generally the longest,
with an average of about 12 hours. You must remember that this is
an average, it is not the expected length of labour. Second and
subsequent labours have an average length of about seven hours.

The speed at which your labour starts does not necessarily give a
clear indication of how it will proceed, either. In the case study
above (in the section on Booking-in) the woman was having
contractions for many hours before she was in established labour,
but her labour was then very quick. It is equally possible for a
labour to be progressing well and then to slow down dramatically.

CASE STUDY: *'When I got to hospital this time [with second baby] I
was already 4cm. I was so pleased with myself, I really thought I was
going to get it right this time. I got to 7cm fine and then I stopped there
for about three hours with these hideous contractions going on and on.
Progress was much slower from then on ... thank God for pethidine!'*

However long the entire labour is, by far the greatest proportion of
the labour is usually spent in the first stage when the cervix is
dilating. The second stage, when you are pushing the baby into the
world can last a few minutes or as much as two to three hours. It is
unlikely to last much more than this because the enormous
pressures and strains put on the baby during the second stage mean
that it is dangerous for this stage to go on indefinitely, and you
would be given an assisted delivery (see below) or a Caesarean
section (see below). The third stage (the delivery of the placenta) is
often very quick because it is frequently drug-assisted.

Backache and Sciatic Pain in Labour

It is very common for women to suffer from backache when they are in labour, indeed pain in the lower back is a common first sign that a woman is going into labour. This is because the contractions in the uterus have a knock-on effect in the entire lower abdomen, including the back. You may be able to ease the pain in your back by staying on the move and by stretching your back out when you are resting.

Backache Labour

If your labour is slow to get going and each contraction feels as if it is actually in your lower spine, you could be having what a backache labour. Here the baby's head is facing forwards, and the pressure from the back of the baby's head is on the back of the uterus and the lower part of your spine (your sacrum) causing considerable pain in your spine during contractions. A backache labour is painful and tends to be longer because the position of the baby's head makes the presenting diameter larger.

Try to find a position to rest in which the pressure on your sacrum is alleviated: standing on all fours or bending over a bean bag may help. You may find that you get some relief if your partner pushes against your sacrum from the outside, countering the pressure produced by the baby's head on the inside.

Most babies will turn into the more normal anterior position just before delivery, but if the baby does not turn, the presenting part of his head will be slightly bigger. There is a higher incidence of assisted delivery in backache labours.

Sciatic Pain

Whether or not you have a backache labour you may find that for all or some of your labour you have acute pain shooting down one or both legs and / or a lack of sensation or co-ordination in the legs. This is caused by pressure on the large sciatic nerves that run down your legs. It may be possible to ease the pain by changing your position, but you are unlikely to be able to be upright or to walk around if you suffer from sciatic pain during labour.

CASE STUDY: *'I moved about a lot in labour but towards the end I just lost my legs completely, they collapsed underneath me ... I wouldn't be able to say if they weren't functioning or if it was just that the pain was so bad that I couldn't walk. Anyway, I had to give up on moving around: I sat on the bed and put the gas and air mask to my face for each contraction from then on. They were very painful.'*

Electronic Foetal Monitoring

When you are first booked in to the hospital you will probably be fitted up with an electronic foetal monitor so that the midwife can check that your baby's heart rate is normal. This gives an indication of how your baby is coping with labour.

How the Electronic Foetal Monitor Works

The most commonly used foetal heart monitor is an external device consisting of electric receptor pads held to your abdomen by an elasticated belt. The pads pick up the foetal heart rate in the same way as an ultrasound scan, and relay the information to the monitoring machine which produces a graph print-out of your baby's heart-rate as well as your contractions.

Once your waters have broken and your cervix has started dilating it is possible to obtain a more accurate reading by attaching the tiny pads of a smaller internal monitor directly onto the top of the baby's head (this sort of monitoring would only be necessary if the external monitoring method could not pick up the heart beat accurately).

What Foetal Monitoring tells you

As your uterus contracts, the blood supply (and hence the supply of oxygen) to the foetus is temporarily cut off or at least diminished. A normal, healthy baby with no complications can cope easily with this temporary drop in oxygen – just as you can hold your breath. If the foetus is very small or weak, however, or if it has an abnormality or a problem such as a knot in the umbilical cord, these regular dips in oxygen levels could pose a threat to the foetus. A serious or prolonged lack of oxygen can cause brain damage or, ultimately, death.

A normal foetal heart rate is between 110 and 150 beats per minute; the upper end of the range is more normal for a baby girl while the lower end is more normal for a baby boy (although the foetal heart rate is not usually considered a useful guide as to the sex of the baby). If the foetus is in distress during labour its heart might begin to slow down under the strain of each contraction or it may race to try and compensate for the lack of oxygen. If your baby's heart-rate implies that the baby is not coping very well with the contractions then you will continue to be monitored during your labour. It may be necessary for staff to carry out further tests on the foetus and possibly even to speed up your labour or give you an emergency Caesarean section.

In most cases, the foetal heart rate will indicate that your baby is coping well with the contractions and it may not be monitored again. Some hospitals like to monitor the foetal heart-rate periodically during labour, perhaps using a hand-held device such as a Pinard, especially if it is a long labour; others like to keep women on the electronic foetal monitor for the duration of their labour. This has the disadvantage of restricting the women's movements. If you feel strongly about wanting to move about when you are in labour you should check what your hospital's policy is on foetal heart monitoring. So long as your baby is showing no signs of distress when you are first admitted to hospital you may well be able to ask for the monitor not to be used continuously.

Eating and Drinking in Labour

Most hospitals advise you not to eat at all during labour because many women feel nauseous or are actually sick when they are in labour. Other hospitals are less cut and dried with their advice, saying that if a woman feels hungry, especially in the early stages, she should follow her instincts and eat.

In general it is not a good idea to eat when you are taking strenuous exercise, and advanced labour is the equivalent of strenuous exercise: the blood is busy circulating to the uterus and the major muscle groups, and any food in the stomach will not be digested efficiently. If food remains undigested in the stomach it becomes very acidic and can cause heartburn and indigestion. By the time you are in advanced labour you are very unlikely to feel hungry anyway, and if you do it should not be long until your baby is born.

If you are hungry in the early stages of labour it is better to have a small snack than to try and tackle a meal which might well be too much for your stomach to handle. This is one occasion when a sugary snack might be a good idea: it will boost your blood sugar levels, giving you a fix of energy but not weighing down your stomach with bulk (take a few sweet biscuits or a banana with you in case you get hungry). One simple way to solve the problem is to sip on a mildly sweet drink such as fruit juice or well diluted squash; this should keep your blood sugar levels up without nauseating you. (Avoid very sugary drinks because they will not really quench your thirst and might make you feel sick.)

Drinking During Labour

It may be important to drink when you are in labour because your body is working hard and – even if you are not obviously sweating – you will be losing a lot of body fluid. During labour you also do a lot of breathing through your mouth which dries the mouth out. Most women do feel thirsty during labour and many hospitals advise women to bring drinks in with them (there are usually vending machines in hospitals and fresh tap water is always available, but if you have a favourite drink you should bring it in with you). As mentioned above, if you sip on slightly sweet drinks you will keep your blood sugar levels up. A little often is better than large quantities, but avoid fizzy drinks at all costs.

Food and Drink for your Partner

Many hospitals are not legally allowed to cater for your partner. Although your partner may be with you all the way when you are in labour, he will not actually be in labour himself and he may be subject to normal hunger pangs at meal-times! It may be possible to get snacks from vending machines, but it is not a bad idea for him to bring a snack with him.

Your Partner's Role in Labour

Throughout this book the word partner is used to mean the baby's father. In many cases the baby's father will be your husband, and he will be with you for the labour and delivery. Whoever your birth companion is (your husband, your mother, a friend) this section will give them an idea of how to help you when you are in labour.

Many men worry that they will not know how to help and will feel powerless while their wives are in labour. It is true that no one can alter the contractions or experience them for you, but your partner can go a very long way to make the whole experience of labour and childbirth a memory that you can cherish rather than try to blot out.

Your partner's most significant role when you are in labour is to give you support, and he can do this in more ways than one:

Physical support: He can actually support you physically, letting you lean on him when you are tired, and helping you to walk about if you want to remain active (you may need someone to lean on when strong contractions come). He can also help you in and out of baths, help you get to the loo, and help you to find comfortable positions to rest in.

Psychological support: He can support you psychologically by encouraging you each time you get through a contraction and telling you that you are doing well; it is impossible to underestimate the value of a little bit of encouragement in labour, especially with a first baby. You are doing something you have never done before and you need people to tell you that you are doing well. He can encourage you by keeping eye contact with you during contractions and by holding your hand throughout. If he puts his hand on your abdomen, he will actually feel the contractions coming, and will be ready to give you all the encouragement you need.

> CASE STUDY: *'He kept saying "well done, good girl" and then worrying that it sounded patronising. He would actually ask: "sorry, do you mind me saying good girl?" and I said "no, it's the best thing you could say". I felt like a child again, a bit frightened and confused, and I just needed reassurance the whole time. It was years since anyone had called me a "good girl", it was very reassuring.'*

Supporting your ideas: Your birth partner can also support your ideas about how you want your labour and delivery to proceed. When you are too tired or in too much pain he can liaise with the midwife, and talk to her about your birth plan. He can make sure that you understand what drugs or intervention you are being offered and why. He can ensure that you have everything you need to keep you as happy and comfortable as possible.

Keeping you comfortable: Your partner is likely to play an important role in keeping you comfortable during labour, not only as mentioned above by making sure you have everything you need and helping you to find a comfortable position. He can also ease aches and pains by massaging you: massage to the lower back can help with backache and massaging of the neck and shoulders can release tension and alleviate tiredness.

If you are very hot he can bathe your face with a cool sponge or flannel. Despite feeling generally hot, some women find that their legs and feet get uncomfortably cold in labour, your partner can rub your feet to warm them and to help relax you.

Helping with breathing: Another important role for your birth partner is to help you to breathe correctly during contractions (see the section on breathing in **Coping Strategies**, below). This will probably be easier for him if he has attended at least one antenatal class or has discussed breathing for labour with you beforehand, but many people have no preparation before being birth assistants, and still manage to be of great help with breathing. It is more helpful for him to keep eye contact with you and encourage you when you are breathing than to give you complicated instructions about how to breathe!

Coping Strategies

Many of the coping strategies for labour in hospital are the same as those used at home (see the section on **Coping Strategies at Home**, above).

Stay on the move: This may become difficult as your contractions become stronger, but the longer you remain active, the more quickly your labour is likely to progress.

Find a comfortable position to rest: This will become increasingly important as your labour progresses and you become more tired.

Breathe through your contractions: However ridiculous you felt practising breathing in your antenatal classes, you will be surprised how much it helps when you are actually in labour. Correct breathing not only makes it easier for you to cope with individual contractions, it means that you are getting enough oxygen so that you do not get dizzy or feel so tired, and it also gives you something other than the pain to concentrate on.

As you feel a contraction coming on let your breath out (some women find it helps to blow their breath out explosively at the beginning of a contraction), then take little shallow breaths during the contraction. This will ensure that you are getting enough oxygen but the small movement of your lungs will not interfere with the contractions of the uterus by pushing down on it. When the contraction passes, take a deep breath, and concentrate on breathing regularly and deeply until the next contraction comes.

> CASE STUDY: *'I'm not convinced that the breathing really made any difference, but it was just something for us both to concentrate on during the contractions.'*

> CASE STUDY: *'It's difficult to say how much the breathing helped, but it definitely made me relaxed, and I was amazed how normal I felt in between contractions.'*

Have a bath: Many hospitals offer labouring women baths to help them to relax. When you visit your maternity unit ask whether women can have baths during labour. Your hospital may have one or several birthing pools and, even if you are not planning to have a water birth, you may be able to use the pool during labour. A birthing pool gives you much more room to move and find a comfortable position than an ordinary bath.

Massage: Your partner may find that you need a lot of massaging to help ease the pain and keep you relaxed. It might be a good idea to take some skin cream or lotion to stop your skin being chafed if firm massaging is helpful.

Distract yourself: Even quite late in the first stage of labour you may find that you can distract yourself to some extent. It is important to remember that you should not be in any pain in between contractions; if you have a favourite tape or a card game to help you feel normal in between contractions it will be easier for you to take the contractions themselves one at a time.

Pain Relief in Labour

There are a number of different kinds of pain relief that are usually available to labouring women in all hospitals. This section is to give you an idea of the different forms of pain relief available, when you are likely to be offered them, and what the benefits and disadvantages of each are.

TENS Machine: TENS stands for transcutaneous electrical nerve stimulation, which means stimulating the nerves through the skin by means of an electrical shock. Electricity has been used in medicine and in controlling pain since the nineteenth century, and TENS machines are used not only for childbirth but also for controlling chronic back pain and arthritis.

The TENS machine consists of four electrode pads that can be placed directly onto the skin on the part of your body worst affected by labour pains, such as the lower back. The four pads are all connected to a control box about the size of a large box of matches, which you use to set off the pulses of current when you feel a contraction coming on. The electrical current not only stimulates your body's production of endorphins, powerful natural pain-killers, it is also thought that it can to some extent block the 'pain signal' that travels from the uterus to the brain.

TENS is most effective if it is used from the very early stages of labour, starting with a tiny current and building to a stronger one as the contractions become more powerful. Used like this, the TENS machine stimulates a steady production of endorphins. The best time to start using a TENS machine is at home when your labour is just starting: it may be possible to hire one from your hospital, and you will need to book one well in advance of your due date in case you go into labour pre-term (it is not considered safe to use a TENS machine before 37 weeks gestation).

The tiny currents produced by the TENS machine have no side-effects (but it should not be used by people with pace-makers) so it is a safe drug-free form of pain relief. TENS will not actually remove any pain, but it may alter your perception of the pain and your ability to cope with it. Some women find that the TENS machine makes absolutely no difference. You may be offered a TENS machine when you first book in to the hospital if you are still in the early stages of labour. It is certainly worth trying because it can be a very useful way of controlling the pain of contractions.

CASE STUDY: *'With my second baby I had a TENS machine right from the beginning. I was fine for a while and then when I thought "oh no, this is too much, give me the epidural now!" they told me I was fully dilated, so it really had seen me all the way to the pushing stage.'*

Tranquillisers: Tranquillisers are not actually used for the treatment of pain relief, but they are very occasionally offered to women, especially first-time mothers, who are in a state of high anxiety about their labour. The possible effects of the tranquillisers on the baby – making him drowsy – are undesirable, but women are sometimes offered tranquillisers if they are very tense and finding it difficult to cope with labour in the early stages. If you prepare well for your labour so that you understand the physiological process, and know the breathing techniques and methods of relaxation, you are unlikely to need tranquillisers. You can prepare for labour by reading books such as this one and by attending antenatal classes.

Pethidine: Pethidine is a powerful sedative drug with pain relieving qualities. It is often used for labouring women because it interferes little with the progression of the labour itself (although if the doses are large, the contractions may become weaker and slightly less frequent). Pethidine is given by injection, usually into the buttocks, or by intravenous injection.

Pethidine can make you feel very sleepy and detached from events; it does not actually relieve the pain, but removes you from it by sedating you. Some women welcome these feelings of detachment, while others say that they feel as if they have lost control of the situation when they are under the effects of pethidine. It is not uncommon for women to complain of nausea, and even to vomit, when they are on pethidine.

You may be offered pethidine even in the very early stages of your labour, or before you are in established labour, if you are already in pain. Pethidine's sedative effect may help you through the pain and may allow you to drift off to sleep in between contractions. As your labour progresses, the midwife will need to gauge how much longer your labour will last before offering or giving you pethidine. This is because the pethidine is transferred to the baby through the placenta and produces the same drowsiness in the baby as the mother. It is undesirable for the baby to be very drowsy when he is born because his sucking reflex may be suppressed and – more importantly – he may even have trouble breathing.

If you are given pethidine four or more hours before delivery, the effects of the pethidine on the baby may have worn off again by the time he is born, and if you are given it less than an hour before delivery the drug may not have had time to reach him; but pethidine given one to four hours before delivery is most likely to cause drowsiness in the baby. This drowsiness in the baby is a major drawback of pethidine, and some babies of mothers who have been given pethidine in labour may need special drugs to help them breathe, and they may be affected by the effects of pethidine for up to three days after delivery.

Another disadvantage of pethidine is that it arrests the digestive system and stops the stomach from emptying. In the minority of women who may go on to need emergency treatment (such as a Caesarean section) under general anaesthetic, there are considerable risks associated with undergoing general anaesthesia with a full stomach.

CASE STUDY: *'When I eventually got to 5cm my contractions became much stronger and more painful. They offered me pethidine, which really depressed me because I knew that that meant they thought I had hours to go. Something told me it wouldn't be long though, and just half an hour later I was fully dilated. I'm very glad that I trusted my instincts and resisted the temptation because it could have been a very different experience if I'd been out of it on pethidine.'*

CASE STUDY: *'I had pethidine because I was adamant about not having an epidural – I don't like any drugs really but I needed more than just the gas and air. The pethidine was fine, I still knew what was going on.'*

Epidural: The full name of an epidural is in fact an epidural nerve block. The pain of contractions can be completely removed by a drug that is injected directly into the epidural space just inside the vertebrae. The drug used is a combination of anaesthetic and analgesic; ideally, the combination will remove the pain, but sensation and some motor power should be maintained. Epidurals are usually not used until a woman is in established labour, and in some hospitals they may not be used if the labour is very advanced (it may simply not be possible to offer the necessary degree of pain relief in time, and it is not desirable for the woman to have little sensation for the second stage of labour when she is pushing).

Epidural nerve blocks need to be set up by a qualified anaesthetist, and the process can take up to 15 minutes; it should not be painful but it can be frightening. An anaesthetist is a fully trained doctor, and you may want to ask your anaesthetist about the process and the effect that it may have on your labour and birth. Once an epidural has been set up, continued pain relief can be achieved by a constant infusion of the drugs, or the drugs may be topped up when necessary by the midwife or the anaesthetist (a woman who has an epidural will have one-to-one attention from her midwife).

Epidurals can block out all the pain of contractions, and this makes them a popular option with many women. Until quite recently, epidurals cut off virtually all sensation and power too, and meant that the woman had to remain in bed for her labour and had to be told when to push for the second stage. Many hospitals now offer much lower dose epidurals which mean that the woman still has bladder control and some motor power; she is still conscious of her contractions and has the urge to bear down. Queen Charlotte's Hospital has pioneered a 'mobile' epidural where very low doses are used, and the woman retains sufficient motor power to walk around during labour.

If a woman has a long labour and needs many top-ups she may find that her legs become heavy and wobbly. Most women who have epidurals recognise the urge to bear down; but if the epidural has been topped up many times or a high-dose drug has been used, the urge to bear down can be lost, and the midwife has to motivate the woman to push, explaining to her how and where to push to deliver the baby.

Only small doses of drugs are used in epidurals and they, therefore, have no side-effects on the baby, but they can cause the mother's blood pressure to drop. Epidurals can slow down the labour, possibly making further intervention – such as an oxytocin drip or an assisted delivery – necessary.

Women considering having epidurals often ask whether they are in danger of being paralysed or whether they will have long-term problems with backache and headaches. These concerns are probably based on evidence of the effects epidurals may have had in a few cases several decades ago. The techniques have improved dramatically: cases of paralysis are now virtually unheard of, and there are extremely rare cases of other temporary nerve damage, but it is difficult to separate them from those that are caused by the delivery itself. In the case of headaches, in a very small minority of cases the dura – the sheath surrounding the liquid that protects the nerves in the spine – may be damaged, and this can lead to a very specific kind of headache that can be treated once diagnosed. Many women may have a tender spot on their back for a few days after having an epidural, but there is no evidence that epidurals are responsible for causing long-term back problems.

Some hospitals can only offer epidurals during the day or if they are booked in advance (because there may not be an anaesthetist on call 24 hours a day), and a few hospitals do not offer epidurals at all. Ask your doctor or midwife about the availability of epidurals in your hospital, and ask whether they provide low dose or mobile epidurals.

CASE STUDY: *'I think anyone who has a baby without pain relief is crazy or a martyr. I had a mobile epidural and it was just wonderful. We wandered up and down serenely and I could top up whenever I needed to. It all started out like that, but then everything went wrong because I couldn't get her out, so I ended up having to have a Caesarean. But at least I was already hooked up to the epidural so they just lay me down, up went the screen, and she came out incredibly quickly.'*

CASE STUDY: *'I had a two-day labour, and I went to hospital after the first day. When I got there I was already so exhausted I wanted them to give me whatever they'd got. The epidural was brilliant!'*

Gas and Air: Gas and air (or entonox) is very commonly used to relieve pain in labour. The gas is a 50/50 mixture of nitrous oxide (laughing gas) and oxygen, and it is inhaled through a mask that the woman herself brings to her face during contractions. Nitrous oxide is a pain-killer although women often say that it does not relieve the pain but makes you feel detached from it, and gives you a feeling of wellbeing. Some women find that gas and air makes them feel nauseous and gives them a dry mouth, and few women like to use it for any length of time. Some women find that they like the 'floating', detached feeling the gas and air produces, while others dislike it and feel that they have lost control of the situation.

One of the great advantages of gas and air is that it has no affect on the baby; once the mixture is exhaled by the mother it is out of her system, and there are no known long-term side-effects of using gas and air.

CASE STUDY: *'I'm not sure that the gas and air made much difference really, or maybe I got used to it, but it gives you something to think about when each contraction comes on and it makes you breathe, which helps.'*

CASE STUDY: *'I really didn't like the gas and air. It made me feel sick and high, I felt as if I was floating, I was losing it.'*

Planning your Pain Relief

When you are thinking about your labour and your birth plan, you need to consider all the forms of pain relief that are available in your hospital. You will learn about pain relief in labour if you attend antenatal classes, but if you have any further questions about methods of pain relief and their side-effects, ask your doctor or midwife, or you could arrange to speak to an anaesthetist. It is important for you to be informed about what pain relief will be available at which stage in your labour so that you understand what you are being offered when you are actually in labour.

You should also bear in mind that every woman's experience of labour and of the various kinds of pain relief is different. Your ideas about what pain relief you think you will use should not be influenced by other people's fear of pain or their ideals of natural childbirth: you must strike the right balance for you between controlling the pain and being in control of the birth of your baby. Giving birth is not a competition, and there should be no feeling of competition about how much or how little pain relief you need. The most important thing is the end result: the baby.

CASE STUDY: *'No question about it: I want an epidural. I mean, people have pain relief when they have a leg amputated or a tooth out. I have no pain threshold so I want that epidural!'*

CASE STUDY: *'I really want to try and do it with as little pain relief as possible. It may all go horribly wrong on the day, but I want to give it a go.'*

Alternative 'Pain Relief'

As well as the 'conventional' methods of pain relief mentioned above there are a number of alternative treatments that may help with pain in labour. It is important to be aware that there is no magical remedy which will make the pain go away: for the massive majority of women, labour is very painful and nothing short of an epidural or a large dose of pethidine will actually take the pain away. Other methods of 'pain relief' are ways of making the process easier to cope with.

Two key elements in making the process easier are: understanding what is happening to your body, and relaxing to let nature take its course. You can understand what is happening to your body during labour by reading books such as this one, by attending antenatal classes, and by talking to your midwife before and during labour. If you understand what is happening to you, you should find it easier to relax which most mothers, midwives and doctors agree tends to make labour shorter and easier. Many of the alternative forms of 'pain relief' are intended to help you to relax.

If you are planning to use an alternative therapy to control your pain in labour, especially if you want to have a therapist present for the birth, you should talk to your hospital about this well in advance. Some hospitals and consultants may be unwilling for you to use alternative therapies, and you will need to clear it with them or possibly look into going to another hospital.

Some of the alternative methods of pain relief have already been mentioned in **Coping Strategies**, above. These include breathing for relaxation, having a bath / using a birthing pool and massage. Other methods of alternative 'pain relief' are discussed here (in alphabetical order).

Acupuncture: (For an explanation of the theories behind acupuncture see the section on **Alternative Therapies and Medicines During Pregnancy** in the chapter **Illness During Pregnancy**.) Acupuncture can be used as an effective form of pain relief in labour (in China some Caesarean sections are allegedly carried out using acupuncture as the only form of pain relief). Some women find that it has no effect at all but most report that it at least 'takes the edge off' the pain. The treatment is thought to work by stimulating the body's productions of endorphins and by normalising the levels of a naturally produced chemical called Serotonin which causes contractions. Acupuncture can also be used to stimulate contractions in slow or erratic labours.

If you are thinking of using acupuncture for pain relief in labour you will need to have preliminary sessions with a trained, experienced therapist and you will have to discuss with your midwife and consultant whether your therapist may attend you in hospital.

Aromatherapy: (For background information on aromatherapy see the section on **Alternative Therapies and Medicines During Pregnancy** in the chapter **Illness During Pregnancy**.) Aromatherapy oils are beginning to gain recognition as useful aids to relaxation, possibly giving some direct pain relief, in labour. Some midwives are actually trained aromatherapists, and more hospitals are receptive to the idea of using aromatherapy oils than a number of other alternative therapies because it is non-invasive, does not interfere with the contractions and usually does not necessitate the presence of a therapist.

Some essential oils are said to have analgesic qualities, and women using them do report that they diminish pain in labour. Perhaps the most useful oils are those that promote relaxation; but invigorating oils are also beneficial if used for the second stage.

If you are thinking of using aromatherapy oils to relieve pain and to help you relax during labour you will need to find a trained aromatherapist who has experience of prescribing oils to women in labour. You should discuss the oils that you are going to use in advance and ensure that the smells are agreeable to you (any therapeutic effect would be nullified if you do not like the smell). When you are in labour, the oils can be inhaled, used by your partner in a massage oil or added to a bath.

Autogenic training: Autogenic training is a system of six exercises intended to achieve deep relaxation rapidly. The system was devised by a German psychiatrist who had observed the benefits of hypnosis on a number of physical and psychological problems in his patients, and who wanted his patients to be able to reach the same state of relaxation by training themselves. The state of relaxation achieved by autogenic training can dramatically improve a woman's experience of labour (although it is questionable whether it actually relieves the pain), and the lack of tension in her body may even speed up the labour. Once you have learned the exercises for relaxation you can use them yourself and there is, therefore, no need to have your 'trainer' with you in hospital.

If you are interested in using autogenic training during labour you will need to go on a course of lessons either in a group or on a one-to-one basis. Be sure to find a qualified instructor who has experience of training pregnant women (some of the exercises used in autogenic training are not recommended for pregnant women). The address of the British Association for Autogenic Training appears at the end of the book. Once you have learned the relaxation exercises you need to practise them regularly to reap the benefits when you are in labour.

Homeopathy: (For background information on homeopathy see the section on **Alternative Therapies and Medicines During Pregnancy** in the chapter **Illness During Pregnancy**.) Homeopathy can be used during labour and childbirth to promote the natural process of birth and to minimise some of the woman's unpleasant symptoms. It certainly will not take away the pain but it can improve a woman's experience of labour and may speed up the labour.

It is possible to buy homeopathic remedies over the counter in health shops, and you could build up a collection of the remedies that are recommended for the feelings you are likely to experience in labour. This is a hit and miss way of using homeopathic remedies: homeopathy is most effective if the remedies are combined specially for you by someone who knows you and your specific symptoms. Ideally, you should find a registered, qualified homeopath with experience of treating pregnant and labouring women, and you should ask your midwife and your consultant whether it would be acceptable to have your homeopath with you in hospital. There are some midwives who have also specialised in homeopathic remedies for use during labour (contact the British Homeopathic Association [see address at back of book] and they may be able to put you in touch with a midwife who has this training).

Hypnosis: (For background information on hypnosis and hypnotherapy see the section on **Alternative Therapies and Medicines During Pregnancy** in the chapter **Illness During Pregnancy**.) Hypnotism produces in the subject a state of deep relaxation, similar to the moments just before falling asleep. Women who successfully achieve this sort of state in labour are likely to have a shorter labour, and to have a less acute perception of pain and of the passage of time; this, therefore, improves their experience of labour. The hypnotised subject also has tremendous powers of concentration, and it may be possible for a woman to concentrate specifically on relaxing, on blotting out the pain, or on the muscular efforts of her contractions and the delivery of her baby.

Hypnosis can be a useful way of improving your experience of labour and delivery, especially as it is non-invasive and can be combined with conventional methods of pain-relief. If you are thinking of using hypnosis to help you control pain in labour you will need to contact a registered, qualified hypnotherapist with experience of treating pregnant and labouring women well in advance of your due date. With time it is possible to learn methods of self-hypnosis so that you do not actually need a therapist with you in hospital. If you do want to have your therapist with you for your labour you will need to clear this with your consultant. If you are intending to use self-hypnosis during labour you should let your midwife know: the calm state that can be achieved by using hypnosis can mask the fact that you are progressing into advanced labour, and your midwife may need to use internal examinations more frequently to check your progress.

Mental relaxation: The fact that relaxation helps a woman to endure and even enjoy her labour has been repeated frequently already. Methods of relaxation that have already been mentioned, such as using breathing exercises, having baths and massage, have concentrated on physical relaxation. It is equally important to relax mentally in order to prolong a relaxed state. If the mind is allowed to continue working at its normal rate and in its normal way it will keep drawing your attention back to the pain, and creating the vicious circle: pain causes fear, which gives rise to tension, which aggravates the pain.

You may be taught methods of mental relaxation in your antenatal classes or you may be able to find a class locally that teaches methods of relaxation. It is possible to teach yourself to clear your mind, and it is worth practising for a number of weeks before you go into labour, to give you the confidence to use the technique when you are in the grip of contractions.

To teach yourself mental relaxation you first need to achieve a state of physical relaxation by lying down in a warm and comfortable place, concentrating on breathing slowly and steadily, and thinking through your entire body – from your toes to the top of your scalp – systematically tensing up the muscles and then letting them go. Once your body is relaxed you are ready to relax your mind by focusing it on one thing: it may be a point on the ceiling, a mental picture of a peaceful place or even a simple phrase of music. Every time another idea comes into your mind, think of discarding it physically (dropping it in a bin or pushing it away), blow it away with a deep breath, and re-impose the single image on which you are concentrating. You could ask your partner to talk you through your relaxation routine, so that he will know how to help you when you go into labour.

Mental relaxation need not cost you anything, it is non-invasive, will not interfere with your contractions or with what the midwife is doing, and it can be used in conjunction with conventional methods of pain-relief.

Reflexology: (For background information on reflexology see the section on **Alternative Therapies and Medicines During Pregnancy** in the chapter **Illness During Pregnancy**.) Reflexology can be used during pregnancy to help a woman to relax and to ensure that the normal functioning of her body, including her uterus, is balanced. A reflexologist can escort you to hospital or can show you and your partner in advance the reflex points on your hands and feet that can be used to achieve a state of relaxation and to stimulate the normal progress of your labour. Women who use reflexology in labour tend to have shorter than average labours and to use less than average conventional pain-relief. It is a useful non-invasive method of relaxation that can be used in conjunction with conventional pain-relief.

If you are interested in using reflexology during your labour, you will need to find a registered, qualified reflexologist with experience of treating pregnant and labouring women in advance of your due date. If you would like your reflexologist to be with you in hospital you will have to clear this with your consultant.

Visualisation: Visualisation – concentrating on visualising a particular image – will not in any way diminish labour pains, but it can be used to promote mental relaxation and to help a woman cope with contractions. When you are trying to relax you may have a store of restful images that you can visualise to help your mind to let go of the here and now. What you choose to visualise is a matter of personal choice: it could be a rainbow, a horse's mane flowing in the wind, waves lapping a Caribbean beach ... the possibilities are endless. By concentrating on the scene you are visualising you will be blocking other thoughts from your brain.

Some women use visualisation to help them understand and cope with their contractions. If you visualise the opening of your cervix, rather like the opening of a tightly furled daffodil, it may help you to get through each contraction. You may find it easier to cope with the remorseless succession of the contractions by visualising them as waves that carry you forward to a destination, or as a series of flights of stairs that you have to climb.

Yoga: Yoga exercises can be used to create a feeling of physical or spiritual wellbeing at any time. Women who practise yoga for some time before going into labour benefit not only from their ability to relax using yoga exercises and breathing techniques, but also from the fact that their bodies are likely to be well-balanced and supple. They are likely to have shorter than average labours. Yoga is, therefore, a useful way of improving your chances of having a good experience of labour, and of relaxing during labour. It is non-invasive and does not interfere with your contractions or the work of the midwife; and it can be used in conjunction with conventional medicine.

In order to reap any benefits from yoga, you will need to attend classes for some time before your due date. It is important that you find a trained instructor who has experience of working with pregnant women and on giving advice about using yoga in labour. If you would like your instructor to be with you in hospital you will need to clear this with your consultant.

The Transition Period

When you come to the end of the first stage of labour, when your cervix is fully dilated, you may enter a strange and often difficult phase called the transition period. Up till now the contractions have been working to efface and dilate the cervix and, now that this has been accomplished, the uterus takes some time to adjust, to 'change gear' for the next phase of your labour when you will push your baby out. At the same time, tremendous hormonal changes are taking place in your body in preparation for birth and lactation, and these hormones can have a profound effect on your emotions.

For some women this change of gear happens almost instantaneously and they do not experience a transition period, for others it is a strange period of suspended animation when they continue to have contractions but they can feel that things are changing. The transition period can last about half an hour, and rarely lasts more than one hour.

Many women feel shaky and confused or frightened during the transition period; they ask to go home and they begin to resent their partner for not being in labour, the baby for causing all this trouble or their midwife for giving so many instructions and making it sound easy! They may feel nauseous and actually be sick, and they often feel jumpy and don't want to be touched. It is useful for your partner to be aware that you may react like this during the transition period, so that he can be sympathetic: he too may be tired and drained by this stage and your reactions may be hurtful to him; the last thing you need in the transition period is to have to worry about his feelings!

As your body prepares for the second stage of labour at the end of the transition period you may become very restless. You may start to grunt involuntarily as you feel the urge to bear down and push your baby out.

CASE STUDY: *'I became very shaky just before I started pushing. I was sitting on the bed and my legs were quaking, it was a horrible feeling.'*

Second Stage of Labour

In the second stage of labour, when your cervix is fully dilated, the purpose of your contractions changes: their tremendous downward force, starting from the top of the uterus, helps to expel the baby from the uterus. Although women can reduce the length of the second stage by bearing down and consciously pushing, the involuntary contractions are believed to be responsible for over 50% of the work of pushing the baby out.

The Urge to Push

You may recognise the beginning of the second stage of labour because you may well have an irresistible urge to push. The baby's head will have begun its journey through the cervix and will be pressing so hard against the back wall of your vagina that it will be applying pressure to the back wall of your rectum. As a result, the urge to push actually feels like a need to empty your bowels; the baby's head feels like a very large, hard stool ... which will be very hard to pass (women have described giving birth as being like passing a water melon!).

You may be conscious of feeling the baby's head for some time before the urge to push becomes overwhelming and irresistible. Some women begin to grunt and strain quite spontaneously when their cervix is ready for the second stage, others have to be told that it is 'time to push'. Once you have started pushing and the baby's head begins to travel through the birth canal (your vagina), the desire to push is increasingly likely to become spontaneous and irresistible.

If you have had an epidural, the anaesthetist will try to time the use of the nerve blocks so that you will feel the urge to push. In some cases, the

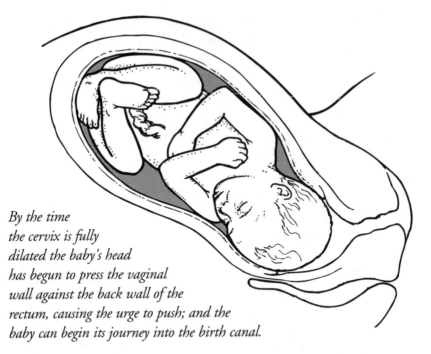

*By the time
the cervix is fully
dilated the baby's head
has begun to press the vaginal
wall against the back wall of the
rectum, causing the urge to push; and the
baby can begin its journey into the birth canal.*

epidural is still very powerful and women have to be told when to push; although the women may feel a little cheated out of the experience of giving birth, their babies can still be born naturally (more than half of the pushing is done involuntarily by the uterus). There is, however, an increased likelihood of assisted delivery with epidurals. Similarly, the doctor or midwife will try to time the use of pethidine so that it wears off in time for the second stage; a woman who has very recently had a dose of pethidine may be too drowsy to participate very actively in the second stage of her labour, and this too can increase her chances of needing an assisted delivery.

CASE STUDY: *'I started to feel her head and to feel as if I wanted to push when I was 7cm. But somehow I knew it wasn't time to push yet. Then I had about half an hour of incredibly powerful contractions and really suddenly the urge to push was just so strong. I looked at the midwife and said "I've got to push, I've got to push". She gave me a quick internal – which I didn't actually feel, there were so many other sensations to think about – and told me "you're fully dilated, go ahead and push!"'*

CASE STUDY: *'Wanting to push was just so strong it was like falling over a waterfall – and we're talking Niagara! – there was nothing I could do to stop myself.'*

How you will Feel

As with so many other aspects of pregnancy and delivery the way that you feel as you go into the second stage of labour can vary enormously. Some women feel that at last they have a real job to do and the end is in sight; others are afraid of what still lies ahead, they worry that they will not be able to push their baby out or that there will be something wrong with the baby. It is not uncommon for women to ask to go home at this stage or to say that they do not want to have the baby at all.

Your physical feelings will change too during the second stage of labour: many women say that they no longer feel pain with their contractions, and this is probably because they are concentrating so hard on pushing with the contractions. Whether or not your contractions hurt less during the second stage, you are now subject to a new sort of pain: the aching sensation as the bones of your pelvis open, and the splitting burning feeling as your vagina and perineum stretch to their limits to allow the baby's head to pass.

CASE STUDY: *'I knew the labour was going to hurt, but what surprised me was how much it hurt when her head was sort of coming through me. There was this incredible bone-aching feeling. I kept looking at my midwife and saying "it hurts down there, it hurts down there!" She must have thought I was crazy, of course it hurts, I was having a baby. But I found it quite a scary sort of pain, as if I was being broken open.'*

CASE STUDY: *'I was frightened when I started pushing. I suddenly had this "now or never feeling'" and I wanted all the pain to be over.'*

Resisting the Urge to Push

Sometimes women feel the urge to push before the cervix is fully dilated, and their midwife will help them to resist the urge. This can be unbelievably difficult, given how irresistible that urge can be (as illustrated by the case studies above). You will only be asked to resist the urge for a very good reason. The most common reason for this is when the cervix is not yet fully dilated. It is possible for the baby's head to start putting pressure on your rectal wall and to give you a powerful urge to push before the cervix is completely ready to allow the baby's head to pass through into the birth canal.

If you begin bearing down and trying to push the baby down the birth canal before the cervix is fully effaced, the pressure put on the cervix may cause it to swell. You can enter a deadlock between the baby's head and the cervix; this can prolong your labour considerably and increase the likelihood of needing further pain relief and other forms of intervention. There is also an increased risk of foetal distress because of the sustained pressure to the baby's head.

Your instinctive reaction to the urge to push will be to take a deep breath and bear down with all your might. If you are told not to push yet, you can to some extent control the actual bearing down by controlling your breathing: by taking very shallow breaths, even just panting, you will not have a good enough lungful of air with which to bear down. Your midwife will keep reminding you to pant when each contraction makes you want to push. Your partner can help you by panting with you so that you concentrate on copying his pattern of breathing instead of following your instinct. Remember to breath slowly and normally in between contractions because panting, especially if you have to do it for any length of time, can cause you to hyperventilate, making you feel sick and dizzy. If you begin to feel dizzy and you can stand having anything over your face, your partner can cup his hand over your nose and mouth when you pant to stop you hyperventilating.

CASE STUDY: *'That was the hardest part of all, not pushing. All I wanted to do was to get the baby out, and she [the midwife] said I couldn't push then. But she kept her face near me the whole time and made me pant each time I wanted to take a deep breath. She was brilliant.'*

CASE STUDY: *'I wanted to push but the front of my cervix was not effaced. I found that the epidural helped me not push, because it sort of took the edge off the urge.'*

Positions for Second Stage and Delivery
Only a generation ago almost all women were delivered of their babies lying on a hospital bed with their legs up in stirrups. This remains the

position in which midwives and doctors have the best view and control of the situation and, if you are advised that you need to be in this position because there are complications and any sort of intervention is needed, it is safest for you and your baby if you follow this advice.

If the second stage of your labour is proceeding normally there are a number of different positions that you can adopt that may make the pushing and the delivery easier for you. You will have learned about positions for labour if you attended antenatal classes, and you may well have discussed positions for labour with your midwife. You may also have adopted a position in the first stage of labour that feels right and in which you want to deliver your baby. Your midwife will be able to suggest positions to you when the time comes if you cannot find a comfortable position.

Many women favour an upright position because the force of gravity can then work with them, and they feel in control of the situation. A few women try a standing position leaning against a wall or their partner, but many women feel too tired or do not have the strength in their legs for this. They also worry that, if the baby is born very quickly, it will fall and injure itself (this is, of course, extremely unlikely to happen because the midwife will be talking you through the entire second stage and the delivery, and will know when the baby is coming).

If a completely upright position does not seem right or is not possible, you can try squatting or half squatting (either by yourself, against a wall, against your partner or supported by one or two other people). Squatting is a popular position for delivery, and is still used by many tribal peoples around the globe.

However much you like the idea of squatting and letting the force of gravity work for you, you may find that your legs give way beneath you; this can be caused by pain in the legs, by the fact that all your muscular efforts and your circulation are concentrating on your uterus, or it may simply be that you feel too tired. Some women compromise by adopting a position on all fours or kneeling against their partner, a bean bag or a pile of pillows.

If you have no strength in your legs at all it is still possible to let the force of gravity help by sitting in an upright or semi-upright position with your knees bent and your hands clasping your knees. This is a popular position with women and midwives: women like it because they say that being able to put their chins onto their chests helps them push, because they can see the baby as it arrives and because they can rest back onto pillows or their partner behind them between contractions; doctors and midwives favour this position because they have a clear view of the vagina and of the baby's head as it arrives, so that they are ready to take action if they have to. Another advantage of this position is that the baby can be delivered directly onto the mother's tummy (see **Where the Baby is Delivered**, below). A variation on this position is to lie on one side, with your upper body supported by pillows.

CASE STUDY: *'In the first stage of labour I had a lot of back pain and some sciatic pain down my legs, I could only really get comfortable lying over a bean bag, stretching out my back ... I even managed to doze off between some contractions, so I decided this would be a great position to have the baby in. But when it came to it, the pain in my legs was so unbearable I couldn't support myself even on the bean bag, so I turned round and sat against it. It was surprisingly comfortable and I could relax back into it between contractions.'*

CASE STUDY: *'I was pushing for a very long time and in the end they had to give me a ventouse. They put my legs up in the stirrups to set everything up, and I actually found that the stirrups were helpful when I was pushing. They gave me something to push against.'*

Bearing Down

Once your cervix is fully effaced and dilated, whether or not you actually have an urge to push, your midwife will tell you that it is time to 'bear down'. You may have learned about bearing down in antenatal classes, and you may instinctively know what to do; in any event, your midwife will talk you through bearing down in time with your contractions to push your baby out. Every contraction helps to propel the narrowest part of your baby's head down through the cervix and along the birth canal.

As you feel each contraction coming on you will probably instinctively take a deep breath in: by filling your lungs you will automatically be putting pressure on the top of your uterus even before you begin pushing. With your lungs full of air you can consciously push down on the top of your uterus. If you are in a squatting position you may find that it helps to squat down further as you push so that the bending of your body works with your pushing. If you are in a sitting position, your midwife will probably tell you to put your chin on your chest when you push.

> CASE STUDY: *'Things suddenly started happening very quickly and the midwife was getting things ready for the baby. Every time a contraction came I wailed "oh no, there's another one coming!" and she would leave what she was doing, put her hand on my knee and say "take a deep breath, chin on your chest and push!"'*

You may well grunt, shout or scream as you bear down. Some books recommend that women should try not to scream but to concentrate their energies on pushing. Actually, the small percentage of your energies which is spent on making a noise is probably not wasted: it may help you psychologically, as if you were vocally underlining your physical effort. If you spend time worrying about not screaming it may throw you off your rhythm of taking a deep breath and pushing in time with the contractions.

If your contractions are very long – and they can last well over a minute in the second stage – you may need to stop pushing, let your breath out and take another breath to continue pushing with the contraction. Once the contraction is past its climax you can drop back and try to catch your breath before the next contraction (they may still be more than a minute apart or they could be as little as 20 seconds apart at this stage).

> CASE STUDY: *'The feeling of pushing was so intense and I was incredibly hot; I was dripping with sweat. I was incredibly focused, I know what people mean by tunnel vision now, I felt as if I was looking at myself down a long dark tunnel because I was concentrating so hard. In between contractions I was exhausted. You think you can't give another push, but then the next one comes along and nothing in the world can stop you pushing.'*

While you are bearing down, your whole pelvic floor needs to be completely relaxed to allow the baby's head to travel down the birth canal. If you have been doing pelvic floor exercises during your pregnancy you will know how to relax the pelvic floor and let it 'bulge' downwards. If you can achieve this while you are pushing your baby out it could make for a quicker, easier second stage.

During the second stage, especially if the muscles of your pelvic floor are very relaxed, you may urinate or defecate involuntarily. Many women actually defecate more than usual just before the onset of labour or in early labour: if you notice that you empty your bowels in early labour you are unlikely to defecate during the second stage. If you do have faeces in your rectum during the second stage of labour they will be pushed out as you bear down. Although women find the idea of this very embarrassing, it is very common and really should be the last thing that you are worrying about in the last few minutes before your baby is born. The midwife will be quite used to it and will simply wipe your anus to keep you clean for your baby's arrival.

As the baby travels down the birth canal, you may be conscious that the focus of your pushing has changed. At first you were pushing down on the top of the uterus, pushing the baby from behind; towards the end of the second stage the pushing comes more from the inside of the vagina, squeezing the baby through.

You may well be able to feel your pelvis opening slightly to allow the baby to pass through the girdle of bone (this can be very uncomfortable as in the case study above in the section on **How you will feel**). In between contractions you may be conscious that the baby is slipping back up so that you feel that half your efforts are being wasted. Although this may seem frustrating, you could ultimately benefit from the fact that your baby travels towards your vagina and then retreats slightly for some time before he is actually born. This allows the delicate skin of the vagina and the perineum to stretch gradually to accommodate the baby's head and means that you will be less likely to tear or to need an episiotomy. If the second stage is progressing very quickly your midwife may tell you to pant during some of your contractions rather than continuing to push in order to allow these tissues to stretch and to minimise the risk of tearing.

CASE STUDY: *'I was pushing for a long time and I was conscious of her slipping back each time. It was demoralising, but the midwife kept saying she was getting there ... I did get away with no stitches, so maybe it was all worth it in the end.'*

CASE STUDY: *'My first baby was born very quickly and I tore quite badly so next time around I warned the midwife that I pushed very quickly. She really tried to pace me and to make me pant through some of the contractions, but I just couldn't stop myself and he was born very quickly ... My memory is probably hazy but I really think I only pushed for three or four contractions ... Yes, I did tear again.'*

While you are bearing down, your midwife will not only be helping you but watching the baby's progress. She will tell you when she first sees the baby's head appearing – although it may retreat again several times before he is born – and when the head is 'crowning', pushing through the vagina. You can put your hand down to feel your baby's head or, if you are sitting upright, you may even be able to see it. This will give you encouragement and incentive to keep on pushing. You need all the encouragement that you can get at this stage, because bearing down is very hard work. You may well be exhausted already by lack of sleep and by the first stage of your labour, and the second stage can take as long as two hours (although it may be much shorter, and certainly is usually shorter with second and subsequent babies).

Pushing Without the Urge

In some cases, women are told to bear down when they do not actually have an urge to push. This may be that for some physiological reason they do not have an instinctive urge to push, or it may be because they have had an epidural or a recent dose of pethidine. Pushing with your contractions can be very hard work, even if you instinctively want to, but pushing without the urge can seem like an insurmountable task. The midwife will help you to time your deep breaths and your pushing with your contractions; even if you do not know when you are having a contraction, she will know either by feeling your abdomen or by checking the read-out on a foetal heart monitor (if you have one fitted). Women who do not have an urge to push may well be able to deliver their babies quite normally, but they do run an increased risk of needing an assisted delivery.

CASE STUDY: *'I was very unlucky because I had a little lip of the cervix which was not effaced or whatever, so I had to pant to stop myself pushing for what felt like ages. That was bad enough and then when they said I could go ahead and push I had completely lost the urge. It was just the hardest work I have ever done in my life, like trying to push a house over with your bare hands.'*

CASE STUDY: *'I didn't realise you had to push. I know it sounds stupid but I thought it all happened naturally. And I don't know if it was because of that but I didn't feel as if I wanted to anyway. The midwife kept telling me that I had to push but I didn't put my heart into it. Then she started worrying about his [the baby's] heart beat, it kept dropping, and it was my husband who said "you have got to get this baby out". I still never wanted to push, but I worked at it harder.'*

What is Happening to the Baby

The second stage of your labour will probably be the most stressful period of your baby's entire life. The adrenaline levels in a newborn baby's bloodstream are higher than he is ever likely to experience again. This is why midwives and doctors are unwilling to let the second stage go on for much longer than two hours, because the demands on the baby's heart are enormous.

The baby has been growing and developing in a relatively stable environment for nine months. Now his head is under tremendous pressure as it pushes down on the cervix, inducing the cervix to dilate. The head then begins to travel down the birth canal, squeezed forward by the contractions and the mother's pushing. The bones of a newborn baby's skull are fairly soft and they are not fully fused together; the different areas of bone can overlap slightly during the second stage of labour to facilitate their passage through the birth canal.

While the baby is being pushed along the birth canal – and, as we have seen, this can be a slow process with the head slipping back in between contractions – his supply of oxygen can be cut off temporarily with each contraction. This intermittent lack of oxygen makes further demands on the baby's heart and circulatory system, and if it is sustained for too long the baby may begin to show signs of distress. Medical staff will keep an eye on how long your second stage is taking, how well it is progressing and how you and the baby are coping with it.

The crown of the baby's head gradually applies pressure behind the vagina and the perineum, forcing the tissues to stretch open to allow the head to pass. Possibly the most stressful moment for the baby is when the head is finally forced through the vagina and is born.

Your Partner's Role During the Second Stage

The second stage of labour is very hard work, and it comes after what may have been a long and exhausting first stage. It is also a time of tremendous anticipation: you know that the end is near, that you will meet your baby soon. You may be eager to know what sex the baby is or frightened that there will be something wrong with the baby, or you may just be longing for the contractions to be over. Your partner probably shares all these emotions with you and can do a great deal to encourage you with your physical labours.

Your partner may well be able to help you find a comfortable position for second stage labour and delivery, and he may even be able to support you in your position. He can keep you going with words of encouragement and praise. He can keep you cool by sponging your brow (you will be surprised how hot you feel), and make sure that you have something to drink if you are thirsty. He can also help you with your breathing, reminding you to take a deep breath before you bear down, and helping you to pant if your midwife has told you not to push with a contraction.

Eye contact or even just a hand to hold can make an enormous difference to a woman's morale and determination in the second stage of labour. Many men come away from delivery suites with one or both hands mauled and battered because their wives have squeezed them so hard during their contractions!

An important aspect of your partner's role during the second stage is to be very understanding. You are in a very stressful situation, you may be exhausted, frightened and confused, and you may not want anyone to touch you. He too may be tired and anxious, but he must not let his feelings get in the way of helping you. If he puts a hand on you to reassure you and you throw his hand off in exasperation, he must accept that you need to be left alone. He also needs to be prepared for the fact that he may come in for some verbal abuse: it is not uncommon for women to harangue their partners, the baby and the midwife during the second stage of labour.

CASE STUDY: *'He was brilliant, I could never have done it without him.'*

CASE STUDY: *'I was pushing for over two hours, and my husband and the midwife kept saying "you can do it, you can do it". In the end they sounded like a couple of parrots. I think I finally managed to make a superhuman effort because I wanted to shut them both up!'*

Assisted Delivery

If the second stage of your labour is taking a long time and / or if your pushing does not seem to be bringing the baby along the birth canal you may need a little bit of help from the midwife or a doctor to assist your delivery. This is because if the second stage lasts more than about two hours the mother is likely to become exhausted and her pushing will become increasingly ineffectual.

There is also a danger that the baby will become distressed because of the sustained pressure on his head and possibly because the supply of oxygen along the umbilical cord is being intermittently cut off by the contractions. Foetal distress is usually gauged by using a foetal heart monitor (see **Electronic Foetal Monitoring**, above). If meconium (the greenish black first stool of the baby) is seen to be seeping from the mother's vagina this can be an indication of foetal distress. If there are signs of foetal distress, your doctor make a small prick in the baby's scalp and collect some blood, by reaching up inside your vagina with a small instrument. The acidity of the baby's blood – an indication of his wellbeing – can be measured from this.

Intervention should not be given for intervention's sake, but the midwife will keep an eye on how long your second stage is taking and how well you and your baby are bearing up to the strains of this most demanding stage before they suggest an assisted delivery. If the doctor or midwife is concerned about the baby's wellbeing, you may be given an episiotomy to allow the baby's head to pass, and/or the delivery may be assisted with forceps or a ventouse. If the baby is considered to be in danger, an emergency Caesarean may be the safest way of delivering him quickly.

Episiotomy: An episiotomy is a deliberate cut to the vagina extending 2 to 3cm (¾–1¼in)into the perineum; it is performed with surgical scissors under local anaesthetic (unless an epidural or other nerve block is already in place). Episiotomies facilitate the passage of the baby's head through the vagina, and they were at one time performed routinely in many hospitals because they speed up the second stage of labour and they are easier to stitch than the tearing which might otherwise occur. It is now considered unnecessary – if not barbaric – to perform an episiotomy unless there is a particular need to do so.

If the mother is very tired and her pushing is becoming ineffectual or if the tissues of her labia and perineum are not stretching sufficiently to allow the baby's head to pass, an episiotomy may be all that is needed to help her give birth to her baby. If there is evidence of foetal distress, an episiotomy may speed up the second stage sufficiently to allow the baby to be born safely without further intervention.

Episiotomies are also useful in a number of special cases such as the delivery of twins and breech babies, or if the baby is very premature (the skull of a premature baby is softer and will be more likely to be injured by sustained pressure during the second stage of labour).

If you need a forceps delivery you may well be given an episiotomy in order to allow the doctor or midwife to place the forceps on either side of the baby's head without tearing you.

CASE STUDY: *'I had an episiotomy but I couldn't feel a thing because I was anaesthetised. It was fine.'*

CASE STUDY: *'I didn't feel the episiotomy because I had an epidural but I – this is revolting – I could hear the snip. It gave me a bit of a shudder, but he came out very quickly after that and I just try not to think about it.'*

Forceps: Special forceps, like large tongs designed to cradle the baby's head, can be used to assist a long second stage or a difficult delivery. As mentioned above, it may be necessary to perform an episiotomy in order to avoid tearing the perineum during a forceps delivery.

Forceps may be used if the second stage is taking a long time and the mother is becoming exhausted, the baby is becoming distressed or the baby's progress down the birth canal is very slow. They are useful in assisting the delivery of large babies and conversely they can be used to protect the more fragile skull of a premature baby from damage that might be caused by sustained pressure in the birth canal. Forceps may also be useful in assisting the delivery if the baby is in the breech position: with breech babies the largest part, the head, is delivered last, and forceps may be necessary to help the mother and to protect the baby's head and neck from damage. Forceps cannot be used if the baby is still above the cervix and the cervix is not fully dilated because they may force the cervix open and damage it.

A slightly different pair of forceps can be used to manipulate the head of the baby so that it is facing your back, the normal position for delivery. If the baby's head is not facing backwards your labour may well be longer and slower and the second stage may not progress well because the presenting part of the baby's head is not the smallest. If the baby can be turned satisfactorily using forceps, further intervention may not be necessary.

Women sometimes worry that forceps could damage them or their babies. It is worth remembering that forceps will only be used when they are needed (that is when some kind of damage – or worse – seems imminent), that they have been used to assist deliveries for about four hundred years, and that they are now so well designed that they can protect the tender head of a premature baby from the rigours of vaginal delivery.

You could be bruised internally by forceps and your baby's head may bear pressure marks or bruises from the forceps for some days after delivery, but the likelihood of further damage to the baby caused by straining with the forceps is very slim. The forceps are not used to tug the baby out against the odds, they are used to assist the delivery, easing the baby forward in time with your contractions and your pushing. If it becomes apparent that the baby is too large or in the wrong position to travel safely along the birth canal you will be given an emergency Caesarean.

CASE STUDY: *'I spent about an hour pushing and they gave me a spinal block so that they could use the forceps. I honestly didn't feel a thing, but in the end he wasn't down far enough anyway so they had to give me a Caesarean.'*

Ventouse: Ventouse is a French word that means suction cup, and the Ventouse does indeed use suction to help draw the baby down the birth canal. A little suction cup is placed on the presenting part of the baby's head, and is held there by the vacuum created by a pump (the other name for a Ventouse delivery is a Vacuum delivery). When the cup is firmly attached to the baby's head it can be used to ease the baby along the birth canal in time with the contractions and the mother's pushing.

The Ventouse is used in much the same way and in many of the same instances as forceps, including easing the baby round into the correct position as it is drawn down the birth canal. Whether forceps or the

Ventouse are used is to some extent a question of the doctor's personal choice, but the Ventouse is becoming an increasingly popular alternative to forceps. Its popularity is largely due to the fact that it is a narrower piece of equipment; it can, therefore, usually be used without the need for an episiotomy, and in many cases it can be applied to the baby's head without extra pain relief for the mother. This means that the Ventouse can be put in place and used more quickly than forceps. It can even be used when the cervix is not quite fully dilated because it can be applied to the baby's head without damaging the cervix, and the gentle pressure drawing the baby forward can be used to dilate the cervix further.

When a Ventouse is used the baby's head does take on a rather unusual shape. The bones of a newborn baby's skull are fairly soft and they are not fully fused together; the suction produced by the Ventouse can draw the top of the baby's head into a point or a rounded lump. This may be disconcerting for the parents, but the lump will disappear over the first few days of the baby's life. Because of the effects of the Ventouse on the baby's head, it may not be used on a very premature baby whose skull is more malleable and delicate than that of a full-term baby.

CASE STUDY: *'I could feel him going back up after every contraction. I knew I had to make an extra effort to push him out, but I had been pushing for a long time and I just knew I didn't have that last push in me ... I felt the cap of the Ventouse go on, which was really uncomfortable, but then it was very quick: I pushed and they pulled and he popped out. He was 8lb 10oz [large for a first baby to a diminutive mother].'*

CASE STUDY: *'Her head was in the wrong position and the pushing was getting nowhere, so they decided to use the Ventouse. I didn't feel it because I had an epidural ... They managed to turn her head but she still wasn't going far, and I had to have an emergency Caesarean.'*

Delivery and Birth

A Burning Feeling

As the moment of delivery approaches the baby's head presses behind the vagina and perineum with each contraction, forcing the tissues to stretch and allow the head to pass. Unless you have had a nerve block or local anaesthetic, you will have a painful burning feeling as the tissues stretch. Some women say that they are not conscious of this feeling and this may be because they are focusing on their contractions and their pushing, or it may be because the tissues are stretched to the point where the nerve endings can no longer send messages to the brain.

CASE STUDY: *'There was a searing hot feeling, now I can see why people compare it to pooing a water melon. I kept putting my hand down to feel her head because I couldn't believe it was hurting so much and the baby's head wasn't there yet. I could feel the whole of my [pubic area] bulging forward.'*

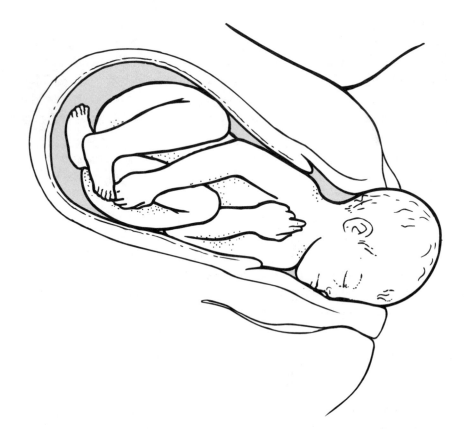

The crown of the baby's head emerges first.

Crowning and Delivering the Baby's Head

Your midwife will tell you when your baby is 'crowning', when the crown of the baby's head is being forced through the vagina. The baby may be crowned several times before one big push finally brings his head into the world. Your midwife may tell you not to push but to pant while the head is being born: if you push too hard you are more likely to tear and to need stitches. You may well then have a rest between contractions before pushing the rest of the baby's body out, and you will be able to feel the baby's head between your legs (this will encourage you and motivate you to carry on).

CASE STUDY: *'Once I had got his head out I was so exhausted, I couldn't believe I was going to have to push any more. The midwife had to ease the rest of him out with the next contraction.'*

Delivering the Baby's Body

Once the baby's head has been born the baby's body swivels round so that he is facing sideways. If the time between contractions allows, the midwife will probably check that the cord is not around the baby's neck which could cause slight strangulation of the baby. If the cord is around the baby's neck, the midwife will try to ease it over the baby's head, or she may swiftly clamp and cut the cord at this stage.

With the next contraction another considerable effort is required to push the shoulders through the vagina, and the rest of the baby's body (which is small in proportion to the head) usually arrives in the same 'push' as the shoulders.

CASE STUDY: *'After all that effort of getting her head out, I had a sort of pause and the final birth was almost an anti-climax. I pushed and there was a funny rushing, slithery feeling between my legs. My body felt about a mile long as she sort of travelled through me and came out.'*

CASE STUDY: *'I'm not the person to ask: she was born very quickly. One minute the midwife said she could just see the baby's head, and with the next contraction she [the baby] was half way across the room ... Well, not literally, but she came out all in one go and she really seemed to shoot out, it felt as if she landed well clear of me! The midwife had actually turned away to pick something up during that contraction, and she turned round to see a baby on the bed. I think she was as surprised as I was.'*

Your Partner's Role in the Delivery

There is a fairly strong divide between the partners who want to have an active role in the delivery of the baby and those who like to stay by the mother's head, encouraging her. The reasons given by the latter are usually to do with not wanting to see their partner's vagina in such a very different situation and role; or it may be that the woman herself does not want to be seen in this way. If your birth assistant is not your sexual partner this sort of squeamishness need not enter into the equation, but many birth assistants – whatever their relationship to the mother – may feel squeamish about seeing too much of the 'working end'.

You should try to discuss in advance how you and your partner feel about his role in the delivery. There is, of course, no accounting for how you will feel on the day, but if you have at least addressed the subject you will both know what you want or expect from each other. It is also worth making a note in your birth plan (if you have one) of the role your partner would like to play in the delivery, or you should let your midwife know your ideas in the early stages of the labour to avoid any embarrassment or disappointment when it comes to the crunch.

Many women feel that at their moments of most extreme exertion, when the baby is being born, they need their partner's support – a hand to hold and eye contact – up at the 'head end' rather than having him actually helping to deliver the baby. Others like to feel that their partner has contributed to the birth of the baby by delivering him.

Some couples are very keen to capture the birth or the moments immediately after the birth on camera, and this becomes the key role of the partner. Just remember that the incredibly powerful emotions that can be associated with the birth of a baby can never be captured on camera, and that the birth is unlikely to be as beautiful visually as it is emotionally. While it is wonderful to have a record of these precious moments, you are very unlikely ever to forget them, and it is a shame to miss them worrying about flashes and f-stops.

CASE STUDY: *'I definitely didn't want him seeing me like that, I wanted him near me – I mean my face – but actually when it came to it he was very curious to see how it all worked … those were his words. And, you know, I was past caring; you could have had a whole BBC TV crew in there and I wouldn't have minded!'*

CASE STUDY [THE FATHER]: *'I wanted to be at the shoulder looking up. I had no intention of seeing the … the coal face, so to speak. Quite soon after [the baby] was born I had to go to the loo and I did this ridiculous Egyptian dance shielding my eyes as I went past so that I didn't see anything.'*

Where the Baby is Delivered

Until quite recently, newly delivered babies were scooped up by the midwives, checked over, weighed, measured, cleaned up and wrapped up before they were presented to their mothers. Many hospitals, midwives and mothers recognise the tremendous benefits of delivering a baby directly into his mother's arms or, better still, onto her tummy nestled between her breasts. The skin-to-skin contact, the natural warmth provided by the mother's body and the rhythm of her heartbeat (which should be familiar to the baby and audible to him if he is between her breasts), all help to soften the blow of arriving from the surrounding moisture and warmth of the uterus into the comparatively cold, dry air. If the baby is delivered straight onto his mother's tummy, her skin will be the first thing that he smells and this – coupled with the physical contact – may be an important part of the bonding process.

Many women welcome the idea of having their baby delivered directly onto their tummies, partly because they know that it is probably what is best for the baby, and partly because they are eager to be the first person to hold this baby that they have carried for nine months and whom they have just brought into the world. Others feel a bit squeamish about the newborn baby before he has been cleaned up a little, or they are so exhausted by the process of giving birth that it takes a while for them to adjust to the idea of handling the baby. Some women are afraid that there may be something wrong with the baby, and that it is safest for him to be checked over by the midwife before he is handed back to her. Even if your baby is delivered straight onto your tummy the midwife will be assessing his wellbeing carefully; she will let you know and take action if there is anything about him that gives cause for concern. If you yourself have any concerns about your baby immediately after delivery, ask the midwife to check that he is all right and ask her to explain anything that seems unusual to you.

If the woman has had a Caesarean and / or if she does not feel up to having her baby delivered straight onto her tummy or into her arms, the baby can, of course, be handed straight to her partner. One important consideration is that newborn babies can lose heat very quickly, and they need to be dried and covered soon after delivery.

CASE STUDY: *'I wanted the baby to be brought straight up onto my tummy, and the second stage was going much more quickly than any of us had expected. I started saying "quickly, undo my buttons!" and my husband started frantically undoing my nightshirt. Afterwards we laughed about it, it was the same sort of urgency like when you're making love. When she arrived I took her straight into my arms, and she hardly cried, she opened these huge eyes and took it all in.'*

CASE STUDY: *'I definitely wanted them to have a good look at her first and check that her airways were clear. A friend of mine nearly lost her baby because he couldn't breathe when he was born, so I was paranoid about that.'*

Breech Birth

Many babies spend at least the first three-quarters of pregnancy in the 'breech position', with their bottoms down. Usually the baby will turn to the head down position at some time in the last two months before delivery. In first pregnancies, because the uterus is firmer, the baby will tend to settle and engage once it has turned. In second and subsequent pregnancies the baby may be able to move around in the more elastic uterus until later in the pregnancy. In about 3% of pregnancies the baby does not turn into the head-down position, and it is the baby's buttocks that engage in the cervix.

There may be a number of complications in labour and delivery, with risks to the baby if he is in the breech position. The buttocks do not constitute such a large, firm presenting part as the head, and the labour may, therefore, be slower and more sporadic; the baby's hips may be damaged during the delivery; and, crucially, the baby's head or neck may be damaged during delivery.

Because of the attendant complications and risks associated with the breech position your doctor may try and manipulate the foetus in the womb into the cephalic position. This is often successful although occasionally can revert to the breech position. If your baby is in the breech position towards the end of your pregnancy, your consultant will consider your case carefully and will decide with you how best to deliver your baby.

If you are keen to try and go ahead with a vaginal delivery your consultant may use ultrasound scans and X-rays to assess whether your pelvis is wide enough for you to give birth to your baby. He may recommend that you have an epidural and that you give birth lying on your back with your feet up in stirrups so that the doctor can deliver the baby safely. You will anyway need some sort of pain relief because episiotomies are performed in breech deliveries to facilitate the passage of the head, and forceps may be used to protect the head as it is delivered.

CASE STUDY: *'My first baby was a breech and I was quite keen to try and have her naturally. The consultant decided that it would be OK. It was a very long labour and in the end her pelvis was dislocated, so she had to be in a cast for a few weeks. She didn't seem to mind but it was very difficult putting nappies on her! I don't think I would do the same again.'*

CASE STUDY: *'I had a very difficult labour with my first baby and second-time-around I was thinking of having an elective Caesarean. When they said he was a breech I was quite relieved, it gave me a really good excuse to have a Caesarean.'*

Delivery of Twins (and Multiple Births)

Twin pregnancies tend to be a little shorter than single baby pregnancies, with an average duration of about 37 weeks (pregnancies involving three or more foetuses are correspondingly shorter). If you start to have contractions much earlier than this you may well be given medication and be kept on complete bed rest in order to prolong the pregnancy and to allow the foetuses to grow and develop more. Twins are usually smaller than the average single pregnancy baby, even if they do go to term; they may, therefore, be less able to cope with the rigours of a long labour.

The wellbeing of the babies and the length of labour will be monitored especially carefully in twin- and multiple-births. It would be unrealistic to expect the births to be intimate events shared by you, your partner and your midwife: because of the possible complications with twin deliveries, your doctor and midwife may be joined by a senior obstetrician and a paediatrician as well as an anaesthetist. There may also be an alarming amount of equipment in the delivery room: as well as all the equipment that may be needed to deliver you, two incubators (or more) will probably be prepared in case the babies need special care when they are born.

During your antenatal check-ups and when you are first admitted to hospital in labour the position of the babies will be noted because this can have considerable bearing on the progress of your labour and the ease of the births. If both babies are lying with their heads down (ie in the normal and most desirable position for delivery), the labour and birth should proceed much as in a single pregnancy, except that shortly after the first baby has been born you will have to do it all over again – you will have only one first stage of labour, but two second stages. The second baby is usually born more quickly than the first; this is mainly because the tissues have already been stretched, but it may also be that he is a little smaller.

The time that elapses between the two births may be a matter of a few minutes, and it is usually less than half an hour. If more than half an hour elapses between the two deliveries there may be concern for the wellbeing of the second baby, and measures may be taken to speed up the second delivery (see the feature on **Assisted Delivery**, above).

Whatever the position of the babies, you may be advised to have an epidural if you are carrying twins, because the labour may be long and there could be complications. If you have an epidural it will be easier for the midwife or a doctor to intervene immediately should the need arise. You may also be asked to give birth in the conventional position, lying on your back with your feet in stirrups so that the midwife can monitor your progress more easily and take action swiftly if and when she needs to.

If the first baby is head down, and the second is in the breech or the transverse position, you may be able to give birth to the first baby 'by yourself', and then have an assisted delivery for the second baby. If the second baby shows signs of distress or if his position makes even an assisted delivery unlikely, you may be given an emergency Caesarean. If one or both babies are known to be in an unusual position you may be advised that it is safest to have an elective Caesarean section.

With twin and multiple births there is a slightly increased risk of postpartum haemorrhage (see below) because of the increased distension of the uterus and the size of the site on the uterine wall to which the placentae were attached. Women carrying two or more babies will usually be routinely injected with syntometrine (see **The Third Stage**, below) in order to speed up the contractions of the uterus so that the site 'closes down' as rapidly as possible and blood loss is minimised.

Water Births

If you have read the sections on **Coping Strategies at Home** and **Alternative Pain Relief in Labour** it will have become apparent that water is a recognised way of promoting a relaxed state during labour, easing the pain of contractions and possibly accelerating labour. Many women have baths at least in the early stages of their labour to help them relax. If a woman finds that the water gives her effective pain relief, she may want to remain in the water for as much of her labour as possible.

During the 1980s, two French doctors, Le Boyer and Odent, became champions of the woman's right to choose what happened during her labour, and of the baby's need to be born into a soothing environment. One of the outcomes of their work was the idea that women could not only labour in water but actually give birth in water. The woman would benefit from the relaxing qualities of warm water for the entire labour, and the baby would be delivered into a warm liquid environment before being brought up into the air.

The idea of the water birth attracted considerable publicity and controversy because it was such a radical break from the conventional managed, monitored labour. There were fears that the baby would 'breath' the water, but the baby appears instinctively not to draw breath when he is submerged. Another concern was that the water would increase the risk of infection to both the mother and the baby; and there is a slightly increased incidence of infection in babies born in water. There is also a danger that the mother will be badly torn (see **Tearing**, below) because the midwife cannot watch the baby's progress in the birth canal and advise the mother when to pant to allow the tissues of her vagina to stretch gradually.

One of the greatest concerns about water births is that, because electrical devices cannot be used in close proximity to water, it is not possible to use electronic foetal monitoring to gauge the wellbeing of the baby. If a hospital routinely fits all labouring women with electronic foetal monitors, the staff are unlikely to welcome the idea of a birthing pool. But many hospitals now recognise that it is not necessary to monitor the foetal heart rate throughout labour if the baby is healthy and the labour seems to be progressing well. If a woman is labouring in water it should be possible to identify the baby's heart beat with a simple stethoscope; if there is any cause for concern the woman should respect the opinion of the midwife or doctor and leave the water so that her baby's wellbeing can be monitored more accurately.

Special birthing pools have been designed to allow the woman enough room to move around and find a comfortable position during labour, and to allow a second person in the pool with her to support and encourage her. Many hospitals, including Queen Charlotte's Hospital, are equipped with one or more birthing pools which may be used for pain relief in labour or for the entire labour and delivery. It is also possible to hire birthing pools (addresses of hire companies appear at the end of the book) for home deliveries or to take to hospital with you if your hospital has agreed for you to do so.

If you are thinking of having a water birth you need to discuss the idea with your midwife and check whether your hospital is equipped with birthing pools or whether they allow women to bring hired pools to hospital. Some hospitals allow women to labour in the birthing pool, but they are not qualified to deliver women in water. It is important that you know what your hospital's policy is, and it is worth asking how much experience the staff have of assisting women in birthing pools: if the staff are experienced they will be more confident and this should boost your own confidence.

CASE STUDY: *'I had both my babies in birthing pools and both times I stayed in the pool for the whole labour. I hired an oval shaped pool, and in the early stages I just lay full length longways in the pool. As the contractions became stronger I felt a bit out of control and I moved so that I was across the pool, and I could hold onto the sides; it gave me something to hold onto, to push against.'*

CASE STUDY: *'I really wanted to have the baby in the birthing pool, it seemed such a lovely soothing way of doing it. I started off in the water, but the contractions started coming so quickly and they were so overpowering that I felt frightened. In the end I didn't feel happy about staying there for the birth.'*

Tearing

It is perhaps not as surprising as it may seem that some first-time mothers are more worried about being torn in childbirth than they are about the labour and the birth itself. This is probably because they can imagine what it is like for skin to be torn, but they cannot imagine giving birth; it may also be that they are worried about the implications of a tear for their sex lives in future.

It is very common for the skin of the vagina and / or the perineum to be torn during delivery. Tearing is more likely to occur if the baby's head is very large, if the second stage progresses rapidly (allowing the tissues less time to stretch) or if the vagina has torn badly previously or has been damaged in any other way. In some of these incidences, the doctor or midwife may decide to give the woman an episiotomy in order to prevent a bad tear (the clean line of an episiotomy is easier to stitch and is likely to heal more satisfactorily than a jagged natural tear). But tearing can happen even when an episiotomy has been performed because the skin can tear on beyond the end of the episiotomy cut. Episiotomies are, therefore, angled so that the line of a possible subsequent tear would cause the least damage.

In many cases, a woman does not even know that she has been torn when she gives birth. This may be because she is experiencing so many different things at once that a skin tear does not really register, or it could be that when the skin is stretched to breaking point the nerve endings are no longer able to send messages back to the brain. Many tears are small and superficial, affecting only the skin, the outer layer of the labia and / or the perineum. These are known as first-degree tears, and the smallest of these may not even need stitching. Longer, superficial tears will need stitching, but they should heal very quickly. First-degree tears are unlikely to cause more than discomfort, and this should not last more than a few days – it is, after all, only a break in the skin, but in a very sensitive area, and one that you do use to sit down (you may find it more comfortable sitting on a pillow for a couple of days).

If the tear is deeper, affecting the muscle tissue below the skin, it is known as a second-degree tear. A second-degree tear will need to be stitched after delivery in order for the muscle tissue to knit and heal well. There may be quite a lot of pain associated with a second-degree tear, and it could take a fortnight or more to heal, depending on just how long and how deep it is. Your stitches will be checked regularly by the midwife, and you may be offered paracetamol or a similar mild analgesic if you are in pain. Sitting may be painful for several days, and you may need a pillow or a cushion to sit on.

A very deep tear, known as a third-degree tear, goes through the skin and muscle tissue right through to the rectum. Third-degree tears are not as common as first- and second-degree tears; they may occur with particularly large babies, very fast deliveries or as an extension of an episiotomy cut. If a third-degree tear is not sutured quickly and expertly, further complications can arise, because excrement may pass from the bowel into the wound and the vagina, causing infection and bowel incontinence. A third-degree tear is likely to be painful for two or more weeks because of the depth of muscle tissue that has been damaged. You will be offered analgesics for the pain and you may be given a special blow-up cushion (like a child's rubber ring) to help you to sit comfortably.

As with every aspect of labour and delivery, women's perception of how much their tears and stitches hurt and for how long varies enormously. If the site of the tear causes you pain you should let the midwife know rather than trying to cope with it stoically: pain should always be investigated because it could indicate that the wound has become infected or that the stitching is too tight and is 'pulling'. It is worth bearing in mind that, even though the actual tear may heal within a week, you may experience discomfort for longer because of internal bruising caused by the birth.

CASE STUDY: *'I've had two [babies] now with just gas and air, and I tore both times, but I didn't know – I had to ask the midwife "did I tear?"both times. No, it's not the actual tearing you want to worry about, it's the stitches.'*

CASE STUDY: *'They used a ventouse and they gave me a local anaesthetic because they were planning to cut me, but that didn't happen in the end – I don't think – but I got a third-degree tear. I didn't feel a thing because of the anaesthetic.'*

Trying to Avoid Tearing

In some cultures, women oil the perineum throughout pregnancy in preparation for the birth, and oiling of the labia and perineum may well help to keep the tissues soft and elastic, therefore limiting the risk of tearing. You may be able to avoid tearing if you listen very carefully to your midwife's instructions during the second stage of labour. She will tell you when to push with your contractions and when to pant and let the baby ease forward naturally; this will allow your labia and perineum to stretch gradually with each contraction (both episiotomies and tearing are more common with first babies, because the skin is stretching for the first time, and the woman is less likely to be able to restrain herself from pushing).

Now that most midwives and obstetricians (and mothers!) agree that episiotomies should not be performed routinely, if you are advised that you need an episiotomy – either because the baby is very large or forceps are needed – this should be seen as a chance to avoid a tear, not an intrusive form of intervention.

CASE STUDY: *'I distinctly remember the midwife saying "pant this time, you don't want to tear do you?" and I tried to pant, but I couldn't help myself pushing … yes, I did have a little tear, but you just don't feel it happen.'*

Cutting the Umbilical Cord

In many hospitals it is policy for the cord to be clamped and cut immediately after the baby has been delivered. The cord is clamped twice about 10cm (4in) from the baby's navel, and it is then cut between the clamps so that the baby is no longer joined to the placenta. One of the reasons this is performed so quickly is that many hospitals routinely inject the mother with a drug called syntometrine during or immediately after delivery in order to speed up the third stage of labour (see below). The cord is cut promptly in order to avoid too much blood being pumped into the baby's bloodstream by the effects of the syntometrine.

It is recognised that the newborn baby can continue to benefit from the oxygen supply provided by the placenta through the umbilical cord even after delivery when he will be breathing for himself. If the cord is not cut immediately the baby will have the benefit of this extra oxygen, and one of the great physiological transitions of birth – switching to breathing with his lungs – may be made easier for him.

If you would like the umbilical cord to be left unclamped until it has stopped pulsating (this indicates that it is no longer pumping blood to the foetus), you need to bear in mind a number of other considerations when you are drawing up your birth plan. The cord cannot be left unclamped if you have the injection of syntometrine, and syntometrine may be necessary to speed up the third stage and avoid the risk of postpartum haemorrhage (see below) if you have had certain kinds of drugs or other intervention. If your labour and delivery proceed with few drugs and little or no intervention, remind your midwife that you would like to avoid having the injection of syntometrine at least until the cord has stopped pulsating and has been cut.

The cutting of the umbilical cord is usually performed by a doctor or a midwife, but – once the cord has been clamped – the actual cutting does not require any medical training. Some men like to cut their babies' umbilical cords as a way of being involved in the birth and possibly as a symbolic gesture, severing the baby from his mother and making him an independent individual. Other couples are squeamish about the cutting of the umbilical cord – it is thick, twisted, rubbery and bluish-white – and prefer to leave the job to 'the experts'.

Third Stage of Labour

Natural Third Stage

After the baby has been born the mother is unlikely to be so aware of what her uterus is doing because she will probably be very preoccupied with her new baby. What actually happens is that the uterus may cease having contractions or have much milder contractions for about ten minutes. This is like a second transition period in which the contractions again change their function, this time from pushing the baby out to shrinking the uterus.

After this transition period the contractions begin again. With each contraction the walls of the uterus shrink in size and the placenta is dislodged by this shrinking action; once the placenta has become dislodged and no longer has a blood supply, the umbilical cord will stop pulsating (see **Cutting the Cord**, above). For a few minutes the woman may bleed from her vagina while the blood vessels, which have been supplying the placenta, flow freely into the uterus. As the uterus continues to contract down these blood vessels are gradually closed off (imagine a woollen sweater shrinking in stages until it is so tightly shrunk that there are no longer any gaps between the stitches).

When the placenta becomes completely detached from the uterine wall you may be able to feel it settle over the cervix, and you should be able to push it out easily with the next contraction. The contractions may be much milder by this stage and it may be difficult to identify when your uterus is contracting and when you should push. If you put your baby to the breast, his sucking should stimulate stronger contractions. A midwife can help to deliver the placenta by massaging your abdomen and pulling very gently on the umbilical cord.

CASE STUDY: *'With my second baby I had no pain relief at all so I felt I should do the whole thing naturally. It was actually very hard work, because I was so tired and I didn't feel the urge to push [the placenta] out. I was suckling the baby, and that didn't seem to be making much difference, and about 30 minutes after he was born the doctor started worrying. He told me to try sitting upright. When I sat up I definitely felt the placenta flop down inside me, one push and it was out.'*

If you have had an epidural or other nerve block or a recent dose of pethidine, it may not be possible to have a natural third stage. Many women anyway choose to have a managed third stage (see below) because it is safer and quicker, and they want to get on with the important business of getting to know their baby! If there is any concern about how long it is taking for your contractions to start up again or how much blood you are loosing, you will anyway be advised to have an injection of syntometrine (see below) to speed up the third stage. You may also be advised to have the much quicker managed third stage if you have been very badly torn; the sooner tears are stitched the more satisfactorily they heal.

Managed Third Stage
In many hospitals women are routinely injected with a drug called syntometrine to speed up the third stage of labour. This is done because it means that any stitching can be done promptly, but mainly because it minimises the risk of postpartum haemorrhage.

Syntometrine is made up of two different drugs: syntocinon and ergometrine. Syntocinon induces uterine contractions quickly, particularly in the upper part of the uterus, so that the uterus shrinks down and hardens, dislodging the placenta and shutting down the blood vessels quickly to avoid blood loss. The ergometrine stimulates strong contractions which last for longer and continue to shrink the placenta and to close in the cervix. There is a very slight risk that the cervix will close before the placenta has been expelled (in this case the placenta may have to be removed manually, a process which can be performed if an epidural is in place or under general anaesthetic).

Most women are unaware of the injection of syntometrine; it is usually injected into the thigh just as the baby's head is delivered or shortly after the baby has been born. It is important that the cord is clamped and cut promptly if syntometrine has been used, because the strong contractions induced by the syntocinon would have the effect of pumping too much blood into the newborn baby. Once the placenta has been dislodged from the uterine wall, the midwife can ease it out by supporting the uterus through the abdomen and pulling gently on the cord.

CASE STUDY: *'I honestly didn't feel the injection at all. If I didn't know I'd had it I wouldn't know, if you see what I mean … I don't remember doing anything about the placenta, I think the midwife must have done all the work for me. I do remember the feeling as it came out, though, soft and floppy.'*

The Placenta

The placenta is a large, shiny dark red organ, weighing about 1kg (2.2lb). It looks not unlike a piece of liver on the side that has been attached to the uterine wall; the other side has a network of blood vessels leading from it to the umbilical cord. Some women like to see the placenta once it has been delivered, but many are either too squeamish or too busy getting to know their new babies to be interested.

The midwife or doctor will certainly examine the placenta to check that it is intact. If any part of the placenta has been retained this could cause postpartum haemorrhage (see below) or infection. The placenta may be weighed and examined in more detail, especially if your baby is very small or seems to have any other problem at birth: the size and condition of the placenta will have a great bearing on the size and wellbeing of the baby.

Stitches

It is very common for women either to be torn or to have episiotomies during delivery, and the incidence is higher with first babies. All episiotomies and all but the most superficial tears will need to be sutured after delivery (as many as 85% of first-time mothers will need stitching, and perhaps 70% of women having second and subsequent babies).

If you have had an epidural or other nerve block it should be possible for the stitching to be done without any other pain relief, and you may not feel anything. If not you will need a local anaesthetic to numb the area of the vagina and perineum that needs stitching. The injection itself can be quite painful and may feel like a sharp sting.

You will almost certainly have to have your legs up in stirrups when you are being sutured, and your legs may become a little cold and uncomfortable. Many women say that having their stitches was the worst part of the whole labour and delivery because it is painful and undignified, it can occasionally take a long time and it means that the mother can not sit up and enjoy her baby straight away.

It is, however, very important that any cuts or tears are stitched promptly and expertly as soon as the placenta has been delivered. The sooner any repair work is done the better the tissues will heal; this is specially important in the case of second- and third-degree tears (and episiotomies, which are usually as deep as second-degree tears) where muscle tissue has been damaged. If the damaged tissue is given the best opportunity to heal well, it should not pose problems with love-making in the future or with future deliveries.

CASE STUDY: *'I had a third-degree tear so they were stitching me up for 30 or 40 minutes. I had my legs up in stirrups for the delivery too, so they had been there a really long time, and they were very uncomfortable. I kept asking if I could take them down just for a minute but it wasn't possible. I had no idea the stitching would go on such a long time. It was the worst bit.'*

CASE STUDY: *'I had an episiotomy so I had been anaesthetised already. It was a deep, long cut, but they stitched me up and it was fine. I don't know what all the fuss is about.'*

Postpartum Haemorrhage

Postpartum haemorrhage, excessive bleeding after delivery, was once responsible for very many maternal fatalities. If the third stage of labour takes a long time or if part of the placenta remains in the uterus or if the uterus does not contract down, the mother could loose excessive amounts of blood. So long as a part of the placenta remains attached to the uterine wall, the uterus will not shrink down completely and blood loss can continue.

The incidence of postpartum haemorrhage is now much lower because the third stage of labour is often managed (see above) so that the blood vessels that supplied the placenta are sealed off promptly, and because the placenta is always checked thoroughly to see whether it is intact. If there is any indication that part of the placenta has been retained it can be removed under general anaesthetic. Even in the few cases of postpartum haemorrhage, the facility for blood transfusion means that it is now very rarely fatal in this country.

There is inevitably some blood loss during and after delivery. There will be some bleeding from the uterine wall and there may also be bleeding from an episiotomy cut or tears to the labia or perineum (or even to the inside of the vagina). Excessive blood loss is an indication that all is not well, and will be investigated immediately by your midwife or a doctor. Cuts and tears will be repaired straight after delivery and should not continue to bleed. You will, however, continue to lose blood for up to six weeks after delivery, but this loss will dwindle gradually and will become brown or pinkish. If at any time you notice an increase in blood loss, or the loss is like bright fresh blood you should let you midwife, doctor or health visitor know immediately.

Caesarean Section

A Caesarean section, when the baby is delivered through a surgical incision in the abdomen and the uterine wall, is performed in over 10% of all births in this country. It is a simple but quite major abdominal operation which can be performed under epidural or general anaesthetic, and it carries no greater risk than any comparable form of surgery. Caesarean sections are often used to minimise certain risks that may be assessed before a woman goes into labour or at any stage in the labour or the delivery.

If a woman and her consultant decide before she goes into labour that she should have a Caesarean this is known as an elective or planned Caesarean. If your midwife or a doctor decides during the labour or the delivery that the baby should be delivered by Caesarean this is known as an emergency Caesarean.

Elective Caesarean

There are a number of reasons why a woman may be advised to have an elective Caesarean:

Abnormal presentation: If the baby is in the breech position (see above) or is lying across the uterus (transverse lie), the consultant may decide that a Caesarean section is the safest way of trying to deliver the baby.

Disproportion: If the baby appears to be very large or the mother's pelvis is very small or an unusual shape, measurements may be taken using X-rays to assess whether or not vaginal delivery would be possible. In some cases of disproportion Caesarean section is the only option.

Elective Caesarean on non-medical grounds: It is not uncommon for labouring women to say 'oh, just give me a Caesarean' at some point without really meaning it, but there are some women for whom labour and vaginal delivery seem a terrifying ordeal which could be avoided by a simple operation. If you feel strongly that you would like to have your baby by Caesarean section even though there may be no medical grounds to justify it, you will probably have to argue your case fairly persuasively with your consultant. Hospitals are unwilling to perform surgery unnecessarily because all surgery has attendant risks and costs (and this latter point is a considerable one). Among other arguments, you will be asked to consider the difficulties of coping with a newborn baby while recovering from major abdominal surgery. When you have discussed your ideas with the consultant and have heard in detail the other side of the argument, you may find that you want to reconsider your decision.

Maternal illness or disability: If the mother is very ill, has a chronic condition or a condition brought on by her pregnancy (such as gestational diabetes or pre-eclampsia) it may be considered that the exertions of labour and vaginal delivery could adversely affect her own and her baby's health, and could even threaten both their lives. In some cases, the mother may have a physical disability which may preclude a vaginal delivery.

> CASE STUDY: *'I knew all along that I would have to have a Caesarean because I had an operation on my back years ago and some of my vertebrae were fused together. I had an epidural so I was conscious throughout, and I saw him being lifted into the air – it's just as miraculous.'*

Placenta praevia: (For background information on placenta praevia see the section in the chapter **When Things Go Wrong**.) Because of the risks of blood loss during labour and delivery with placenta praevia, most consultants will recommend a Caesarean section.

Previous Caesarean section: It was once considered that a woman who had had one Caesarean section would only ever be able to have babies delivered this way, and in some cases this does hold true because the site of the scar and the nature of scar tissue in the uterine wall mean that the uterus is unlikely to withstand labour without damage, possibly threatening the life of the mother and the baby. In most cases, however, a trial of labour (see below) can be appropriate. If you have already had a Caesarean section your consultant will advise you as to what is best for you.

> CASE STUDY: *'I had to have an emergency section with my first baby because he was huge and he literally got stuck. The next time they kept an eye on the size of the baby and she was much smaller, so they said it would be quite safe to have her normally. I did, and it was wonderful.'*

Small-for-dates baby: If the baby is very small, even when the pregnancy reaches term, the consultant may recommend that he is delivered by Caesarean section in order to spare him the stress and potential damage of labour and delivery.

Twins and multiple births: The decision to perform an elective Caesarean in a twin pregnancy depends mainly on the health, presentation and size of the babies. If the babies are very small and vulnerable, and / or if they are both in an abnormal presentation, a

Caesarean section is likely to be recommended in order to avoid a long and difficult labour and traumatic delivery.

If you are to have an elective Caesarean it is important that you understand fully the reasons why this is the safest way for your baby to be delivered. Discuss the reasons with your midwife or your consultant. Some people are just as frightened of abdominal surgery as they are of labour and delivery (perhaps more so: childbirth, after all is natural and surgery is not); in any event it may be easier for you to contemplate your Caesarean if you understand the procedure itself and if you talk to other women who have had Caesarean sections.

Women are sometimes a little relieved when they are advised to have an elective Caesarean, others feel disappointed that they will not have an active part in the birth of their baby. If you feel that the operation is cheating you out of your chance to give birth to your baby, you should try to remember that you have taken the responsible decision to have your baby delivered in a way that is safest for you and for him. It may again help to talk to other mothers who have had Caesareans; they will soon help you to realise that the end result will be the same: you will have a baby.

Trial of Labour

In some cases, it may be possible for the woman to have what is called a 'trial of labour', she may be allowed to go into labour spontaneously and to try to have a vaginal delivery, but with the epidural set up and all the equipment on hand should the need for a Caesarean become urgent.

Emergency Caesarean

Some of these considerations are niceties that are not available to women who need emergency Caesareans during labour. An emergency Caesarean may be necessary if certain reasons for elective Caesareans have gone undetected until the mother goes into labour. These may include:

Abnormal presentation
Disproportion
Placenta praevia
Small-for-dates baby

An emergency Caesarean may also be necessary if the labour fails to progress, if there is evidence of foetal distress, if an assisted delivery has failed or if the umbilical cord is prolapsed.

Prolonged / ineffectual labour: If progress in labour is slow or if a labour is very long, the doctor or midwife may try to speed up the process with the use of syntocinon to promote contractions. In some cases, however, the cervix stops dilating, inhibiting a vaginal delivery, and in these cases, Caesarean sections are needed.

As with an elective Caesarean, women who have emergency Caesareans can feel that they have been cheated out of one of the most intense experiences of their lives: the delivery of their baby. Some women feel as if they are inadequate or that they have failed their baby or their partner. It will help you to come to terms with what happened to you if you understand fully why the operation was needed. Make sure that you understand the reasons: if it is clear to you that the operation was performed to save your life or your baby's, you may have more positive feelings about it. Talk to other women who have had Caesareans, and talk to women who have had other forms of intervention: think of the Caesarean as just another form of assisted delivery, rather than a complete absence of involvement on your part. The most important thing is that you do have a baby to show for it, a baby that your body alone nurtured for nine months.

CASE STUDY: *'I really felt as if I had missed out on something. It just didn't seem fair. I think I was quite depressed about it, but he was a big baby and I'm very small, and I gradually came round to feeling proud that I had managed to grow this huge baby inside me, and it was hardly surprising that I couldn't get him out. With the second one they monitored his growth and they said that I would have to have a Caesarean again, and it didn't matter that time, because I was prepared for it.'*

Foetal distress: If there is evidence of foetal distress during labour, it may be that an emergency Caesarean is required to deliver the baby before he suffers any long-term effects from stress and lack of oxygen. Foetal distress is usually gauged by monitoring the foetal heart rate (see **Electronic Foetal Monitoring**, above). If the baby's heart rate implies that he is not coping well with the stresses of labour, the doctor may take a blood sample from his scalp to gauge the acidity of his blood. If this reading gives cause for concern, a Caesarean will almost certainly be recommended.

CASE STUDY: *'My first child has cerebral palsy, and they think it may be because I had a difficult labour. This time I was referred to Queen Charlotte's because they have the expertise ... At 5.30 the baby's heart rate dropped so they did a scalp sample. It was OK. They did another scalp sample half an hour later and it was a bit iffy. They wanted to let me carry on another half hour and do a third sample before deciding to go ahead with a Caesarean, but I wasn't taking any risks, I couldn't see the point of doing a third sample and they agreed to do a Caesarean straight away.'*

Failed assisted delivery: In some cases of very difficult deliveries even forceps and vacuum extraction can fail to deliver the baby by the normal route, and the baby may become 'stuck'. It may be that a Caesarean section is the only way of freeing the baby and delivering him safely.

CASE STUDY: *'They tried a ventouse but it wouldn't work, so they said I would have to have an emergency Caesarean. It was fine because I had an epidural anyway, but then the trouble started ... she was so stuck that I had a lot of internal bleeding and suddenly the room was full of people and I was conscious of all these pairs of hands working inside me. I had this really lovely anaesthetist, she was here all the time [indicating just above her head] talking to me and explaining. Eventually, I had to have a general anaesthetic while they sorted me out.'*

CASE STUDY: *'They tried to use forceps but the baby was not down far enough so I had to have a Caesarean. I'd had an epidural anyway so up went the screen and out came the baby. It seemed to happen very quickly.'*

Prolapsed umbilical cord: This is a rare occurrence in which a loop of umbilical cord prolapses out of the cervix before the baby has begun travelling through the cervix. The prolapse can sometimes be seen hanging out of the vagina or it may be felt by the midwife doing an internal examination. In the case of a prolapsed cord an emergency Caesarean must be performed; if the delivery were allowed to continue normally the pressure of the baby's head as it passes through the cervix would crush the umbilical cord, therefore cutting off the supply of blood and vital oxygen to the baby. If the baby's oxygen supply is cut off for any length of time (as it would be in this incidence) the baby can suffer brain damage or may die.

How a Caesarean is Performed

The first five or ten minutes of the operation are taken up with the process of setting up the operation. If you already have an epidural fitted, the amount of drugs used will be raised to ensure complete lack of feeling for the operation. Queen Charlotte's Hospital is one of many hospitals that can now offer an epidural Caesarean even in an emergency (some hospitals are not adequately equipped or staffed to offer emergency epidural Caesareans round the clock). If for any reason it is not possible for the operation to be performed using an epidural you will be given a general anaesthetic.

Your pubic hair will be shaved, you will be fitted with a catheter to collect urine during the operation, and you will be put on an intravenous drip to replace fluids lost during the operation. Your abdomen will be cleaned and a screen of fabric will be set up so that you cannot watch the operation. The surgeon will make an incision in your lower abdomen, usually a horizontal line just above the top of your pubic hair, and the amniotic fluid will be drained off using a suction pump.

Now the surgeon will lift the baby gently from the uterus, either using his hands or forceps, and the cord will be clamped and cut. The baby can be handed straight to his mother or father in some cases and in others he will be checked over thoroughly before being handed to you or your partner. If there is any question about the baby's wellbeing or if the operation was performed because of concerns about the baby, he may have to be resuscitated or put in an incubator.

Once the baby has been delivered you will be given an injection of syntocinon to induce contractions of the uterus. These contractions dislodge the placenta, which can then be removed, and shrink the uterus down so that the blood vessels are sealed off. This whole process will probably only take about 15 minutes, but the operation is not over yet: you have an incision in your abdomen which cuts through muscle tissue including the very special muscles of your uterus. If you are to recover fully and to have future pregnancies, the incision must be stitched expertly. The stitching of a Caesarean incision can take about 30 minutes. The outer layer of the incision, the skin of the abdomen, may be repaired using tiny metal clamps or conventional sutures.

The operation will probably last about 45 minutes in all. The surgeon or the anaesthetist may well talk you through the procedure so that you feel involved, and you will be able to watch the baby being lifted out above the screen. Your partner may be able to accompany you into the operating theatre (but he will have to wear theatre clothes, a cap and a surgical mask as precautions against infection).

Once your incision has been repaired you will be taken to a 'recovery' area and then to the postnatal ward. You may well be kept on the drip and the catheter for several hours (some hospitals leave the catheter in for the first day or so). Your stay in hospital will be longer than for most women who have had vaginal deliveries because a Caesarean section is a major form of abdominal surgery. Your stitches will probably be removed on the fourth or fifth day and, if your consultant is satisfied with your recovery so far, you may be allowed to go home then. (There is more information about recovering from a Caesarean in the **Postpartum** chapter).

The Newborn Baby

When your baby finally arrives you may be a little taken aback by his appearance: he is likely to have traces of blood, mucus and vernix over him; he may appear long and thin or short and plump; his colour could be white, grey, purple or red; he could still have traces of lanugo hair over his body and he may have anything from no head hair at all to a great shock of hair; and he may come out fighting and screaming or be quiet and inactive.

New parents are always eager to check that 'everything is there', and that their baby is normal. First-time parents are often alarmed by the shape of the baby's head. A newborn baby's head can be a strange shape because the soft plates of bone in a baby's skull can overlap to facilitate their passage through the birth canal; this is not harmful to the baby, but it can take several hours for moulded plates of the skull to realign. If you had a forceps or ventouse delivery, any marks left on your baby's head or body will usually disappear in the first few days of his life. Parents are also often surprised by the size of a baby's genitals, especially a boy's testes; the hormones surging round the mother's bloodstream during pregnancy have been filtering into the baby through the placenta, and they may cause swelling of the genitalia and even a show of blood in some baby girls. The swelling is not harmful to the baby and should go down in the first few days after delivery.

The First Cry

It is a myth that a baby has to cry when he is born, although a very large percentage of them do. The shock of birth is likely to produce some reaction from a baby unless he is sedated by the effects of pethidine, and that reaction is usually to cry. The now outdated ritual of doctors slapping newborn babies' bottoms to make them cry was just a way of ensuring that they breathed. Despite its small size a newborn baby can have a surprisingly impressive cry; others, especially very small or premature babies, will have a much quieter cry. Some babies can cry for several minutes after delivery, others will have an initial shriek of shock but will then settle.

Tests and Procedures

Ensuring that the baby breathes: After your baby has been delivered, the midwife's first priority is to ensure that he is breathing; in most cases this will be obvious because he will cry. If the baby is not crying the midwife will check to see whether he is breathing. If he is not breathing she will take action rapidly: clearing his airways of mucus with a catheter, and resuscitating him with oxygen. A member of the medical team should be able to talk you through the procedure and keep you informed of your baby's progress. If there is any further doubt about your baby's ability to breath on his own, he may need to spend his first few hours in special care.

Apgar score: While the midwife is looking over the newborn baby she will be assessing his wellbeing; about one minute after delivery she will make a note of his condition in the form of a score known as the APGAR score. The baby is given a mark of 0, 1 or 2 on each of the following five categories: heart rate, breathing, movements, skin colour and reflex response, so that scores can range from 0 to 10. A very low score indicates that the baby is in need of resuscitation, a score of seven or more means that the baby is doing well. A second Apgar score is taken five or ten minutes later to check the baby's progress. The midwife will probably not need to hold the baby to assess his Apgar score, she will be able to gauge it from experience just by watching him in your arms.

Weighing and measuring: After asking the sex of your new baby the second thing your friends and family will want to know is his birthweight. Within the first hours of your baby's life he will be weighed, and his length and head circumference will be measured. The baby's birthweight is a benchmark for his growth from now on. Most babies lose a small amount of weight in the first few days of life as they make the massive physiological switch from being nourished by the placenta to digesting milk taken orally, but they usually regain their birthweight by the end of the first week of life. Their weight gain from then on can be charted against the expected weight gain for a baby of the same birthweight.

The baby's birthweight in relation to his length and head circumference is a useful guide to how well he has gained weight in the uterus. If, for example, a baby's length and head circumference would normally be associated with a much higher birthweight, the baby has failed to gain weight in the last weeks of pregnancy. This could be because the placenta began to deteriorate and he may well put on weight very quickly in the first few weeks of life to compensate for this. A healthy baby's weight should follow approximately the same curve as his length.

Cleaning, drying and wrapping: Until quite recently it was traditional for the newborn baby to be whisked from the mother at birth, weighed measured, cleaned, dried and wrapped before she was able to hold him. It is now accepted that the best place for a newborn baby to be is nestled between his mother's breasts (unless he is in need of resuscitation), and the niceties of cleaning him up can wait till later. It is, however, important that a newborn baby is covered and dried as quickly as possible. Newborn babies are not equipped to maintain body heat efficiently, and they can lose heat very rapidly. Delivery rooms are usually kept warm (as many women notice at their expense during the exertions of the second stage of labour!), and the midwife may dry and cover the baby snugly while he is in your arms in order to cut down on heat loss.

It does not matter if the mucus and blood that may have been smeared on your baby's body at birth dry on him. You will probably be shown how to bath him in the next day or so, and it is more important that you spend some time with him now.

Vitamin K: Almost all babies born in this country are routinely given with vitamin K shortly after delivery. This vitamin plays an important role in the clotting of blood, and is given in case the baby has a vitamin K deficiency which could have serious repercussions. Vitamin K is water soluble which means that it will do your baby no harm because excesses can easily be excreted in his urine.

How you Feel

The words most frequently used by newly-delivered mothers are 'happy', 'proud', 'tired' and 'relieved'. Most women do feel happy and proud when their baby is born, but there is nothing wrong with you if you feel simply relieved that it is all over, or just overwhelmed or bewildered by the whole proceedings. In general, women who have understood what has been happening – or have had it explained to them throughout labour and delivery – have more positive feelings after delivery, whereas those who had little understanding of the process or needed a great deal of intervention are more likely to have ambivalent feelings.

You will almost certainly be physically tired and perhaps emotionally drained, and in some cases this will make you feel flat and exhausted. On the other hand, many women find that they have a surge of energy when their baby is born; this may be because of the surge of endorphins (the body's own painkillers) and adrenaline in the body or it may be simply an emotional reaction to the triumph of having a baby. Your feelings of tiredness will, of course, also be affected by how long your labour has been and what drugs you have been given.

Despite the warmth of the delivery room, it is not uncommon for women to feel cold and shivery after delivery. This is partly because the body is finally relaxing after hours of exertion, and partly because of the massive changes taking place in the mother's circulation now that it is no longer supplying the placenta. You may find that your legs shake and that your feet are especially cold; it is a good idea to ask for a thick blanket to keep you and the baby warm.

CASE STUDY: *'I can't describe the feeling ... you want me to describe the feeling? I don't know, I mean I've never tried bungee-jumping or bob-sleighing, but I think the rush they get probably doesn't come close ...*

actually, that's probably why it's men who come up with all these dangerous sports, because they can't have babies!!'

CASE STUDY: *'I was just so glad it was all over, and all I wanted to do was have a bath. [The baby] was very sleepy, which suited me fine, because I wanted a breathing space to sort myself out.'*

As well as how you feel in yourself you will have a whole new dimension of feelings: those you have for the baby. You may be astonished at your own capacity for emotion, a complete new realm of feeling opens up (second-time parents often worry that it cannot be possible to love a second child as much as the first but the human capacity for emotion is astonishing, and yet another realm of love is created with each successive child). The great majority of women are instantly captivated by their babies, and if not besotted at least fascinated. There is, however, nothing wrong or unusual about a woman who feels bewildered or indifferent when confronted with her baby: not every woman has a surge of maternal love for the baby or bonds with him straight away. The bond will grow in time as you learn how to care for him, and he becomes an irreplaceable part of your life.

CASE STUDY: *'I'm very proud of him, but he doesn't do much for me at the moment. [Hides head in hands] That sounds awful, but it was the same with his sisters; it happens gradually over about the first month and then I just love them to bits.'*

CASE STUDY: *'She's gorgeous, she's just gorgeous. We both wanted a girl so badly that we'd persuaded ourselves it was going to be a boy, and when she popped out it was just this wonderful surprise. She's wonderful.'*

Stillbirth

Stillbirth is the term used when the baby dies in the womb before birth, at any time after the twenty-fourth week of pregnancy. It happens in less than 1% of pregnancies and it is probably the greatest fear of pregnant women. A stillbirth can range from the foetus dying in the uterus pre-term so that labour has to be induced; to the pregnancy going to term and the baby being lost at some stage during labour up to the birth.

Causes of Stillbirth

One of the most common questions asked by parents bereaved by a stillbirth is 'why did it happen?' Sadly, it is not always possible for doctors to answer this question satisfactorily, because there may have been a number of contributory factors. The most common explanations for stillbirths are:

Abnormalities in the foetus: The foetus may have had congenital abnormalities and deformities which meant that it could not thrive or develop normally.

Asphyxia: The foetus may die in the uterus because it is deprived of oxygen if the placenta begins to fail in the latter weeks of pregnancy or during labour, or if the umbilical cord becomes trapped between the baby's head and the cervix during delivery.

Obstetric cholestasis: Recent research has shown that stillbirths could be caused by a liver malfunction in the mother called obstetric cholestasis. This condition can cause severe itching in the mother, especially on her hands and feet due to a build-up of bile salts. It is believed that these bile salts may cause the death of the foetus.

Premature delivery: If the mother goes into labour prematurely, the small, vulnerable pre-term baby may not survive the stresses of labour and delivery.

Sometimes parents are keen to have an answer to this question as a way of apportioning blame: did the mother take too much exercise during pregnancy? Was the doctor too slow in deciding to opt for an emergency Caesarean? In fact, only in very extreme cases could the mother's actions cause her baby to be stillborn, and babies very rarely die as a result of negligence or procedural errors during the labour and delivery. There will hardly ever be a question of blame in a case of stillbirth, which may prove little comfort to the parents.

Other couples feel that they may find it easier to come to terms with their loss if they understand how and why it happened. Unless there is a very obvious explanation for the baby's death, an autopsy will probably be carried out. You will be asked for your consent and, although the idea of the autopsy may be painful to you, you may welcome the opportunity for an answer to your questions.

This is, however, not just a straightforward question of the cause of the baby's death, it is a philosophical question too: whether or not the cause of the stillbirth has been discovered, the parents will want to know why this had to happen to them rather than any other couple. It can take a long time for couples to reconcile themselves to their loss, and they may find that they take comfort from talking to families who have had a similar experience (organisations who can put you in touch with bereaved couples are listed at the end of the book). It may also be very helpful to talk to a trained bereavement councillor (Queen Charlotte's Hospital is one of a number of hospitals that have bereavement councillors specifically to help couples who have lost babies).

Stillbirth before labour: In most instances of stillbirth, the foetus dies in the uterus before the woman goes into labour. She may notice that the foetus is no longer moving or the midwife may fail to find a heartbeat at an antenatal check-up. If there is concern about the foetus, an ultrasound scan or an electronic foetal heart monitor can confirm whether or not the foetus has died.

If the foetus dies the mother has to be induced (see **Induction**, above) to be delivered of the baby. It is difficult to imagine having to go through labour in the full knowledge that the baby will be dead, but some women who have had this experience say that they still have a feeling of pride, and that they feel they have at least some memories to attach to the baby: every labour is different, and the memories they have of this labour and the pregnancy are all that they have to remember this baby by. It is possible to have an elective Caesarean in cases of stillbirth, although hospitals are usually unwilling to perform surgery unnecessarily. The body takes longer to recover from a Caesarean, and – although it seems an easier option – it may be more difficult to adjust to emotionally because the woman has been less involved in the birth of the lost baby.

Stillbirth during labour or delivery: It is mercifully rare for babies to die during labour and delivery, because the use of foetal monitoring means that midwives are usually aware of a problem before it becomes life-threatening. This fact makes it all the more difficult for bereaved parents to come to terms with the terrifying absence of a baby after the nine months of pregnancy, the hours of labour and the exertions of delivery.

Stillbirth of one twin: It is possible for a woman who is carrying twins to have one normal healthy baby, but to lose the other twin. Even if the stillborn foetus dies earlier in the pregnancy, this may not always be diagnosed because the surviving twin's heartbeat and movements can mask the fact that the second foetus is not thriving or is already dead. Obviously, the surviving baby is a source of great joy and comfort to his parents, but he cannot compensate for the loss of his twin. It is all too easy for friends to dismiss the parents' grief, believing that – because 'they've got a baby anyway' – they will not feel so bereaved, but parents of twins feel the loss just as keenly as parents who have lost a single baby (you would not expect someone who lost one of two brothers in a car crash to recover significantly more quickly than someone who lost an only brother).

> CASE STUDY: *'I was carrying twins and I had a normal check-up at 33 weeks, and everything was fine. The next day, though, I went into labour. When I got to the hospital I went to have a bath, and while I was having the bath I had the most excruciating pain in my tummy and the whole outline of my tummy changed shape. I was violently sick too. For some reason the placenta of one of the twins had come away. They checked immediately for his heartbeat; and there was a very faint trace and then he died. He was blocking the route for the second twin so I had to have an emergency Caesarean to deliver the second twin safely.'*

Adjusting Emotionally

Seeing and holding the baby: Even if a woman feels squeamish about the idea of holding a dead baby, many women find that they take great comfort from at least seeing their stillborn babies. The baby will still be warm from the warmth of the mother's body, he may well be perfectly formed with a calm expression on his face as if he is sleeping. If the baby had physical abnormalities the staff will warn the parents before offering to show him to them. His abnormalities may shock the parents but they will help to explain his death to them, and they may feel comforted that their baby's natural death may have spared him from a difficult and painful life.

If the parents can spend a little time with him and think of him as an individual, they will find it easier to mourn him. Some couples like to take photographs of the baby to add to the all-too-few memories they will have of him.

Religious services: It is sometimes possible to arrange a small service of blessing for the baby in the hospital shortly after delivery. Many couples also like to arrange a funeral service, and to have a grave – or other site – that they can visit.

Registering the birth: Although it seems absurd that the parents have to register the baby's birth and death simultaneously, these certificates will reinforce what has happened and they may help the parents to try and make some sense of it. Many couples find that the naming of a stillborn baby helps to give him an identity, and registering his birth in his own name will make him seem more real to them.

Talking about feelings: Women who have had stillborn babies often feel guilty, inadequate or even tainted, and they may shun the help and support of others. It may be difficult to talk to other people at a time of bewilderment and unhappiness, but talking can help a woman to come to terms with what has happened to her. Friends, family, the family doctor or the community midwife may be able to listen and give the support she needs, but there are also organisations for bereaved parents which may be able to help and, as mentioned above, some hospitals have specially trained bereavement councillors.

> CASE STUDY: *'It didn't sink in straight away. For the first three days I was still a bit under the effects of the anaesthetic, and they began to worry because I hadn't cried. They were brilliant, they made sure we named him, photographed him, took his footprint and some of his hair. Then it hit me about four or five days later. On the fifth day we had a little service and it really hit me then. For a long time I would just break down for no reason, I still cry now [three and a half years later] for no reason sometimes, and I know that it's because of the baby I lost.'*

Adjusting Physically

The emotional adjustments to stillbirth are not helped by the fact that the body is also having to adjust to the end of the pregnancy and the absence of a baby; these physical symptoms act as painful reminders of the baby. Even though there is not a baby to stimulate the production of milk, women who have had stillborn babies do produce milk; this can be physically as well as emotionally painful. The hospital staff can give advice about how to soothe engorged breasts, and a course of pills may be prescribed to dry up the milk supply. The uterus gradually shrinks back to its pre-pregnancy size, and there is some blood loss from the site of the placenta for several weeks after delivery. There will almost certainly be some weight to lose after the pregnancy, too, and this can be particularly dispiriting.

One major physical and emotional adjustment after a stillbirth is that the woman may have nothing to do – especially if this was her first baby – because she will have arranged her life so that she would be free to enjoy and look after her baby. Some women even find that their arms ache from the instinctive urge to hold the baby. In the first few days the sheer shock and the necessary arrangements will fill the void, but by the end of the first week the baby's absence will be painfully obvious. It is in the weeks and months that follow that the bereaved couple most need the support of friends, family, employers and support groups.

Will it Happen Again?

Part of the reason that couples are so eager to understand why a stillbirth has happened is that they want to know whether the same thing will happen to them again. If the baby was stillborn because of a congenital abnormality there is a chance that any subsequent babies could have the same abnormality. In these instances, each case is investigated thoroughly and the couple will be given genetic counselling.

There may be other causes of stillbirth, such as failure of the placenta towards the end of the pregnancy, which might be repeated in subsequent pregnancy. With specialised monitoring in future pregnancies it should be possible for any threat to the baby's life to be minimised. The great majority of stillbirths are caused by what can only be described as very unlucky series of circumstances, and it would be really extremely unlucky – and the odds would be very slender indeed – for those same circumstances to occur again.

Starting Again

If a woman's reaction to a stillbirth is that she wants to try for another baby straight away, she may well be ready physically to conceive again in a matter of weeks (some doctors advise waiting three or four months so that the menstrual cycle can settle again, others are more concerned that the woman should do what she feels is right). On the other hand, it may be many months before a woman feels ready emotionally to go through another pregnancy. There is no right time, and every couple faced with this problem will react slightly differently. Whatever their decision, it is worth remembering that the next pregnancy will inevitably give them a nine-month period of adjustment, and that the next baby will never replace the one that they lost but he will help to ease the pain.

Time Alone with your New Baby

Once your baby has been checked over, dried and wrapped, you have had any stitches you need, and the midwife is happy that you are comfortable, they may leave you alone to get to know and enjoy your new baby before you are moved on to the postnatal ward. Most women welcome this opportunity and this quiet time with their partner and the new member of the family who will change their lives so fundamentally, but some – especially first-time mothers – feel a little frightened at the thought of being left alone with this colossal new responsibility. Some, like the woman in the case study above (see **How you Feel**), are tired and unsettled by the birth, and they like to use this time to gather their thoughts by themselves.

> CASE STUDY: *'All I wanted was a cup of tea, and that's exactly what I got. It was very civilised, and I looked across at [my husband] sipping his tea, and I thought "we're a family now!"'*

The First Feed

If you are planning to breastfeed your baby, this quiet time is the perfect opportunity to give your baby his first feed, especially as it is recommended that the baby is given his first feed within an hour of being born. This is because most babies are born very alert thanks to the surge of adrenaline in their bloodstream, and the rooting and sucking reflexes are at their strongest in this first hour. If the baby is fed now the pattern of rooting, latching on and sucking should be established satisfactorily. After this first hour, the adrenaline in the baby's bloodstream will have dissipated; he may become drowsy and less responsive, so that attempts to feed him are less effective. If he is then allowed to sleep off the birth – and newborn babies sleep a great deal to recover from the labour and the birth – he may be very hungry when he wakes, and his frenzied crying may make the first feed a frustrating experience for him and his mother.

As with every other aspect of having a baby, there will be a different 'right time' for everyone. If the mother is tired and drained after delivery, and the baby is happy to take in the new world around him, then she should not feel pressured to feed him until after she has recovered a little. It can take several attempts for the mother and the baby to 'synchronise watches' and settle down to a successful first feed.

Do not be tempted to think that, because breastfeeding is natural, it will be simple. If you have any worries about feeding your baby – whether it is with this first feed or at any other time – the hospital staff should give you all the help and support that you need.

Chapter 6

Postpartum

If you have a Domino delivery and in hospital you and your baby are fit and well, you will probably be allowed to go home within six to twelve hours of delivery. The tests and check-ups carried out on you and your baby will be done at home by your community midwife if you have a home delivery or a Domino.

If you are staying in hospital you will be transferred to the postnatal ward, and you will stay there for between one and six days depending on how well you and the baby are doing, and on whether or not you have a Caesarean section.

For many first-time mothers this can be a time of misgivings and uncertainty: you suddenly realise that this is the beginning, not the end, that the pregnancy was just a warm-up exercise, and that you now have the most enormous responsibility in the shape of your new baby.

The Postnatal Ward

Once your baby has been delivered, you have had a little time to recover from the delivery and the staff are satisfied that 'both mother and baby are doing well', you will be taken to the postnatal ward. Most maternity units around the country have rooms of four or six beds as well as a number of single rooms for very special cases and for private patients. (Depending on the size and type of the unit, there may be one ward kept specifically for women who have had Caesarean sections.)

In the rooms, each bed has rails and curtaining around it to afford mothers some privacy, but these offer no sound proofing from the cries of other babies in the night! 'Rooming in', a practice where the baby remains next to you, is encouraged in most units. Transparent plastic cot are used so that you can see him even when you are lying down and resting. If your baby is in an incubator to maintain his body temperature, it may be possible for him to be in the ward with you (babies who need more specialised care will be kept in the neo-natal unit, and parents are usually free to visit them at any time). Most women like to keep their babies next to their own beds at all times, and very few hospitals now routinely remove babies to a nursery at night.

Some hospitals have a nursery where you can bathe your baby or sit and feed him, others have a mother's room where you can feed uninterrupted, and baby bathing is carried out at the bedside. In some hospitals it may be possible to leave your baby in the nursery while you have a bath or catch up on sleep but policy on the use of the nursery and how much responsibility the staff take for the babies varies from one hospital to another. The staff will discourage you from being away from your baby for any length of time because of the security risks.

Security in Hospital

There has always been a danger that two babies could be 'mixed up' in hospital, and the wrong family sent home with the wrong baby. This was a more common anxiety a generation or so ago, when babies were routinely removed to the nursery in between feeds. Now that mothers are encouraged to keep their babies next to them at all times and to feed on demand according to the individual baby's needs, this is a less likely eventuality. Most mothers know that they would recognise their own baby 'in a million', but there was a case of 'swapped' babies in this country as recently as 1993.

In order to avoid this sort of mistake – which could have profound and devastating psychological effects on the parents and, later, the child – most hospitals fit one of the baby's wrists and / or one of his ankles with a plastic-covered name-tag. These tags have adjustable closing devices so that they can be closed to fit snugly round any size of wrist or ankle. Once they have been closed it should not be possible to re-open them. The staff will probably show you the name-tags in place and ask you to let them know if anything happens to one of them. You may also be given an arm bracelet matching your baby's birth details. It should be possible to bath your baby without the writing becoming smudged, and the tags should fit sufficiently tightly to preclude their slipping off. If your baby does lose a name-tag, let the hospital know immediately and they will give him another one. The staff will snip them open carefully with scissors just before you leave hospital.

A far more sinister security risk in hospitals is the very slender chance that someone could come into the ward, posing as a visitor or a member of staff, and take a newborn baby. These incidents are mercifully rare, and the babies are almost invariably found and returned to their mothers safely, but this rarity does not make the possibility any less terrifying for new parents or any less of an anxiety for the hospital staff. Almost all large hospitals are now equipped with closed-circuit television, and have trained security guards on duty twenty-four hours a day. Some have also introduced a system of electronic tags that can be attached to the baby's name-tag or clothing, and which bleep when the baby is taken outside the ward (on the same principle as the anti-shoplifting tags used in clothes stores).

Any problems of security with newborn babies are minimised if mothers keep their babies with them at all times. If you are concerned about security in hospital ask your doctor or midwife about the security measures taken in your local hospital.

Sleep in Hospital

Sleep becomes a precious commodity in a postnatal ward. Most women lose at least one night's sleep in labour and delivery, and they are tired by the exertions of delivery. Now they are adapting to feeding and to a routine imposed on their sleep patterns by the baby. You may find that you are exhausted after the birth but that you are too exhilarated to get the sleep that you need: you may be 'buzzing' for a day or so after your baby is born. When you do manage to fall asleep you are very likely to be woken by your baby for a feed before you have even begun to catch up on your sleep.

Even if your own baby sleeps at great length, you may be woken repeatedly in the night by the others in your room. If you are not able to sleep because of your own turmoil of emotions or because of the noise in the ward, it is still important that you get plenty of rest. In hospital someone else is there to worry about the cooking, the washing and the cleaning; you should make the most of this brief opportunity to rest and relax by listening to music or watching television and allowing yourself to drift off to sleep as often as possible. It will probably be many weeks – or even months – before you have an uninterrupted night's sleep again, so it is worth getting used to grabbing a few minutes' sleep when you can.

However much of a high achiever you may normally be, do not be tempted to think that you are being lazy and doing nothing. You are recovering from one of the most prolonged and demanding undertakings of the human body, you are still undergoing considerable physiological and hormonal changes and (if you are breastfeeding) you are manufacturing your baby's food.

CASE STUDY: *'Towards the end of the pregnancy I was up a lot in the night and I lost two night's sleep in labour. When he was born I was so tired I said something about "oh, I'm just so looking forward to having a proper night's sleep". The midwife opened her mouth to say something, but maybe she thought it would be too discouraging to say. Anyway, I now know she was going to say that that was probably the last thing I was going to get now I'd got the baby.'*

CASE STUDY: *'I just got frantic for sleep in hospital. My baby kept me up for the first two nights, then she slept but I was so exhausted and there was so much noise in the ward that I couldn't really sleep for the next two nights. I can honestly say that I got more sleep in my first 24 hours back at home than in my entire stay in hospital.'*

Care of the Newborn Baby

Even if you have had a baby before or have learnt about caring for the newborn in your antenatal classes, you may find that you are all fingers and thumbs when it actually comes to handling your tiny new baby. The staff in hospital will give you all the help and advice you need: in some hospitals a midwife will show you how to bathe and dress the baby, and will talk you through changing nappies. Queen Charlotte's Hospital is one of many hospitals that have trained breastfeeding councillors to help you with specific feeding problems during your hospital stay and beyond.

Crying

Newborn babies do cry, all babies cry, but the newborn baby certainly does not have the guile to cry just to attract your attention: his cry is a response to some kind of discomfort. The discomfort may be hunger, cold, heat, a wet nappy, a dirty nappy, tiredness or pain. You are 'programmed' to respond to the cry, and to try to remove the discomfort. As your baby gets older you will learn to distinguish between the various cries, and to know which ones need immediate attention. When the baby is tiny you may feel overwhelmed if he cries a great deal (some cry inconsolably when they are bathed or dressed whereas others seem to relish the attention). If you are worried about how much he cries, talk to your midwife or health visitor about it, and try to identify the reasons for his crying. If your nerves are at breaking point, it is safer to leave the baby to cry on his own for five minutes while you calm down and have a cup of tea (with the radio turned up to blot out the sound if necessary!) than for you to try and settle him when you yourself are overwrought.

Feeding

In the first few days of your baby's life the midwife will make sure that you are confident about feeding your baby. She may suggest various positions for breastfeeding until you find a position that suits you and your baby. She may watch you feeding to get an idea of how well the baby latches onto the breast and how efficiently he sucks. This will vary enormously from one baby to another, and will change as the baby gets older.

You will be shown how to wind the baby half way through and at the end of each feed so that he can burp up any air trapped in his stomach during the feed (it is not always necessary to wind breastfed babies). This can either be done over the shoulder or over the knee, and it is advisable to have a towel or cloth ready to catch any milk that comes up with the wind.

You will also learn the difference between 'possetting' and being sick: babies will often possett a certain amount of milk shortly after a feed (this may be because they have ingested more than the capacity of the stomach, or it may be brought up with wind). This may look like a large quantity, but it is not significant (unless it happens copiously after every feed and the baby fails to put on weight).

When a baby is properly sick, bringing up foul-smelling curdy fluid some time after a feed, this could indicate that he is ill and you should discuss this with your GP or health visitor. Sickness could indicate that something in the milk disagrees with the baby. If you are breastfeeding your baby, you may notice that he is sick after you have had certain foods, and you should try to cut these foods out of your diet for a few weeks and re-introduce them gradually. If the baby is bottle fed and is sick repeatedly, you may be advised to try a different formula.

Bowel Movements

In the first twenty-four hours of your baby's life he should have his first bowel movement which is called meconium. Meconium is a very dark greenish black and it is very sticky; it may be quite difficult to clean the baby's bottom and the baby may cry at the shock of this first bowel movement and the thorough washing you are giving him! As the milk begins to work its way through the baby's digestive tract the meconium will become lighter green and more fluid, and – over the next day or so – will give way to the bright yellow yoghurt-smelling stools that are typical of very young babies. If you are worried about the colour, volume, consistency or frequency of your baby's stools, speak to your doctor, midwife or health visitor.

Holding and Eye Contact

An important aspect of caring for your baby has nothing to do with practical considerations, it is the love and attention that you give him. It has been shown that babies and children are more likely to thrive physically and psychologically if they have love but an inadequate diet than if they have an adequate diet but are not brought up in a loving environment. Your baby craves contact with you and with other human beings, he is programmed to explore human faces with his eyes and to learn the contours of your face (his range of focus is about 20cm [8in], so that he can focus on your face when he is at your breast). Most mothers are fascinated by their babies and do not need to be told to hold their babies and to make eye contact with them. If you are feeling unsure of yourself or the baby, try holding the baby about 20cm (8in) from your face and talking to him, and watch his eyes as they travel around your face. It may also help to watch him in someone else's arms and to see him respond to them too; you will realise that the burden of responsibility need not lie entirely on you.

Jaundice and Phototherapy

It is very common for newborn babies to be slightly jaundiced and to have the typical yellowing of the skin associated with this metabolic disorder. Jaundice can also make babies very sleepy, and this is undesirable because it means that they do not feed well. Some jaundice needs to be treated with phototherapy: when the baby is sleeping he can be put under a sun lamp (with a protective mask over his eyes), and the ultra-violet rays promote the excretion of excess bilirubin in the bloodstream which causes jaundice. Feeding is also an important concern in the treatment of jaundice. The baby who needs phototherapy may require more frequent feeds.

Tests Carried Out on the Baby

In the first few days of his life your baby will be checked over by a paediatrician or midwife, and a number of tests will be carried out on him to ensure that he is developing normally. The following things will probably be checked:

Ears: The baby's ears and his reflex response to loud noise.

Eyes: The baby's eyes and his reflex response to bright light. It is not uncommon for newborn babies to have bloodshot eyes as a result of the pressures on the head during delivery. This should clear in the first few days after delivery. Newborn babies are also prone to minor eye infections, and you will be taught how to keep your baby's eyes clean.

Fontanelle: The diamond-shaped gap between the unfused plates at the front of the baby's skull will be felt gently to check that there is a tough layer of membrane under the skin protecting the delicate brain beneath. First-time mothers are often afraid that they will hurt their babies if they touch the fontanelle, but it is not as vulnerable as it appears. If the fontanelle seems to dip into a concave shape the baby may be dehydrated. If the fontanelle suddenly seems to be bulging out above the surrounding plates of skull, let your doctor, midwife or health visitor know.

Genitals: The genitals of a newborn baby can be swollen by the effects of hormones transmitted through the placenta from the mother's bloodstream. Baby girls may have a whitish jelly-like discharge or a show of blood, and baby boys may have very large testicles. The doctor will check that the testes have descended into the scrotal sack.

Heart and lungs: The doctor will listen to the baby's heartbeat and his breathing using a stethoscope.

Hips: Every newborn baby will have his hips checked in case one or both of the hip joints is dislocated. The foetus can actually grow with dislocated hips and the earlier this is discovered and remedied the better the outcome will be. This can be one of the more traumatic tests for the mother because many babies find it disturbing and scream. The doctor will lie the baby on his back on a firm surface, splay the legs with the knees bent (in a frog-leg position) and rotate the top of the thigh in the hip joint. If there is any limitation to or abnormality in this movement, further tests will be carried out with ultrasound.

Motions: The doctor will ask whether the baby has yet passed any meconium (see above) and whether the meconium is being replaced by normal stools.

Spine: The doctor will hold the baby facing down in the palm of his hand; he will look at the baby's spine, and will run the end of a finger gently down his spine, to assess whether or not it is straight and intact.

Urine: The doctor will ask whether the baby has yet urinated, and he may ask whether the urine was very watery or dark. Some babies pass an orange coloured substance in their first days. It is very common and quite harmless, but if you have any concerns, discuss them with your midwife.

Tests for Reflexes

As well as checking your baby's reflex reactions to noise and light, the doctor will probably test him for the following reflexes, which are usually present in the newborn but some of which are lost in the first few months of life:

Babinski (gripping) reflex: This is the baby's reflex to grab hold of things with the hands and, to some extent, the feet (it is believed that our ancestors were covered in long body hair and that the newborn infant, as with some species of ape, clung to the mother's hair with hands and feet). The doctor may stroke the palms of the baby's hands and the soles of his feet with a finger or a pencil to see whether his fingers and toes curl over to grasp it. If a finger is put in the palm of each of the baby's hands he should grip so tightly that he can be lifted clear of the cot so that he is carrying his own bodyweight.

Moro (scare) reflex: The doctor may make a loud noise or may even cradle the baby in his hand and drop his hand swiftly to check whether the baby displays the characteristic reflex of throwing his arms and legs up and out, and then bringing them in together in a grasping action (as with the Babinski reflex, it is believed that the Moro reflex is an illustration of how a newborn primate could save himself by responding to any shock stimulus by reaching up and grasping for his mother).

Rooting reflex: The doctor will ask whether your baby seems to be 'rooting' well: if he is held next to your breasts and the nipple or any other part of your breast touches his cheek, the baby should turn towards the breast to suckle. The doctor may stroke the baby's cheek to see whether he turns towards this stimulus.

Sucking reflex: In newborn babies sucking is a reflex not a voluntary action, without this reflex they would not eat and would not survive. Premature babies sometimes have a much weaker sucking reflex or none at all, and they may find it easier to feed from a cup than from the breast (although this should not preclude them from having breast milk if their mothers express their milk). Some babies need to be fed with a tube. The doctor may ask whether your baby is sucking well, and he may check the sucking reflex by stroking your baby's lip.

'Walking' reflex: As well as the Babinski and Moro reflexes – which seem to identify humans very closely with our more primitive ancestors – the newborn baby has an astonishing reflex that is very peculiarly associated with *homo sapiens*: if you hold a newborn baby upright on a flat surface so that his feet just touch the surface, he will make very distinctive, slightly exaggerated stepping or walking motions. Doctors probably enjoy this test more than any other for the look of amazement on first-time mother's faces.

Tests for Illness or Abnormality

Guthrie test: Every baby in this country is screened for a metabolic disorder called phenylketonuria, an inability to digest protein. This test is known as the Guthrie test and is performed in the first week or ten days of the baby's life. It involves taking a few drops of blood from the baby by pricking his heel, so that the blood can be tested for certain substances. Although the condition is very rare, affecting about one in every 700 babies, it can be very damaging, causing severe mental retardation. It is worth having this simple test because, if sufferers are identified early enough they can be treated with a special diet and they can develop perfectly normally.

Bilirubin: It is not uncommon for newborn babies to have jaundice. If the jaundice is severe, or if it persists the baby will be given a series of blood tests to assess the levels of a substance called bilirubin which causes jaundice. The levels of bilirubin indicate whether jaundice requires treatment with phototherapy.

Blood group: Your baby's blood group will probably be noted from the blood sample taken in the Guthrie test (see above). If you have Rhesus negative blood and your baby has Rhesus positive blood you may be given an injection to pre-empt the possibility of Rhesus incompatibility in future pregnancies (see the section of **Blood Groups** in the **Preparing for Pregnancy** chapter).

Blood sugar levels (hypoglycaemia test): If your baby is very small or has a low birthweight, he may be given a blood test to assess whether his blood sugar levels are low. This is known as the hypoglycaemia test because hypoglycaemia is a condition in which blood sugar levels are low (this can have a number of causes). If his blood sugar levels are low, the baby will need extra feeds and, in some cases, breastfeeding may have to be supplemented with bottle feeding if lactation is not fully established.

Changes in your Body

A woman's body undergoes some major changes after delivery, and she needs to understand and adapt to these changes as well as coping with a new baby: even going to the loo can become a major issue (see below). The hospital staff, or visiting midwife or health visitor should be able to give her the advice and support that she needs, to answer any questions and to offer pain relief if necessary. For about the first ten days they will systematically check or ask you about the following things every day: stitches and bruising, urinating and bowel motions, blood loss, contracting down of the uterus, and breasts and milk production. For the first few days your temperature and blood pressure will also be taken as indicators of how your body is coping with this period of transition, and because they could act as a warning if you have any sort of infection.

Your Tummy

The gradual growth of your abdomen during your pregnancy gave you a chance to get used to its changing size and appearance. Some women are shocked by how large their tummies still look after delivery, and many are alarmed by the slackness of the skin which has been stretched and has now been allowed to fall back. Although your tummy may still be much bulkier than your pre-pregnancy shape, this is not all caused by fat stores. Much of this bulk is simply stretched skin, and the skin's natural elasticity will firm it up again gradually. This firming-up process depends to some extent on your age, your general level of fitness, how much weight you normally carry and how much exercise you take after having the baby.

> CASE STUDY: *'I was huge, eight months pregnant, at Christmas time, and my sister-in-law gave me a piece of skimpy underwear for Christmas with a card saying: "it does all go back!" I was quite encouraged by this, but when [the baby] was born my tummy was like a water bed, and I thought it would never "go back". She was right, though, it does.'*

Your Uterus

After the third stage of labour the uterus continues to contract more gently for several days or weeks as it gradually shrinks back to its pre-pregnancy size and position. This process is usually faster in women who are breastfeeding because the baby's suckling stimulates uterine contractions. The midwife will assess the position of your uterus every day by gentle abdominal palpation to check that it is contracting down.

Afterpains

The milder uterine contractions that continue after delivery are often painless, but some women experience considerable pain as the uterus continues to contract. These are known as afterpains, and they are more common with second and subsequent babies, the more the uterus is stretched, the harder it has to work to return to its pre-pregnancy shape. Afterpains are also more likely to affect women who are breastfeeding, and they will be most noticeable during feeds because the baby's suckling stimulates the contractions. If you have very uncomfortable afterpains, let the hospital staff know, and they will probably offer paracetamol or another mild analgesic to ease the pain.

Lochia

The site of the placenta on the uterine wall will continue to bleed a little for several days or even weeks after delivery. This blood loss and the discharge that may accompany it is called lochia. In the first few days after delivery it may be quite heavy bleeding, and the blood may be bright and fresh, perhaps with small clots. Bleeding is often heavier and does not last so long in women who are breastfeeding, because of the extra stimulus to the contracting uterus. The bleeding will gradually become lighter within the first week after delivery; it will turn a rusty red and then a pinkish colour, before stopping altogether up to six weeks after delivery.

You should use sanitary pads to absorb the blood, and it may be advisable to take a pack of disposable knickers to hospital with you. Tampons should not be used because they can increase the risk of infection, and they are, anyway, unlikely to be adequate in the first few days. The hospital staff will ask you about your blood loss, and you should let them know if you are worried by the volume of blood you are losing, if the volume suddenly increases or if you lose a large clot. If you do lose a large clot, keep the sanitary towel it is on, in case the staff ask to see it; it could indicate that there are still fragments of the placenta in the uterus.

CASE STUDY: *'I was very surprised by how much blood there was. You need big thick STs and granny knickers which you don't mind throwing away because they'll get covered in it. Nobody told me there would be so much blood.'*

Stitches

Tears, episiotomies and the stitches needed to repair them can be the greatest source of discomfort to newly delivered women. If the wound was deep you may be in considerable pain: you may be given a special cushion to sit on or advised to sit on pillows, and you may be offered paracetamol or a similar mild analgesic for the pain. It is important to keep the area clean and dry, but be careful not to drag your flannel or towel over the stitches; dab them gently instead.

As the wound knits together, the stitches may tickle or they may give you a gentle tugging sensation. If the stitches themselves feel very uncomfortable or seem to be 'pulling', let the staff know: in a very few cases, the stitches are too tight and will have to be removed, and the wound stitched again.

The staff will check your stitches at least once a day, and will tell you how to look after them. You need to keep the area scrupulously clean, washing frequently and wiping from front to back when you open your bowels. You should also avoid strenuous lifting or sudden movements which could cause the stitches to tear: this can be very painful and you would then require further repair work (it may seem self-evident that you should avoid heavy lifting, and there may not be an opportunity for it in hospital; but you could be caught out the day you go home when you automatically pick up an ebullient toddler or a wagging dog who rushes to meet you).

Any internal stitches in muscle tissue will have been 'dissolving stitches', made of a material which is dissolved into your own tissues. Superficial stitches in the skin may or may not need removing within about ten days. This should not be painful – it is usually described as tickling – but it might be if you tense up at the thought of it. Whenever your stitches are being checked, or when they are being removed, you can use breathing exercises to help you relax and make the process easier.

CASE STUDY: *'I know it's not really important but I felt really self-conscious about having my stitches checked. Well, it seemed normal that everyone should be looking between my legs for the delivery, but in the cold grey light of dawn it was embarrassing.'*

Bruising

Many women have internal and external bruising in and around the vagina after delivery, especially if the second stage of labour was very long or explosively quick. The midwife will keep an eye on external bruising and, if you are in a lot of pain, she will offer you mild analgesics such as paracetamol; sometimes anti-inflammatory drugs are used. This bruising can take considerably longer to heal than a tear, and it may be several weeks before you feel comfortable inside or are able to make love.

CASE STUDY: *'My baby was born very quickly and they said that I was badly bruised ... I felt uncomfortable but I thought it was just all part of having a baby. When I got the all-clear at my six weeks check, we tried to make love that night, but I couldn't, it just hurt terribly. I went back to the doctor and she looked internally and said that I was still recovering from internal bruising. I couldn't believe it, that was six weeks afterwards. In the end it was more than three months before I felt comfortable and confident to try again.'*

Urinating

Most women have no problem passing urine after delivery, but if you have torn or have had an episiotomy you may be very anxious that urinating will hurt the wound. Urine is salty and it does sting wounds, but there are ways of getting round this: the staff may advise you to run a warm shallow bath, and to sit in it to urinate (you will need to throw off years of prejudice about 'doing that sort of thing in the bath'!); once you are feeling more confident, you can take a jug of warm water with you to the loo and pour the water so that it runs down past the urethra as you urinate. The urine will immediately be diluted so much that it does not sting. If you have any problems passing uring following delivery, let your midwife know immediately.

It is very important that you do not cut down on your intake of fluids as a way of avoiding urinating too frequently. You will be losing fluids rapidly in the form of lochia, sweat (newly delivered women tend to sweat more than usual because of the hormones in their bloodstream) and – if you are breastfeeding – milk.

Opening your bowels

The first bowel movement after delivery is something that new mothers may worry about almost more than anything else, especially if they have had a lot of stitches. The thought of straining against the stitches is frightening: women worry that it will hurt, which it can do, or that they will tear their stitches (it is actually very rare for a woman to tear her stitches in this way).

The problem is compounded by the fact that you will probably have had a disrupted pattern of meals because of your labour and this – as well as certain hormones – increases the likelihood of being constipated. In order to avoid constipation you should eat foods rich in fibre, especially fruits and vegetables, and drink plenty of fluids. This should help to ensure that the first stool is soft enough to be passed without straining. The actions of swallowing and digesting food, and movement of the whole body (even just walking up and down the hospital corridor) will help to stimulate the muscles in the bowel.

The midwife will ask you every day whether or not you have opened your bowels, and she may be able to give you laxative suppositories if you have not opened your bowels after two or three days (the longer a stool remains in the bowel the drier and harder it will be). It is important to remember to wipe your anus thoroughly from front to back after opening your bowels, especially if you have passed a loose bowel motion.

CASE STUDY: *'I was really worried about it [opening bowels], everyone was, it became quite a topic of conversation. But it was nothing like as bad as I thought it would be.'*

Your breasts

Your breasts will have been producing colostrum, the first milk, for many weeks now (some women have leaks of colostrum during pregnancy), and the production of colostrum will be stepped-up after delivery, stimulated by hormones that are automatically triggered at delivery and by the baby's sucking. Colostrum is an especially rich milk that contains many antibodies and, even if you have decided not to breastfeed your baby for any length of time, it is worth giving him the benefit of these antibodies for the first few days of his life.

On about the third or fourth day the milk itself will 'come in'. In fact, the milk-producing glands simply draw more fluids and nutrients from your bloodstream and switch to producing milk instead of colostrum, but such is the volume usually produced that it does feel as if it has 'come in' from somewhere else. Some women do not notice this transition, while others are very aware of the milk coming in. The day on which the milk comes in will vary slightly from one woman to another, and it might be altered by the feeding pattern of the baby: if you are not breastfeeding, the milk-producing glands will have less stimulation and the milk may not come in for four days; if your baby is very hungry and feeds every hour or two, he may stimulate the glands sufficiently for the milk to start coming in on the second day.

Your breasts are likely to be very tender when your milk first comes in. You will be able to feel the individual chambers containing milk under your skin; they may be very hard. The skin will feel stretched and sore, and it may feel hot. The skin of the nipples may also be stretched and flattened. If your breasts are very uncomfortable, and feeding the baby does not relieve you for long, the midwife will show you how to soothe your breasts with warm flannels, in a basin of warm water or by expressing a small amount of milk by hand. The best way to ease the congestion is to feed the baby, and it is very important that you should not use bottles at this stage: if the breasts stay full for too long they will automatically produce less milk to meet the low demand.

If you are not breastfeeding your baby, your breasts may be full and tender for several days. Most hospitals advise against expressing milk to ease them, because drawing-off milk acts as a stimulus for further milk production. You may have heard of pills prescribed to dry up the milk, but these powerful hormones can have a number of side-effects, and most hospitals are unwilling to use them. If you wear a supportive bra and take mild analgesics you should not be too uncomfortable, and your breasts will go back to normal in a few days.

If your baby is too weak to suckle well, or is being fed through a tube, you may want to keep up your supply of milk and collect your milk to give to the baby in a bottle or through the tube. You can do this by using a breast pump; many hospitals have electric breast pumps and, although women may feel a little like dairy cows when they are using them, they are not painful to use.

The first few minutes of a feed can be quite painful in the early days, especially if the breasts are very engorged. If you find that you are in a lot of pain, try not to take a deep breath and brace yourself before your baby latches on. The baby will feel your arms tensing around him, and this may alter the way he latches on, and it certainly will not remove any pain for you. Use the breathing exercises you learnt for labour to help you relax when you are feeding your baby. If you are worried about any aspect of feeding your baby, speak to the midwife.

CASE STUDY: *'... She was premature and very sleepy with jaundice so she really didn't suckle well at all. They said it would be easier for her to suckle from a bottle so I have to use the breast pump to express off my milk. I really hate it, but it does the job ... I put her to the breast at the beginning of the feed so that she gets used to that then, when she gets frustrated, I feed her with my milk out of the bottle.'*

CASE STUDY: *'My baby kept me awake for all of the second night wanting to suckle the whole time. Then, while she was sleeping, the milk came in, and it was just so painful, there was so much of it. I'm normally a 34AA and that afternoon I went up to 39 inches round the bust. They were holding the bra up not the other way round, they felt like rocks and they chafed the skin on the inside of my arm.'*

Recovering After a Caesarean Section

If you have had a Caesarean, you may be surprised how much the operation has taken out of you: a Caesarean represents major abdominal surgery, you will have a deep wound, you may be suffering the after-effects of a general anaesthetic and a long labour, and you will be coping with a new baby. It is especially important that women who have had Caesareans make the most of their stay in hospital to rest and recover from the operation. They will, anyway, be kept in hospital for longer (probably four to six days instead of two to four days), and the staff may help out with bathing, dressing and changing the baby. Some units now have special cots which are attached to the side of the bed, so you can have easy access to your baby.

Your scar: It may appear quite small on the surface but it is a deep wound, crossing layers of muscle tissue. They are very painful, and an aspect of recovering physically and psychologically from a Caesarean is having adequate pain relief (see below). It will be more comfortable to wear waist high underpants so the waistband will not chafe the wound.

The scar may look ugly, and you could be quite shocked by it (some women do not like their partners to see the scar even if they were present for the entire operation), but you will have to take experts at their word when they tell you that, in all but the very rare cases when complications arise, these scars heal very satisfactorily and can be almost imperceptible once they have healed.

The wound will 'weep' fluid and / or blood for about 24 hours, and there may be a small tube to drain fluid into a bottle for the first day or so after the operation. The wound will be dressed, and the staff will check and change your dressing regularly. You should not hesitate to call for help if you notice an increase in fluid draining either through a drain or onto the dressing.

The external incision may be sutured with dissolving stitches (which do not need removing), or with metal staples or silk stitches. These will be removed on about the fifth day. People often worry about having stitches removed but this need not be painful if you are sufficiently relaxed and do not watch the process. It might be worth using a few breathing exercises to give you something else to think about while your stitches are removed.

Pain relief: If you had an epidural Caesarean, the epidural may be left in and topped up for several hours after the operation to give you continued pain relief. Once the epidural is removed, or if you had the operation under general anaesthetic, you will need to take pain relieving drugs. These can be injected or taken orally. There is little point in 'trying to be brave' about having analgesics after a Caesarean; your body has a great deal of recovering to do and you will be encouraged to get up and move around as soon as possible to promote your circulation and the natural healing process: this will be easier if you have adequate pain relief. You will probably be given anti-inflammatory medication for the first three days as well as mild analgesics. You should not worry that the drugs will affect your baby if you are breastfeeding, the doctors will choose drugs that have a minimal effect on the baby. If you are finding it difficult coping with the pain, or if you notice any sudden increase in pain, let the staff know.

Changes in your body and check-ups: Many of the changes in your body are similar to those experienced by women who have had vaginal deliveries (see **Changes in Your Body**, above) with the exception that you will have a debilitating scar in your abdomen as well as all the other discomforts (people assume that women who have had Caesareans have 'got off lightly' in terms of pain and injury in and around the vagina, but if you have an emergency Caesarean after a failed forceps delivery, you will have a stitched episiotomy and possibly a very bruised vagina as well as the stitches in your abdomen. Your tummy may take longer to go back to its pre-pregnancy shape after a Caesarean section because the scar and the damaged muscle tissue will preclude you taking very much exercise. Your uterus will go down in the same way, you will lose lochia and your breasts will produce milk. All of these things as well as your temperature and blood pressure will be checked at least daily by the midwife.

Urinating: Passing water itself should not be as painful as it may be for a woman who has had a vaginal delivery (unless you had an episiotomy before having your Caesarean), but it may be difficult for you to get to the lavatory and to find a comfortable position in which to pass water. Your catheter may be left in for a day or so after the operation so that you do not have to get up to pass water, but most hospitals encourage women to move around as soon as they can, and the need to pass water is as good an excuse as any. There may be loos in the hospital with handle bars on either side to help you lower yourself down and lift yourself back up again.

Bowel movements and wind: Constipation is a common problem after having a baby (see **Opening your Bowels**, above) and it is even more common after Caesarean section. The fact that movement of the whole body facilitates the functioning of the muscles in the bowel is one of the reasons that women are encouraged to get up as soon as possible. You may well suffer from quite painful wind, and it may be several days before you can pass a motion. Again it may be difficult for you to sit down on the loo, and you may find that you have no muscles in your stomach to push, or you may be afraid of tearing your stitches if you push. Ideally, you should not need to strain to pass motions; stick to high fibre foods and plenty of fluids as described above. If you do not pass a motion for several days you will be given a laxative suppository.

Getting comfortable: Many women who have had Caesarean sections are surprised by just how debilitating it is to have lost the use of their tummy muscles, and alarmed by how painful a simple sneeze can be. Queen Charlotte's is one of many hospitals that have obstetric physiotherapists who can give very specialised advice about how to cope with sneezing, coughing and laughing, how to get in and out of bed comfortably, how best to sit, and lie down and what positions to adopt for feeding the baby.

The midwife will encourage you to move around as soon as possible and will help you to find comfortable sitting, lying and feeding positions. Unfortunately, it is not true to say 'if it hurts, you are not doing it right':

many simple actions may well hurt, but you must do them slowly and use your breathing exercises to relax yourself – tension will only increase the pain.

It is tempting for women who have had Caesareans to sit, stand and walk in a slightly bent position, as if they were protecting their wound. This will put unnecessary strain on your back, and also on the back of the scar as the abdominal organs weigh down on it under the force of gravity. Try to keep your back upright and lift yourself up and down using the palms of your hands and the flexion in your knees.

Changes in your Moods

Many women feel happy and energised when their baby is born, and they may continue to feel so with few fluctuations in their mood. It is, however, very common for women to experience quite dramatic mood swings, especially in the early days, and you should certainly not feel that there is anything wrong with you if you do not feel happy the whole time. Your body undergoes tremendous hormonal changes in the first few days after delivery: it suffers the withdrawal of the pregnancy hormones, and a surge in the hormones that promote lactation. The body is also repairing itself and you are likely to be very tired (which affects levels of certain hormones). It is, therefore, hardly surprising that women experience mood swings and crises of confidence in the first few days – or even weeks – after having a baby.

If you felt tired and flat after delivery, it may be some days before your mood gradually picks up. If you were euphoric after delivery, you may come down with quite a bump when the exhaustion hits you. In any event, it is important to get as much sleep and rest as possible to allow your body every opportunity to recover and adapt.

Newly delivered mothers can be prone to tearfulness and irritability; their confidence may be especially fragile so that the slightest negative remark causes great distress. In general, women who have had a very difficult labour and delivery are more likely to be tearful and unsure of themselves than those who have had relatively easy births, but this is by no means always the case.

You may find that you want to keep yourself to yourself, and you should be able to curtain off your area of the room so that you can get to grips with your feelings and your new baby in your own time. Some women find that they are desperate for contact with other people, perhaps as a source of reassurance and support. Other mothers may be happy to sit and chat with you, especially in the nursery or mothers' room, which can act as a sort of 'common room'; and if you have any specific concerns or questions the staff should be able to help.

CASE STUDY: *'The breastfeeding was really painful, and when I asked one of the nurses for help she asked to watch me put him to the breast and she said straight away "ah, he's not latching on properly!" I should have been happy and relieved she had found the answer to my problems, and she was really helpful, but I felt as if I'd had my wrist slapped for being a "silly girl", and I was really tearful about it.'*

Baby Blues

It is very common, although certainly not universal, for women to reach a bit of low about three or four days after the baby is born. This is known as the 'baby blues' and it often coincides with the time when the milk comes in; it is probably due to the fact that hormonal changes are at their most intense at this time. It is also thought that the baby blues are a reaction to the psychological effects of the birth: after all the build-up of the pregnancy and the excitement and exertion of delivery, the aftermath can feel like an anticlimax, however thrilled the mother is with her baby. Once the first buzz of euphoria has passed, the mother begins to realise how tired she is and just how tiring and demanding her new responsibility is.

The baby blues, if they affect a woman at all, usually only last for a few days, although they may intensify a little when she goes home because of the added demands and responsibilities of being out of hospital. If the symptoms persist for longer than a few weeks, it is very important that you talk to people about them. Your partner, your mother, close friends or a local support group may be able to help and boost your confidence. If you feel as if you want to talk about your feelings in confidence, talk to your doctor, midwife or health visitor.

These feelings are in some ways a self-perpetuating myth: the more tearful and anxious you are, the less you will sleep; the less you sleep, the more listless and tearful you become. This will ultimately damage your confidence still further and you may start to have the feelings of guilt, pointlessness and self-loathing that typify the onset of depression.

Postnatal Depression

Postnatal depression will affect at least one woman in ten (the real figure is probably higher than this, but not all cases are diagnosed or reported). It does not always follow on directly from the baby blues: it may be triggered at any time in the first year of the baby's life. As mentioned in the section on **Baby Blues**, above, if your feelings of tearfulness and inadequacy persist for more than a few days or weeks it is very important that you have some sort of help.

Symptoms of Depression

Some typical symptoms of depression include tiredness and an inability to sleep, listlessness, feelings of guilt and hopelessness, lack of appetite, lack of interest in sex, withdrawal from social contact and an inability to concentrate. Except for a very small minority who suffer from the far more serious postnatal psychosis, many depressed mothers are meticulous in the care that they give to their babies, but they will do it all as a chore with a deadpan face, not giving the baby the eye contact that he craves (research has shown that the emotional and intellectual development of the baby can be impaired by prolonged exposure to a very depressed carer).

Treatment of Depression

Depression can be a dangerous, long-term illness if it is not identified and treated correctly and promptly. It is crucial that you understand that there should be no stigma attached to depression; it is caused by an imbalance of certain chemicals in the brain rather as diabetes is caused by an imbalance of insulin. If you understand this it may be easier for you to ask for the help that you need.

Once depression has been identified it can be treated with drugs and / or counselling. Anti-depressants take about two weeks to take effect as they raise the levels of the deficient chemicals in the brain; some anti-depressants are regarded as safe to use if you are breastfeeding. If you are very keen to avoid using anti-depressants, you may find that tranquillisers or sleep aids help: by allowing the body to relax and the mind to give in to sleep, tranquillisers give the metabolism an opportunity to synthesise more of the deficient chemicals.

Counselling is usually a very important part of the treatment of postnatal depression. Psychiatrists and psychiatric nurses will not only understand the chemical changes that are causing your condition, they will also recognise all the symptoms and feelings that you are experiencing. They are trained to talk to you and to let you talk about your feelings so that you come to understand them better, and to realise that some of them are not really you but are being imposed on you by your depression.

Self-help

There are a number of ways that you can try to extricate yourself from the onset of depression if you think you recognise some of the symptoms listed above. First of all it is important that you minimise your responsibilities, do not overburden yourself with chores that are not really necessary, and this will cut down on your feelings of guilt and inadequacy.

Talking to people is a very good way of dealing with feelings of depression. Some women are unwilling to talk to their partners because one of the symptoms – or causes – of their depression is that they feel their partner is not giving them enough support. Many women are also afraid that their parents will not understand their feelings of depression, saying 'in my day, we just pulled ourselves together'. Friends, especially women who have had babies themselves, should be a good source of support and shoulders to cry on. If you cannot think of anyone you want to talk to there may be a local mother-and-baby group, or you may be able to contact an organisation (addresses appear at the end of the book) that can give you the support you need and put you in touch with someone local who can help you.

If possible, spend some time away from the baby, especially if he cries a great deal. This should be possible even if you are breastfeeding and you do not feel up to expressing milk: if you can find someone who will come in and look after the baby while you catch up on some sleep or go round to a friend's house nearby, they can call you when the baby needs feeding. Many women are afraid of social contact when they are depressed: if your partner tries to 'buck you up' by taking you out and arranging for lots of people to come round, try to explain to him that the strain of seeing lots of people is not what you need at the moment.

Try to do something that boosts your morale and makes you feel good about yourself. It need not be something complicated or expensive; it might just be watching a feel-good film, having your favourite meal or having a manicure (many beauticians come to the customer's home), but if it makes you feel happy and takes you out of yourself for a short time it may help.

Taking exercise is a very good way of overcoming the early stages of depression. When you take even light exercise the adrenaline and endorphins that circulate in your body make you feel well and happy; as your mood lifts, the brain begins to synthesise the deficient chemicals, restoring normal levels. Try to find out whether your local leisure centre or swimming pool has a creche, and try to join a gentle exercise or yoga class. They may have classes specifically designed for women who have just had babies.

Having Visitors

Most women are happy to see their partners and their parents at any time after having a baby, but it may be a day or two before they want any other visitors. For the first day after your baby is born you are likely to be very tired and bruised, but you may feel ready to see visitors as early as the following day. If you do not feel ready to have visitors when you are in hospital make sure that your friends know this when you, your partner or a mutual friend rings to tell them the news that you have had your baby.

Even after you have gone home and have started settling in to a routine, there may be times that you feel you cannot cope with having visitors. Once you are back in your own home, visitors can actually be quite hard work: you may want to keep the house tidy, to dress the baby up, and to have drinks and biscuits ready for them. Try to forget about little details like this: your friends are really there to see you and the baby, not the shine on the furniture, and you should know them well enough to tell them to make a cup of tea for themselves and for you!

If you are very tired and you really need some sleep, let those closest to you know that you need some time to yourself; there is nothing wrong with disconnecting the telephone and the doorbell for a few hours after a feed to catch up on sleep. The rest you get more than justifies a little disappointment for your friends.

Leaving Hospital

However long your stay in hospital, you may either be dreading going home or longing for it. Some women feel afraid of the responsibility of going home with their new babies or they worry about all the extra demands that will be made on them when they return home; others are very keen to get away from the institutionalised atmosphere – and food! – and to get on with their own lives with their babies.

The length of your hospital stay will depend on how straightforward your labour and delivery were and on how well you and the baby are doing. Before you are discharged from hospital you and the baby will have a final check-up to assess your recovery. You will be asked whether your lochia is beginning to become lighter in volume and turning from red to rusty brown; your abdomen will be checked to ensure that the uterus is shrinking back; your stitches will be checked; and you will be asked how the feeding is going, and whether your breasts are comfortable (if you are breastfeeding). Your temperature and blood-pressure may also be taken, and you may be given a blood test to check whether you are slightly anaemic (in which case iron tablets may be prescribed).

The baby will be weighed to assess how well he is putting on weight. Many babies are actually lighter than their birthweight when they leave hospital, but it is quite normal for a baby to lose about 10% of his birthweight in the first few days of life while he sleeps off the birth and makes the transition to feeding orally. (His weight will be monitored by the community midwife once you return home, until he has at least regained his birthweight.) His temperature and blood pressure may be taken, and the doctor may listen to his heart and lungs with a stethoscope.

During these check-ups talk to the doctor or the midwife about any concerns you have or any questions you need answered. Once you and your baby have been given the all-clear there may be two more important things that the staff talk to you about: firstly they may not let you take the baby out of hospital until they are satisfied that you have a suitable car seat for him, and they are likely to ask you what method of contraception you intend using now.

Contraception

Making love may be a very long way from your mind when you are tired and sore from delivery; but some couples are very eager to make love again. Whatever your feelings about sex at this stage, the desire may creep up on you before you have put any thought into a method of contraception. It is far better to be prepared than disappointed!

It is worth bearing in mind that, however eager you feel about making love, it may cause you some discomfort or pain, and the first few attempts may even have to be abandoned. The lining of the vagina is not so well lubricated after childbirth because of hormonal changes, and you may find that it helps to use a lubricating jelly. Taking things slowly and not having high expectations will help too.

It is very important to realise that women are often very fertile immediately after having a baby. This is especially true if they are not breastfeeding, but it may also be the case if you are breastfeeding. Neither can you assume that you will not conceive if your periods have not started again: because ovulation takes place before menstruation, it is quite possible to conceive before you start menstruating again.

In the first few weeks after delivery there are certain methods of contraception that cannot be used, for example the cap or an intrauterine device. If you would eventually like to be fitted for one of these devices, discuss it with your doctor when you go for your six weeks check. In the meantime, make provision to use another kind of contraceptive such as condoms.

If you want to use the contraceptive pill, the type of pill you use will depend on whether or not you are breastfeeding. The combined oral contraceptive is not suitable for breastfeeding women, whereas the progesterone-only pill is. Your doctor will explain to you when to take your first pill (brands differ), and how long it will be before the pill offers complete protection. In the interim you should use another kind of contraceptive such as condoms.

Condoms are perhaps the best answer for the early weeks after delivery: you do not have to remember to take a pill every day, but they offer the protection you need as and when you need it. Condoms offer higher protection if used in conjunction with a spermicidal cream.

At Home with your Baby

Many women are happy, proud and excited – if a little daunted – when they come home with a new baby, especially if it is their first. If you are worried about any aspect of taking your baby home, discuss it with your doctor or midwife before you leave hospital. You will anyway continue to have daily visits from your community midwife until the baby is ten days old or until he has regained his birthweight (if this is later), and then you will be visited regularly by the health visitor until he is one month old. After that, you can attend baby clinics in your local surgery as often as you like to check on his progress. When the baby is six weeks old you will have a thorough 'MOT' to assess your recovery from the pregnancy and delivery.

You should feel free to talk to your midwife, your health visitor or your GP during one of these check-ups or at any other time about any problems you are having with the baby or with feeding him. If you feel that you are not coping well with the demands of motherhood, if your baby cries a great deal, or if you are having trouble establishing your breastfeeding, there are organisations and support groups that can put you in touch with someone local to you who can give you the help and encouragement you need (some addresses are listed at the end of the book).

The important thing to remember when you take your baby home is to get plenty of rest: your body is still recovering and doing internal repair work; and caring for and feeding the baby make considerable physical and emotional demands on you. Go to bed in good time in the evenings and to rest at least once during the day. Newly-delivered women are actually entitled to domestic help from social services. This service is strictly means tested, but the very fact that it exists means that it is recognised that you will need help in the early days: try to find someone who can come in once a day to help out with chores, or to take the baby (and any older children) out for a walk while you catch up on some sleep.

Reducing the Risk of Cot Death

Sudden Infant Death Syndrome or cot death occurs when a baby dies for no discernible reason. Although this only happens to one in every 1400 babies, it is so devastating that the syndrome itself and any research into the factors which may cause it attract considerable media attention. There are a number of ways in which you can reduce the risk of a cot death:

Temperature: We all instinctively want to keep newborn babies warm, but it is very important not to let them get too hot. Overheating is associated with an increased risk of cot death. The baby's room should not be kept at more than 20°C, and the baby should not be dressed up too warmly.

Sleeping position: Always put your baby down to sleep on his back. As the baby gets bigger and stronger he will be able to roll and to assume whatever sleeping position he favours, and this should not be discouraged. But while he is tiny he should sleep on his back.

No smoking: Do not smoke near your baby or subject him to smoky environments. Smoky rooms are implicated in many incidents of cot death. If you or a member of your family or close circle of friends cannot give up smoking, try to ensure that you or they smoke only outside, or in a well-ventilated room far from the baby, and that ashtrays are emptied after each cigarette.

Mattresses: A few years ago it was believed that cot mattresses might release toxic gases which could cause cot deaths. These claims have never been substantiated, and there is no evidence that a foam or PVC-covered mattress can harm your baby. Some foam mattresses have holes in the head area to reduce the risk of suffocation if the baby rolls onto his front. The Foundation for the Study of Infant Deaths says that, so long as a mattress is clean and firm, it should be safe to use. Be wary of buying a second-hand mattress because it will be difficult to assess how clean it is.

Enjoying your Baby

Despite being tired and uncomfortable in the early days, you should have plenty of opportunities to enjoy your baby. Some people feel that newborn babies – even their own – are boring, but most of us are enthralled by these tiny little miracles, and we coo hopelessly over every yawn and hiccup.

You are likely to feel tremendously proud of your baby, and you may be able to 'waste' many an hour just watching him. This is not wasted time: the more pleasure you take in your baby, the more secure and happy he will feel. When he is about a month old (unless he was very premature) he will reward you with his first social smile. Babies do smile in their sleep and when they are awake right from their first days, and these are true smiles in that the muscle actions are the same, but what every mother waits for is the first smile directed exclusively at her. Babies instinctively study faces methodically, looking at the eyes, up and round the hairline and then down to the nose and the mouth and back up to the eyes. One day your baby will mimic the smile he sees on your lips, and then look back up to your eyes with a smile on his face – he will truly be smiling at you.

Glossary

AFP test A test to assess levels of a protein called alpha-feto-protein in the mother's bloodstream during pregnancy. High levels of AFP may indicate that the foetus has a neural tube defect such as spina bifida.

Afterpains The muscular pains experienced by some women after delivery as the uterus continues to contract regularly

Amniocentesis A procedure for testing for genetic abnormalities (such as Down's Syndrome) in the foetus. A small amount of amniotic fluid is drawn off for testing by inserting a hollow needle through the abdominal wall into the uterus.

Amniotic fluid The clear fluid that surrounds and protects the foetus throughout pregnancy. It is contained within the membranes of the amniotic sac, and is also known as the liquor or waters.

Analgesic Pain relief.

Anaemic Having low levels of haemoglobin in the red blood cells, which can cause lethargy, tiredness and dizziness. It may be caused by iron deficiency.

Antenatal Before the birth.

ARM Artificial rupture of the membranes. A surgical procedure for inducing or accelerating labour by shipping a surgical hook into the cervix and rupturing the amniotic sac.

Assisted delivery Any procedure, such as an episiotomy, forceps delivery or vacuum extraction, that assists or accelerates delivery.

Birth canal The vagina.

Booking clinic The first and usually the most detailed antenatal check-up attended, usually in about the fourteenth week of pregnancy although this will depend on when the woman discovers that she is pregnant, and it may vary from one hospital to another. It includes taking a full medical and obstetric history.

Braxton Hicks contractions The mild and occasionally uncomfortable contractions of the uterus that take place throughout pregnancy but are usually not felt, if at all, before the third trimester.

Breech presentation / delivery Position in which the baby is presenting and / or delivered with its bottom, rather than its head, first. There are a number of variations on the breech position.

Caesarean section Delivery of the baby by means of a surgical incision through the mother's abdominal wall and into the uterus.

Cephalic The usual and most desirable presentation of the foetus in the latter weeks of pregnancy with the head down.

Cervix The firm muscular neck of the womb that usually has an aperture of a few millimetres to allow sperm and menstrual blood to pass. During pregnancy it holds the baby in the uterus, and during labour it dilates to allow the baby to be born.

Chromosomal abnormalities Unusual configurations of the genetic material contained in the sperm or egg which may be duplicated when cell division of the fertilised egg begins, and can give rise to congenital abnormalities in the foetus.

Chorionic villus sampling (CVS) A test for certain congenital abnormalities in which a small sample of the placenta is removed by inserting a tube through the cervix or by inserting a needle through the abdominal wall and into the uterus.

Colostrum The first milk, which contains many antibodies as well as nutrients. It is highly nutritious and helps prevent infections in your baby. It is produced by the breasts during pregnancy and in the first few days of the baby's life. Colostrum may leak from the breasts during pregnancy.

Conception The moment of fertilisation, when the nucleus of the sperm cell and the nucleus of the egg cell fuse to form the genetic material for a complete human being.

Congenital abnormalities Variations on the normal development of the foetus which may be serious and life-threatening, such as a heart defect, or may be more superficial, such as extra digits on the hands and feet.

Contractions The regular flexing or tightening of the muscles of the uterus. Contractions actually occur regularly throughout pregnancy and after the baby is born but are felt most intensely during labour.

Cot death The sudden unexplained death of a baby usually within the first three months of life. Also known as sudden infant death syndrome (SIDS).

D & C Dilation and curettage. A procedure used to ensure that all the 'products of the pregnancy', such as any fragments of placenta, are removed after a miscarriage. The cervix is dilated and the lining of the uterus is scraped. D & Cs are performed under general anaesthetic.

Dilation The opening up of the aperture of the cervix caused by contractions of the uterus.

Domino Scheme A scheme for antenatal care and short-hospital-stay deliveries available through most hospitals around the country. Antenatal check-ups are carried out in the woman's own home (her domicile), she is escorted into hospital by her community midwife, and is discharged from hospital as soon as possible after delivery (**Dom**icile **in** **out**)

Ectopic pregnancy A pregnancy in which the fertilised egg implants itself anywhere other than on the lining of the womb. In the commonest form of ectopic pregnancy implantation occurs in the fallopian tube. This is known as a tubal pregnancy. Very few ectopic pregnancies can be carried to term.

EDD Estimated day / date of delivery. The day on which a pregnancy is likely to come to term, estimated by calculating from the first day of the last menstrual period, or by assessing the age of the foetus from an ultrasound scan. Also known as the due date.

Effacement The flattening and thinning of the cervix caused by contractions of the uterus. The cervix is usually fully effaced before it begins to dilate.

Embryo The name given to the developing baby up to and including the seventh week of the pregnancy.

Endorphins Naturally-occurring pain-killers made by the body. Endorphins are chemically similar to morphine. They are released into the blood stream and block or relieve pain in response to certain stimuli.

Engagement The lowering into the pelvis of the baby's presenting part, usually the head. In first pregnancies, the baby's head may engage as early as the thirty-sixth week, but in later pregnancies it may not engage until as late as the onset of labour.

Entonox The mixture of nitrous oxide and oxygen that can be inhaled to control pain during labour and delivery. Also known as gas and air.

Epidural A form of nerve block in which a drug is injected through a tube into the lining around the spinal column. It can offer mild to complete anaesthesia (lack of feeling) from the waist down, and is frequently used as pain relief for labour and delivery.

Episiotomy A surgical cut made to the perineum, under local or epidural anaesthetic, to facilitate the delivery of the baby's head and / or the use of forceps.

Fallopian tubes The tubes on either side of the uterus that fan out near the ovaries. When a ripe egg is released by one of the ovaries the tiny hairs that line the fallopian tubes help to waft the egg along the tube towards the uterus.

Fertilisation The moment when the nucleus of the sperm cell and the nucleus of the egg cell fuse to form the genetic material for a complete human being.

Foetal distress Signs of stress, such as an abnormally slow heart-rate, detected in the foetus. The foetal heart rate can be monitored during labour using electronic monitoring devices. If the foetus is found to be distressed, intervention such as an assisted delivery or a Caesarean section may be recommended.

Foetus The developing baby from the eighth week of pregnancy, when the embryonic period comes to an end, until the day it is born.

Forceps delivery A delivery assisted with surgical forceps. The forceps are designed to cradle the baby's head and can be used to ease the baby along the birth canal in time with contractions.

Fundus The top of the uterus. The height of the fundus (the distance in centimetres from the pubic bone to the top of the fundus) can be a useful guide to the dating of the pregnancy and the growth rate of the foetus.

Gas and air The mixture of nitrous oxide and oxygen that can be inhaled to control pain during labour and delivery. Also known as entonox.

Genetic counselling Advice and support offered to parents concerning the implications of chromosomal abnormalities and hereditary diseases that may be present in one or both parents.

Gestation The duration of a pregnancy from the first day of the last menstrual period until the birth of the baby.

Height of fundus see Fundus.

Hormone A chemical 'messenger' or 'catalyst' synthesised by glands and other parts of the body to perform specific functions and trigger changes in the metabolism.

Hypertension High blood pressure.

Incompetent cervix A cervix that is malformed or has been damaged so that it is no longer able to remain closed for the duration of a pregnancy, it may open suddenly during pregnancy and the foetus's chances of survival will be very slim.

Induction Any method of encouraging the onset of labour.

Jaundice A metabolic disturbance in which the body is unable to excrete excesses of bilirubin, the waste product of broken down red blood cells. Jaundice is very common in newborn babies.

Kick chart A record of movements made by the foetus charted over several days or weeks.

Lactation The process of producing milk.

Lanugo The fine hair that covers the foetus's body from about the third month of pregnancy. Some babies are born with lanugo hair still on their bodies.

Large-for-dates baby A baby that is larger than the expected or average size for a baby at that stage in the pregnancy. This could imply that the dating of the pregnancy is inaccurate.

LMP Last menstrual period. The acronym LMP is often used as an abbreviation for the date of the first day of the last menstrual period, which is used in calculating the estimated day of delivery.

Lochia The blood and discharge lost from the vagina for up to six weeks after delivery.

Meconium The baby's first bowel movement.

Nitrous oxide The gas, nick-named laughing gas, which is combined with oxygen and can be inhaled to give pain relief during labour and delivery. The mixture is known as gas and air or entonox.

Oedema Retention of fluid in body tissue, most noticeable in the fingers and at the wrists and ankles.

Ovulation The time at which a ripe egg or ovum is released by the ovary.

If the woman has unprotected sex on the days just before or just after ovulation, fertilisation can take place.

Pelvic floor The muscles that run under a woman's pelvis in a figure-of-eight formation, forming a sling that supports the rectum, the vagina and the bladder.

Pethidine A drug with powerful analgesic and sedative qualities that is sometimes used during labour.

Perineum The small area of skin between the aperture of the vagina and the anus.

Placenta The organ that develops on the uterine wall and filters oxygen, nutrients and antibodies from the mother's bloodstream to supply the foetus (via the umbilical cord), and transmits waste products from the foetus into the mother's bloodstream to be excreted. When the placenta is delivered it is also known as the afterbirth.

Placenta praevia A pregnancy in which the placenta is attached unusually low down on the uterine wall, covering all or part of the cervix. Placenta praevia may cause heavy bleeding in late pregnancy, and Caesarean section may be the safest method of delivery.

Placental Abruptio A rare complication in which the placenta (or a part of it) becomes detached from the uterine wall before the end of the pregnancy (it may occur during delivery). This can cause bleeding into the uterus, tenderness in the abdomen and sometimes abdominal cramps. If the entire placenta comes away, the supply of oxygen and nutrients to the foetus will be cut off and the foetus will die.

Post-mature A baby born after 42 weeks gestation.

Postnatal After the birth.

Postpartum haemorrhage Dangerously heavy bleeding in the hours or days after delivery from the site on the uterine wall to which the placenta was attached.

Pre-eclampsia Pregnancy-induced high blood-pressure. This condition, which can threaten the lives of both mother and baby if it is not detected and treated, occurs in about 10% of pregnancies. Several of the tests carried out at antenatal check-ups are designed to pick up on symptoms of pre-eclampsia.

Presentation The position in which the foetus is lying in the uterus.

Pre-term, premature A baby born before 37 weeks gestation.

Pudendal block A local anaesthetic to the perineum used for episiotomies, delivery and stitching of episiotomies or perineal tears.

Rubella German measles.

Show A one-off discharge from the vagina which may be seen in late pregnancy and which usually indicates that the onset of labour is imminent. The show is actually a plug of mucus which has been sealing off the aperture of the cervix during pregnancy, and it is dislodged by uterine contractions.

SIDS Sudden Infant Death Syndrome: the sudden, unexplained death of a baby, usually within the first three months of life. Also known as Cot death.

Small-for-dates A baby that is smaller than the expected or average size for a baby at that stage in the pregnancy. This could imply that the dating of the pregnancy is inaccurate or that the foetus is not thriving or growing normally.

Spontaneous abortion Another term for miscarriage.

Stillbirth The birth of a dead baby any time after the twenty-fourth week of pregnancy.

Stirrups A pair of slings placed round a woman's ankles and raised about 70cm (28in) above the hospital bed and 100cm (39in) apart to facilitate difficult deliveries and the stitching of episiotomies and tears.

TENS Transcutaneous Electrical Nerve Stimulation. A way of relieving pain using very low electrical currents.

Term The end of the average gestation, the due date.

Threatened miscarriage Signs of a miscarriage, such as vaginal bleeding and some abdominal discomfort. A threatened miscarriage may not culminate in a miscarriage.

Transverse lie An unusual presentation in which the baby lies horizontally across the uterus.

Trimester A third of the pregnancy. Each trimester of the pregnancy constitutes about three months.

Tubal pregnancy The commonest kind of ectopic pregnancy in which the fertilised egg implants in the wall of the fallopian tube.

Ultrasound scan A way of building up an accurate image of the foetus and the placenta in the uterus using sound waves.

Uterus The womb. The muscular walls of the womb offer protection for the foetus and the placenta; they grow steadily throughout the pregnancy and contract back down during labour and delivery, eventually resuming their pre-pregnancy size and position some weeks after delivery.

Vacuum / Ventouse delivery A method of assisted delivery in which a suction cup is applied to the crown of the baby's head, and the baby is then eased along the birth canal in time with the mother's contractions.

Vernix The thick whitish grease that covers the baby's skin during pregnancy and is believed to protect the skin from bloating with amniotic fluid. Vernix usually disappears towards the end of pregnancy although many babies are born with traces of it still in folds of their skin.

Useful Addresses

The following organisations may be able to give you information and support either over the telephone, by sending you leaflets or by putting you in touch with someone in your area who may be able to help you. It is usually better to make contact by telephone in the first instance, but if you are writing always enclose a stamped addressed envelope.

General Support and Information

Association for Improvements in the Maternity Services (AIMS)
40 Kingswood Avenue,
London NW6 6LS
0181 960 5585
40 Leamington Terrace,
Edinburgh EH10 4JL
0131 229 6259

Life
Life House, Newbold Terrace,
Leamington Spa,
Warwickshire CV32 4EA
01926 421587

Maternity Alliance
45 Beech Street,
London EC2P 2LX
0171 588 8582

National Childbirth Trust (NCT)
Alexandra House, Oldham Terrace,
London W3 6NH
0181 992 8637

Wellbeing
27 Sussex Place, Regent's Park,
London NW1 4SP
0171 723 9296

AIDS and HIV

National Aids Helpline
0800 567 123
Northern Ireland: 0800 137437

Body Positive
51B Philbeach Gardens,
London SW5 9EB
0171 835 1045 (office hours)
0171 373 9124 (evenings)

Alcohol
see Smoking, Alcohol and Drug
Addiction

Alternative / Complementary
Therapies

Association of Reflexologists
27 Old Gloucester Street,
London WC1N 3XX
0990 673320

19 Benson Road, Henfield,
West Sussex BN5 9HY
01273 492385

British Acupuncture Council
Park House, 206 Latimer Road,
London W10 6RE
0181 964 0222

**British Association for Autogenic
Training and Therapy**
c/o Jane Bird, 18 Holtsmere Close,
Watford, Herts

British Chiropractic Association
29 Whitley Street, Reading,
Berkshire, RG9 0EG
0118 975 7557

British Homeopathic Association
27a Devonshire Street,
London W1N 1RJ
0171 935 2163

British Hypnotherapy Association
67 Upper Berkeley Street,
London W1H 7DH
0171 723 4443

**British Society of Medical and
Dental Hypnosis**
73 Ware Road, Hertford,
Herts SG13 7ED
0181 905 4342

British School of Osteopathy
 275 Borough High Street,
London SE1 1JE
0171 930 9254

**British Society for Experimental
and Clinical Hypnosis**
c/o Dr Michael Heap, Centre for
Psychotherapeutic Studies, 16
Claremont Crescent,
Sheffield S10 2TA
0114 262 0468

British Wheel of Yoga
1 Hamilton Place, Boston Road,
Sleaford,
Lincs NG34 7EF
01529 306851

Institute for Complementary Medicine
PO BOX 194,
London SE16 1QZ
0171 237 5165

The National Insitute of Medical Herbalists
56 Longbrook Street,
Exeter EX4 6AH
01392 426022

The Osteopathic Information Service
Premier House, 10 Greycoat Place,
London SW1P 1SB
0171 799 2559

Relaxation for Living
Foxhills, 30 Victoria Avenue,
Shanklin, Isle of Wight PO37 6LS
01983 868166

Shirley Price Aromatherapy
Essentia House, Upper Bond Street,
Hinckley, LE10 1RS
01455 615466

The Society of Homeopaths
2 Artizan Road,
Northampton NN1 4HU
01604 621400

Breastfeeding

Association of Breastfeeding Mothers
PO BOX 207, Bridgewater,
Somerset TA6 7YT
0181 778 4769
La Leche League (Great Britain)
BM 3424,
London WC1N 3XX
0171 242 1278

Diabetes

British Diabetic Association
10 Queen Anne Street,
London W1M 0BD
0171 323 1531

Cot Death
see Miscarriage, Stillbirth, Cot Death and Bereavement

Disability

Disability Action
2 Annadale Avenue,
Belfast BT7 3JH
01232 491011

Disabled Living Centre
Musgrave Park Hospital,
Stockman's Lane,
Belfast BT9 7JB
01232 669501 ext 2708

Drugs
see Smoking, Alcohol and Drug Addiction

Fertility Problems

Child
Charter House, 43 St Leonards Road,
Bexhill-on-Sea, E. Sussex TN40 1JA
01424 732361

Hereditary Diseases and
Congenital Abnormalities

Association for Spina Bifida and Hydrocephalus (ASBAH)
ASBAH House, 42 Park Road,
Peterborough PE1 2UQ
01733 55988

Northern Ireland Spina Bifida and Hydrocephalus Association
Graham House, Knockbreacken
Healthcare Park,
Belfast BT8 8BH
01232 798878

Scottish Spina Bifida Association
190 Queensferry Road,
Edinburgh EH4 2BW
0131 332 0743

BLISS (Baby Life Support Systems)
17–21 Emerald Street,
London WC1N 3QL
0171 831 9393

Cleft Lip and Palate Association (CLAPA)
138 Buckingham Palace Road,
London SW1 9SA
0171 824 8110

Contact a Family
170 Tottenham Court Road,
London W1P 0HA
0171 383 3555

Cystic Fibrosis Trust
Alexandra House, 5 Blyth Road,
Bromley BR1 3RS
0181 464 7211
20 Bryansburn Road, Bangor, Co
Down BT20 3SB
01247 272781

Down's Syndrome Association
155 Mitcham Road, Tooting,
London SW17 9PG
0181 682 4001
Scottish Down's Syndrome
Association
158–160 Balgreen Road, Edinburgh
EH1 3AU

Genetic Interest Group (GIG)
Farringdon Point, Farringdon Road,
London EC1M 3JB
0171 430 0090

Haemophilia Society
Chesterfield House, 385 Euston
Road, London NW1 3AU
0171 380 0600

Muscular Dystrophy Group of Great Britain and Northern Ireland
7–11 Prescott Place,
London SW4 6BS
0171 720 8055

National Society for Phenylketonuria and Allied Disorders
08456 039136 (general enquiry)
0131 445 4514 (information and leaflets)

REACH (The Association for Children with Hand or Arm Deficiency)
12 Wilson Way, Earls Barton, Northants, NN6 0NZ
01604 811041

SENSE (National Deaf-Blind and Rubella Association)
11–13 Clifton Terrace,
London N4 3SR
0171 272 7774
The Manor House, 51 Mallusk Road, Mallusk, Co Antrim BT37 9AA
01232 833430

SCOPE (Advice to parents of children with cerebral palsy)
6 Market Road,
London N7 9PW
0171 636 5020

Brunell House, Ynys Bridge Court, Gwaelod-y-Garth,
Cardiff CF4 8SS
01222 813913

Toxoplasmosis Trust
Room 26, 61–71 Collier Street,
London N1 9BE
0171 713 0599

The UK Thalassaemia Society
19 The Broadway, Southgate Circus,
London N14 6PH
0181 882 0011

Home Births

Independent Midwives Association
Nightingale Cottage, Shamblehurst Lane, Botley, Hampshire SO32 2BY

Miscarriage, Stillbirth, Cot Death and Bereavement

Compassionate Friends
53 North Street,
Bristol BS3 1EN
0117 953 9639

Foundation for the Study of Infant Deaths (Cot Death Research and Support)
14 Halkin Street,
London SW1X 7DP
0171 235 0965

Miscarriage Association
c/o Clayton Hospital, Northgate, Wakefield,
W Yorks WF1 3JS
01924 200799

Stillbirth and Neonatal Death Society (SANDS)
28 Portland Place,
London W1N 4DE
0171 436 5881

Multiple Births see
Twins and Multiple Births

Obstetric physiotherapists

**Association of Chartered
Physiotherapists in Women's
Health**
c/o Chartered Society of
Physiotherapy
14 Bedford Row
London WC1R 4ED
0171 242 1941

Pre-eclampsia

Pre-Eclampsia Society (PETS)
17 South Avenue, Hullbridge,
Essex SS5 6HA
01702 232533

Single Mothers

**Gingerbread Association for One-
parent Families**
16–17 Clerkenwell Close,
London EC1R 0AA
0171 336 8183

Gingerbread, Northern Ireland:
169 University Street,
Belfast BT7 1HR
01232 231417

Gingerbread, Wales:
Room 16, Albion Chambers,
Cambrian Place,
Swansea SA1 1RN
01792 648728

**National Council for One Parent
Families**
255 Kentish Town Road,
London NW5 2LX
0171 267 1361

One Parent Families Scotland
13 Gayfield Square,
Edinburgh EH1 3NX
0131 556 3899

Smoking, Alcohol and Drug
Addiction

Alcoholics Anonymous (AA)
PO BOX 1, Stonebow House,
Stonebow,
York YO1 2NJ
01904 644026

Drinkline
0345 320202

Dunlewey Substance Advice Centre
1A Dunlewey Street,
Belfast BT13 2QU
01232 324197

Narcotics Anonymous
202 City Road,
London EC1V 2PH
0171 730 0009

Northlands
13 Pump Street,
Londonderry BT48 6JG
01504 263356

Quit (Smoking)
Victory House, 170 Tottenham
Court Road,
London W1P 0HA
0171 388 5775

Quitline (Smoking)
0800 00 22 00
Wales: 0345 697500

SCODA (Standing Conference on Drug Abuse)
Waterbridge House, 32–36 Loman
Street,
London SE10 0EE
0171 928 9500

Scottish Drug Forum
Shaftesbury House, 5 Waterloo
Street, Glasgow G2 6AY
0141 221 1175

Stillbirth
see Miscarriage, Stillbirth, Cot
Death and Bereavement

Stress, Depression and Loneliness

Association for Postnatal Illness (APNI)
25 Jerdan Place,
London SW6 1BE
0171 386 0868

CRY-SIS
BM CRY-SIS,
London WC1N 3XX
0171 404 5011

MAMA (Meet-a-mum Association)
26 Avenue Road,
London SE25 4DX
0181 771 5595

Parentline
Endway House, The Endway,
Hadleigh, Benfleet,
Essex SS7 554782
01702 5547822 (admin)
01702 559900 (Helpline)

Parents Advice Centre
Franklin House, 12 Brunswick
Street, Belfast BT2 7GE
01232 238800

Parents Anonymous
6–9 Manor Gardens,
London N7 6LA
0171 263 8918

Samaritans
0345 909090

Terminations / Abortions

SATFA (Support around Termination for Abnormality)
73–75 Charlotte Street,
London W1P 1LB
0171 631 0285

Twins and Multiple Births

The Multiple Birth Foundation
c/o Queen Charlotte's and Chelsea
Hospital, Goldhawk Road, London
W6G OXG
0181 383 3519
**Twins and Multiple Births
Association (TAMBA)**
PO BOX 30, Little Sutton,
S Wirral L66 1TH
0151 348 0020
Out of hours: 01732 8680000

Water Births

**Birthworks (Hire of birthing
pools)**
Unit 3F, Brent Mill Trading Estate,
South Brent, Devon TQ10 9YT
01364 72802

**Splashdown (Hire of birthing
pools)**
17 Wellington Terrace, Harrow-on-
the-Hill,
Middlesex HA1 3EP
0181 422 9308

Index